Neurocritical Care Pharmacotherapy

Neurocritical Care Pharmacotherapy

A Clinician's Manual

Eelco F. M. Wijdicks, MD, PHD, FACP, FNCS, FANA

Professor of Neurology, College of Medicine
Chair, Division of Critical Care Neurology
Consultant, Neurosciences Intensive Care Unit
Saint Marys Hospital
Mayo Clinic, Rochester, Minnesota

Sarah L. Clark, PHARMD, RPH, BCPS

Assistant Professor of Pharmacy, College of Medicine
Neurosciences Clinical Pharmacist
Senior Manager of Pharmacy, Clinical Practice
Saint Marys Hospital
Mayo Clinic, Rochester, Minnesota

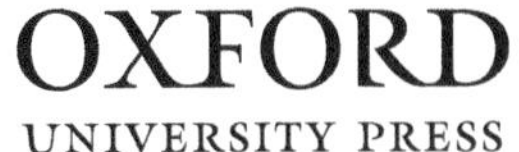

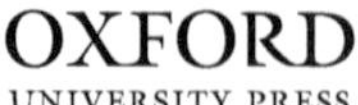

Oxford University Press is a department of the University of Oxford. It furthers the University's objective of excellence in research, scholarship, and education by publishing worldwide. Oxford is a registered trade mark of Oxford University Press in the UK and certain other countries.

Published in the United States of America by Oxford University Press
198 Madison Avenue, New York, NY 10016, United States of America.

CIP data is on file at the Library of Congress
ISBN 978–0–19–068474–7

The science of medicine is a rapidly changing field. As new research and clinical experience broaden our knowledge, changes in treatment and drug therapy occur. The author and publisher of this work have checked with sources believed to be reliable in their efforts to provide information that is accurate and complete, and in accordance with the standards accepted at the time of publication. However, in light of the possibility of human error or changes in the practice of medicine, neither the author, nor the publisher, nor any other party who has been involved in the preparation or publication of this work warrants that the information contained herein is in every respect accurate or complete. Readers are encouraged to confirm the information contained herein with other reliable sources, and are strongly advised to check the product information sheet provided by the pharmaceutical company for each drug they plan to administer.

9 8 7 6 5 4 3 2 1

Printed by WebCom, Inc., Canada

To Barbara, Coen and Kathryn, Marilou and Rob (EFMW)

To Byron, Noah, Audrey, and Austin (SLC)

Contents

	Preface	xi
1.	Drug Delivery, Monitoring, and Interactions	1
	Bioavailability of a Drug	1
	Drug Administration Routes	4
	Drug Interactions	7
	Drug Errors	8
	Pharmacogenomics	9
	Neuropharmacology and Critical Care Pharmacology	9
2.	Analgosedation and Neuromuscular Blockers	12
	Deciding on Sedation	12
	Sedative Drugs	13
	Analgesics	19
	Neuromuscular Blockers	23
	Neuromuscular Blockers in ICU Practice	24
	Reversal of Neuromuscular Blockers	28
3.	Agitation and Delirium	31
	Causes of Delirium	31
	Clinical Features of Delirium	33
	Pharmacologic Treatment of Agitation	35
	Neuroleptics	36
	Benzodiazepines	40
	Preventive Drugs	43
4.	Pain Management	47
	Grading Pain	47
	Types of Pain in the Neurosciences ICU	49
	Drugs for Pain	50
	Control of Specific Headaches	51
	Patient-Controlled Analgesia	63
5.	Osmotic Therapy	66
	The Constants of Brain Volume	66
	Hyperosmolar Fluids	68
	Osmotic Agents in Clinical Practice	73

6. Antiepileptic Drugs	77
Seizures in the ICU	77
Treatment Protocols	77
Antiepileptic Drugs Used in ICU Practice	80
Interactions and Adjustments	90
7. Anticoagulation and Reversal Drugs	93
Heparin and Warfarin	94
Factor Xa Inhibitors	100
Thrombin Inhibitors	105
Hemorrhage from Anticoagulants and Drug Reversal	108
Reversal of Vitamin K Antagonists in Life Threatening Bleeding	108
8. Antifibrinolytics and Thrombolytics	115
Basic Mechanisms and Targets	115
Antifibrinolytics	116
Fibrinolytics	119
Thrombolytics	122
Post-Alteplase Care	123
9. Antiplatelet Agents	127
Clinical Trials on Antiplatelet Agents in Stroke	127
Current Recommendations for Antiplatelet Agents	128
Antiplatelet Agents	129
Glycoprotein IIb/IIIa Inhibitors	135
Testing Platelet Function	138
Antiplatelet Agent Resistance	138
Discontinuation of Antiplatelet Agents Before Procedures	139
Clinical Urgency While on Antiplatelet Agents	139
10. Immunosuppression and Immunotherapy	142
Corticosteroids	142
Plasma Exchange	150
Intravenous Immunoglobulin	151
Checkpoint Inhibitor Immunotherapy	156
Other Therapeutic Targets in Autoimmune Neurology	157
11. Antimicrobial Therapy for Central Nervous System Infections	162
Bacterial Meningitis	162

Viral, Fungal, and Parasitic Infections 165
The Pharmacology of Antibiotics 167
Antivirals 178
Antifungals 180
12. Vasopressors and Inotropes 185
Mechanisms of Action 185
Vasopressors 186
Inotropes 191
Use in Clinical Practice 194
13. Antihypertensives and Antiarrhythmics 199
Definition of Hypertension and Blood Pressure Goals 199
Current Practice of Antihypertensives 201
Control of Blood Pressure After Urgent Control 216
Antiarrhythmic Drugs 216
14. Fluid Therapy 223
Regulation of Fluid Status 223
General Principles of Fluid Management 224
Fluids and Administration 225
Types of Fluids 228
Fluid Management Principles in the Neurosciences ICU 230
Volume Depletion and Acute Resuscitation 231
Fluid Overload and Prevention 232
15. Drugs to Correct Electrolyte Disorders 234
Common Electrolyte Replacements 234
Disorders of Sodium and Water Homeostasis 235
Drugs to Manage Sodium Disorders 240
16. Antidotes with Overdose 247
Toxins and Major Laboratory Abnormalities 247
Neurology of Drug Overdose 248
First Treatment Considerations 249
Commonly Used Agents for Detoxification 250
Major Toxidromes 251
Toxic Dysautonomias 257
17. Drugs Used to Prevent Complications 260
Prevention of Deep Venous Thrombosis 260
Prevention of Hyperglycemia 264

Prevention of Stress Ulcers 264
Prevention of Infections 272
Prevention of Constipation 275
Prevention of Cerebral Vasospasm 277
18. Drugs Used to Treat Withdrawal Syndromes 280
Alcohol Withdrawal Syndrome 280
Initial Approach to Drugs for Alcohol Withdrawal 282
Approach to Refractory Withdrawal Delirium 284
Opioid Withdrawal 287
Stimulant Withdrawal 289
Baclofen Withdrawal 290
Nicotine Withdrawal 292
19. Treatment of Brain Injury-Associated Symptoms and Signs 295
Control of Nausea and Vomiting 295
Control of Hiccups 300
Control of Secretions 302
Control of Constipation and Dysmotility 303
Control of Fever and Shivering 304
Control of Rhabdomyolysis 306
20. Drugs Used in Neurorehabilitation 309
Neurostimulants 309
Drugs for Post-Stroke Depression 316
Treatment of Spasticity 320

List of Graphs 329
Index 333

Preface

More than anything else, knowing how to prescribe neurotherapeutics appropriately and effectively is a core requirement for clinicians treating patients with an acute neurologic illness. Once acutely ill neurologic patients are admitted, the number of drugs on their pharmacy profile quickly increases. Most disorders need specific neurotherapeutics, but there are also less neurospecific medications used to treat or prevent complications associated with mechanical ventilation and immobilization. The treatment of the critically ill neurologic patient is unique and involves drugs infrequently used in other intensive care units (ICUs), such as antiepileptic drugs, antifibrinolytics, thrombolytics, osmotic agents, neurostimulants, or acute immunotherapy agents such as intravenous immunoglobulin and plasma exchange. Interactions with drugs are thus also different. Many other drugs used in medical and surgical ICUs are administered, so clinicians must recognize the changes in vital signs and organ function in the acutely ill neurologic patient in order to optimize medication delivery.

Rounds in the neuroscience ICU always involve a spate of questions and queries to pharmacists. Neurointensivists closely consult with critical care–trained pharmacists who, in major medical institutions, are important members of the multidisciplinary neurosciences ICU and emergency department healthcare team. They are available to answer medication-related questions and to provide important clinical drug monitoring for patients.

Electronic monitoring tools have changed the landscape, and today virtually every drug side effect is at the physician's fingertips. Thus, this book must be different; it cannot just provide an endless list of potential complications of drug administration. Here we list the side effects that are clinically relevant——those that would lead a physician to consult the pharmacist. It is far more important when using these drugs to have a practical understanding of their indications, monitoring, and immediate and lingering effects, and most importantly to have a good understanding of the most commonly prescribed drugs. It is better to know a lot about a few drugs.

The book opens by setting the stage: How do these drugs work and what does the body do with the drug in the acutely ill neurologic patient? How are these drugs best used, administered, and monitored in practice? How do we most effectively practice medication reconciliation? Each of the commonly used neurotherapeutics is discussed in great detail to allow for its efficient use and to allow clinicians to recognize drug-related problems. This book provides not only the tools needed to order and monitor the most commonly prescribed neurocritical care drugs, but also vital information about how they are prepared and how this may delay administration and thus affect drug choice. Fluid administration is needed not only for systemic resuscitation but also for "brain resuscitation" and thus is also included.

This book is deliberately constructed differently. A clinician's manual should be eminently readable and should quickly inform the reader. The amount of information in a small book is inherently curtailed but should be presented logically. Thus we decided to use bullet points and quick-glance boxes and graphs rather than more time-consuming narrative text. Each statement was carefully vetted and rewritten multiple times. Pharmacy books are often awash in acronyms; we tried to avoid them. Ultimately, what we want to know is what drug to use and at what dose, what to expect, what complications could occur, and what we should do if it does not work. Yet, this manual cannot provide all the answers on how to move from one drug to the next ("if this drug does not work, try that one") and often the best sequence is unknown.

These simple principles have guided us in writing this manual, and we hope we have found a good number of knowledge nuggets that will inform physicians and pharmacists. We wanted to write something the reader has not read before, and we wanted to avoid presenting facts that are much less relevant to clinicians.

We created graphs of the most commonly used drugs and included four essential pieces of information: order to the patient (how long does it take to get the drug into the patient); starting dose (how much is needed initially); half-life (how long does it work); and clearance (which organ predominantly clears the drug). All drugs with a graph are listed at the end of the book with abbreviations explained.

This book is the product of a fine joint effort. Writing the book together created an unprecedented opportunity to critically look at each other's specialty (including misconceived orthodoxy) and to come up with a body of work we both agree on. It became quickly clear that small books need much more work than large books. We are grateful to our spouses (and children) who unflinchingly supported us while we were going through yet another round of writing and editing. Some credit should go to the loyal dogs at our feet that provided a necessary state of serenity.

We have many others to thank. First and foremost, Lea Dacy edited this unusual book with great care and suggested changes along the way. We are grateful to several of our experienced hospital pharmacists who provided heavy scrutiny and valuable input. (Jan Anderson, Jeffrey Armon Erin Barreto, Caitlin Brown, Gabriel Golfus, Megan Leloux, Scott Nei, Whitney Bergquist, Andrea Nei, Erin Nystrom, Narith Ou, Christina Rivera.) Jim Rownd masterfully created the illustration on the cover. We thank Craig Panner, associate editorial director with Oxford University Press for US Medicine books Neurology and Clinical Neuroscience for suggesting this work and the staff at Newgen KnowledgeWorks Pvt Ltd (Devasena Vedamurthi) for providing all that was needed to smoothly see it through production.

We compiled this small but chock-full manual to serve the needs of any healthcare provider managing patients with acute neurologic disease and to offer the necessary assistance. We hope this book works for you.

EFMW
SLC

Chapter 1

Drug Delivery, Monitoring, and Interactions

It is not a question but a certainty—drugs can be used to treat, salvage, and protect the brain; and there is a growing pharmacopeia. In the neurosciences intensive care unit (NICU), the medication profiles of patients can rapidly expand even during a short stay. Orders include daily prescribed medications and as circumstances arise (*pro re nata*).

Generally, once a drug is infused or absorbed and becomes active, major physiologic changes occur. This is conceptualized as pharmacokinetics and pharmacodynamics. *Pharmacokinetics* is the study of the way drugs move through the body; in other words, the absorption, distribution, metabolism, and elimination of drugs. This is often thought of as "what the body does to the drug." *Pharmacodynamics* is the study of the effects of drugs on the body—"what the drug does to the body" (1).

The nature of critical illness is a major factor. The more pertinent issues in neurologic critical care patients are difficulties with routes of administration (e.g., patients with dysphagia), absorption impairment (e.g., ileus caused by barbiturate use), and drug interactions (e.g., complex interactions with new antiepileptic medications). Furthermore, acute brain injury may change the body's response to medications. These changes may be neurology-specific (e.g., disruption to the blood–brain barrier or exaggerated response to drugs in dysautonomia), or more general such as the acute stress-induced sympathetic response affecting the absorption of the drug (e.g., gastric atony).

Bioavailability of a Drug

Practicing physicians may appreciate some understanding of the typical pathway of an administered drug and the factors that influence it. The main components that determine pharmacokinetics and pharmacodynamics are shown in Box 1.1. These parameters are mostly of interest to pharmacists but have clinical relevance if a drug–drug interaction or unexpected abnormal metabolism requires further explanation.

An orally administered drug is absorbed, distributed, metabolized, and eliminated, and several factors may change it (Fig. 1.1). When drugs are administered intravenously, bioavailability reaches 100%. One can assume that at five times the half-life, the mean plasma concentration of the drug is constant and at a plateau for drugs with zero-order kinetics (i.e., the rate of drug elimination is constant over time). Assuming there is no organ system

Box 1.1 Pharmacokinetic Parameters

- **Area under the curve:** plasma drug concentration related to time; the body's exposure to a drug after administration
- **Bioavailability:** portion of the drug reaching the systemic circulation
- **Clearance:** rate at which a drug is removed from the body
- **First-pass effect:** drug concentration that is removed prior to reaching the systemic circulation; refers to the intestinal and hepatic metabolism of drugs
- **Elimination Half-life:** amount of time required for the drug concentration to decrease by 50%
- **Steady state:** time when the drug has reached full therapeutic effect and elimination and intake are at the same rate; typically achieved after four to five half-lives
- **Therapeutic window:** range between effective dosing and the presence of adverse effects

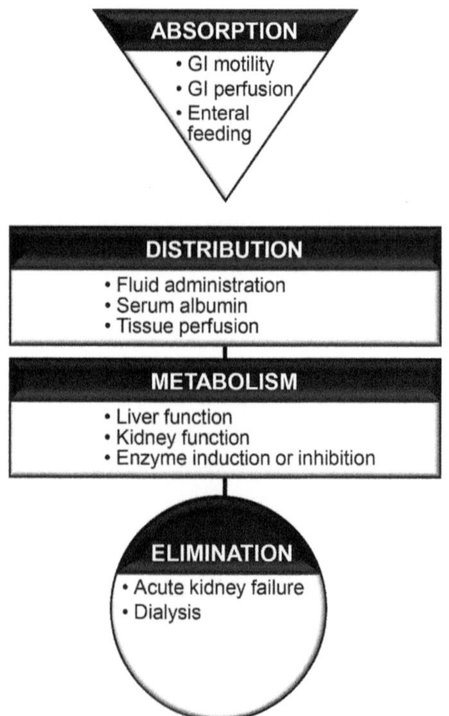

Figure 1.1 Pathway of a drug and factors that matter (GI = gastrointestinal)

dysfunction, the reverse occurs, with the plasma concentration decreasing to zero in five half-lives. Metabolism in patients with hypothyroidism and hypothermia is reduced, including other factors that can be less precisely assessed are advanced age, morbid obesity, and chronic liver disease. Renal replacement therapy changes the clearance of many antibiotics and also the clearance of certain antiepileptic drugs (Chapter 6) and cardiovascular medications.

Drug absorption is ultimately influenced by the drug's solubility and by gastric motility, gastric perfusion, or enteral feeds (2). Enteral administration is the most common preferred route for drug administration. It is the safest and most convenient route and considered more economical than others. Unfortunately, dysphagia is common after an acute brain injury and precludes the patient's ability to swallow medications. Nasogastric tube placement for enteral nutrition will influence the absorption of drugs (e.g., phenytoin or carbamazepine suspension, nimodipine, carbidopa/levodopa, certain antibiotics). In some instances, enteral administration is not appropriate and intravenous administration is the preferred route (e.g., uncooperative agitated patients, profuse vomiting). However, unfortunately many drugs for neurologic conditions cannot be administered in an intravenous formulation.

A loading dose (intravenously or orally) is advised for drugs when an immediate therapeutic concentration is needed (e.g., antibiotics, antiplatelet agents, anticoagulants, antiepileptic drugs). This approach is used for drugs with longer half-lives, in particular when waiting for a steady state to be achieved would be detrimental to the patient's care. In drugs with a very short half-life (e.g., propofol), where the time to steady state occurs rapidly, a loading dose is not essential.

Once administered, drug distribution follows a two-compartment model: (1) the intravascular volume and rapidly perfused tissues and (2) distribution in other tissues. Lipophilic drugs (e.g., barbiturates) distribute more readily in fat tissues and thus can accumulate in obese patients. Pharmacokinetic changes are common in obese patients and there are differences in dosing. Total body weight is usually used for most sedatives, anticoagulants, and most antimicrobials, but ideal body weight is recommended for other medications (e.g., acyclovir, IV immune globulin) when the patient is overweight. Doses can be modified further in the presence of adverse events (i.e., toxicity) or inadequate clinical response (i.e., underdosing).

Distribution through the blood–brain barrier (BBB) and into the cerebrospinal fluid is restricted (3). Tight junctions between the epithelial cells prohibit many drugs from diffusing through the BBB into the central nervous system. These tight junctions break down with acute brain injury, allowing medications easier access to the central nervous system. This is best exemplified by the use of antibiotics needed to treat bacterial meningitis, which are molecularly too large to penetrate the BBB readily (4). Other factors that improve the ability of a drug to penetrate the BBB include molecular weight (e.g., <400–500 Daltons), drugs that are unionized, and basic molecules with minimal hydrogen bonding. Permeability plays a role in distribution of the drug: Greater lipophilicity is better for penetration into the central nervous system but is also dependent on cerebral blood flow.

Generally, the distribution of a drug is dependent on fluid administration, protein-binding affinity (albumin for acid drugs and glycoprotein alpha for basic drugs), and tissue perfusion. The heart, brain, and kidneys are readily perfused and receive the highest drug concentration after administration. In most patients with acute neurocritical illness, fluid administration remains constant except in patients requiring frequent osmotic diuretics or those who have been resuscitated in a setting of polytrauma. Liver function, renal function, and enzyme induction or inhibition all influence metabolism; these components are generally intact unless a systemic complication intervenes. In some drugs, hepatic clearance is much less sensitive to changes in the hepatic blood flow (e.g., phenytoin). However, the most important factor that influences hepatic function is the use of targeted temperature management, which decreases the metabolic clearance of many drugs including midazolam, fentanyl, phenobarbital, phenytoin, and neuromuscular-junction blockers. The pharmacokinetics in induced hypothermia are substantially changed, often approaching a 10% decrease in drug clearance with any decrease of 1°C—this factor is often underappreciated by clinicians.

Once a drug is distributed and reaches equilibrium between the tissues and the plasma, the unbound or "free" fraction links to the receptor. This implies that the bound (albumin) fraction is inactive, and therefore decreasing the bound fraction increases drug availability. Monitoring free drug levels is especially important when albumin body stores are unknown and with drug interactions between highly protein-bound drugs (e.g., valproic acid, phenytoin, warfarin). Hypoalbuminemia can be seen in elderly or malnourished patients or in patients with prolonged critical illness.

Drug elimination in neurocritical illness changes in patients with acute renal failure or those receiving renal replacement therapy. Glomerular filtration changes in acute kidney injury but mostly after sepsis, prolonged hypotension, and use of vasopressors. Any of these changes can result in altered elimination of antibiotics such as beta-lactams and carbapenems (1). Moreover, acute kidney injury can result with the use of certain antibiotics (e.g., vancomycin, aminoglycosides, beta-lactams).

The glomerular filtration rate (GFR) is an important metric and can be calculated as follows:

$$\text{For males: } C_R CL(\text{ml/min}) = \frac{(140 - \text{age})(\text{weight in kg})}{72 \times \text{serum creatinine}}$$

For females: the above result should be multiplied by 0.85.

Most pharmacists would then adjust the dose using the following formula:

$$\text{Measured GFR/normal GFR} \times 100 = \text{Dose adjustment in \%.}$$

Drug Administration Routes

Determining the appropriate route (oral, rectal, intravenous, or interosseous) remains a critical question, and some guidelines follow.

Oral Administration

- Timing of administration: Poor timing may lead to subtherapeutic drug levels and suboptimal clinical response. Antacids markedly reduce absorption because many drugs require low gastric pH for absorption. Food may affect antimicrobials. Other examples are carbidopa/levodopa and high-protein meals (decreased drug absorption) and carbamazepine suspension and nimodipine. Spacing remediates these problems.
- Enteric tube binding: Enteral phenytoin is notorious for binding to tube feedings, and the enteric tube requires frequent flushing. Clogging in tubes can also be solved by flushing with carbonated drinks such as Coca-Cola.
- Sustained/extended-release formulations: Crushing pills prior to administration results in suboptimal disease management or adverse effects. Crushing pills with enteral feeds may alter the absorption of medications, and removal of the pH-protectant coating of the medication results in lower drug concentration. Crushing these pills may also result in supratherapeutic drug concentrations.
- Oral disintegrating tablet: Sublingual mucosa allows for rapid absorption and instant bioavailability. This option could be the solution for patients with poor medication adherence and with dysphagia.
- Liquid formulations (to replace tablets/capsules for ease of administration): Many liquid formulations contain sorbitol, which in high doses can predispose patients to diarrhea, lactic acidosis, and electrolyte abnormalities.
- Pill size may increase the risk of aspiration when a patient experiences dysphagia (5,6).

Intravenous Administration

- This is the preferred route of administration if a quick effect of the drug is needed
- This is the preferred route of administration when gastrointestinal absorption is inadequate
- There is a greater risk of medication errors and adverse events if medications are not administered appropriately.
  - The use of "smart pumps" with warnings embedded in them (e.g., soft and hard stop warnings) helps prevent medication administration errors.
  - Controlling access to high-risk drugs (keeping them not readily accessible on the nursing unit and requiring a double-check prior to preparing and administering them) is another method to prevent drug administration errors.
- Propylene glycol is a commonly used solvent, found in lorazepam, diazepam, phenobarbital, phenytoin, and barbiturates. Accumulations of propylene glycol have been associated with hypotension, metabolic acidosis, neurotoxicity, and acute renal failure.
- Be aware of particulate matter or crystallization in the bag or tubing when administering drugs intravenously.

Peripheral Versus Central Intravenous Catheter

- Catheter line compatibilities and diluent compatibilities: Assistance from a clinical pharmacist is needed if information is not readily available.
- Drug concentration is used to determine the choice of central versus peripheral route and the rate of administration (e.g., Potassium Chloride10 mEq/hr infusion, unless central line and cardiac monitoring, then 20 mEq/hr is allowed).
- Drug osmolarity is used to determine central versus peripheral route (e.g., peripheral infusion with hypertonic saline 3% or more is for emergent use only).
- Recognize high-risk vasopressor agents (e.g., 24-hour norepinephrine drip with peripheral access, 12-hour epinephrine drip with peripheral access).

Tubing (Choice and Replacement)

- 0.2-micron in-line filter (e.g., mannitol 20% or greater, parenteral nutrition)
- 1.2-micron in-line filter (e.g., fat emulsion)
- Vented tubing (e.g., nitroglycerin, propofol, tPA, tranexamic acid, acetaminophen)
- Dedicated line (e.g., propofol, fat emulsion, clevidipine, intravenous immune globulin)
- No filter (e.g., propofol, intravenous immune globulin, amphotericin liposome, amphotericin B lipid complex, amphotericin B, nitroglycerin)
- Change every 12 hours: propofol, clevidipine
- Change every 24 hours: fat emulsion
- Change others within 24 to 96 hours or per hospital policy

Rectal Administration

- Faster onset, higher bioavailability than oral administration
- Typically fewer side effects than oral administration
- Used in patients experiencing vomiting or gastric irritation
- When enteral or injectable routes are inappropriate or unattainable (e.g., actively seizing patients)

Interosseous Administration

- Bedside drilling in tibia
- For immediate administration of fluids or bicarbonate
- Equivalent to intravenous access in terms of drug delivery
- Transient fluid resuscitation method until intravenous access can be established

Miscellaneous Routes of Administration

- Intranasal (e.g., midazolam for status epilepticus)
- Intraventricular (e.g., tPA for intraventricular hematoma, antimicrobial agents for ventriculitis)
- Intra-arterial (e.g., verapamil for symptomatic cerebral vasospasm)

Drug Interactions

It is important to understand how drug interactions could occur in order to prevent or recognize them. Drug interactions, which are to be expected in critically ill patients, are often the result of polypharmacy rather than just from two drugs. Drug interactions can lead to medical complications, the most recognized of which are electrolyte abnormalities, hypotension or hypertension, sedation, and cardiac arrhythmias. With current computer databases and warning programs, clinical pharmacists often identify these drug interactions early and help prevent adverse events or drug interactions.

Drug interactions can be caused by pharmacokinetic interactions (drug A affecting the absorption of drug B) or by pharmacodynamic interactions (drug A having an additive effect with drug B). Additional important principles are (1) additive toxicity (e.g., two nephrotoxic agents); (2) additive effect (e.g., similar mode of action); and (3) multiple drugs, unknown patient history, and unstable patients.

For example, drugs prolonging the clearance of sedatives and analgesic agents are shown in Table 1.1.

Some drugs inhibit the metabolism of benzodiazepines and increase their effects. Calcium channel blockers and cytochrome P450 inhibitors (e.g., erythromycin, fluconazole) all prolong sedation, whereas cytochrome P450 inducers (e.g., phenytoin, carbamazepine) increase the metabolism of midazolam, potentially resulting in inadequate sedation. Barbiturates (e.g., phenobarbital) lead to added respiratory depression when administered concomitantly with midazolam.

Antiepileptic drugs are commonly associated with drug–drug interactions since many of them act upon the cytochrome P450 metabolic pathway, are highly protein-bound, and have a narrow therapeutic index for safety. Many antiepileptic drugs are cytochrome P450 enzyme inducers and decrease the International Normalized Ratio (INR), so higher warfarin doses are needed to achieve a therapeutic target. However, valproate acts as an enzyme inhibitor and increases the INR in patients receiving warfarin. Many antiepileptic drugs decrease the effect of commonly used drugs such as corticosteroids and tricyclic antidepressants because of their inducing effects. The newer second- and third-generation antiepileptic drugs have significantly fewer drug–drug interactions associated with their use and thus have a more

Table 1.1 Drugs Prolonging Clearance of Sedatives and Analgesic Agents

Drug	Interfering Agent
Midazolam	Diltiazem, erythromycin, fluconazole, verapamil, conivaptan
Lorazepam	Valproic acid
Propofol	Lidocaine, valproic acid
Morphine	Cimetidine, azithromycin, itraconazole, glycoprotein inhibitors
Fentanyl	CYP3A4 inhibitors
Diazepam	Cimetidine, erythromycin, fluoxetine, CYP3A4 inhibitors

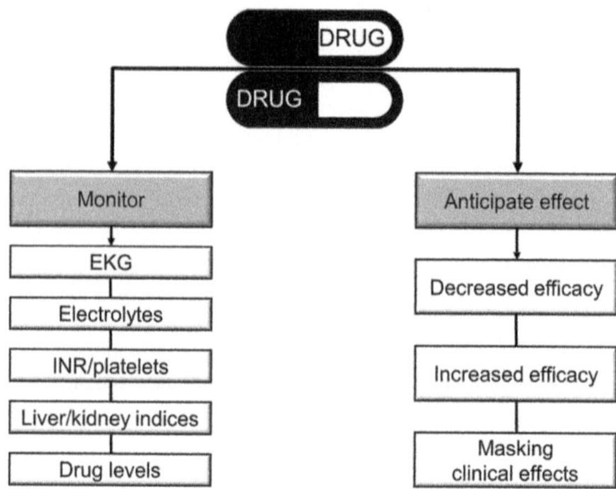

Figure 1.2 Drug interactions (EKG = electrocardiogram; INR = International Normalized Ratio)

predictable therapeutic response. There is less interaction between the direct oral anticoagulants (e.g., dabigatran, apixaban, rivaroxaban, edoxaban) and antiepileptic medications, but data are limited. A summary of anticipated consequences and monitoring suggestions with drug-drug interactions is shown in Figure 1.2.

Drug Errors

Errors may occur in all levels of hospital care including unrecognized medication nonadherence (7,8). One major factor is poor healthcare resources (e.g., high patient volumes, high patient acuity). Unfamiliarity with drug product is another common error, especially when there are different doses for different indications. Errors are also commonly associated with failure to adjust a dose in elderly patients and in patients with developing organ failure. Often there are "look-alike—sound-alike" drugs (e.g., tra*mad*ol, tra*zod*one), which unknowingly get started and lead to more problems (9–12). Having a clinical pharmacist review medications with the medical team and awareness of the patient's condition is critical to help prevent these kinds of errors. Another important point to remember when using infusions is that most infusions are dosed in mg/kg per hour or mcg/kg per minute—except for dexmedetomidine, which is dosed in mcg/kg per hour.

In the United States each year, there reportedly are 450,000 medication errors and 7,000 deaths due to medication errors, 25% of which are deemed preventable. The intensivist, the clinical pharmacist, and the nurse all have specific roles in ensuring the "five rights" of medication administration: right dose, right patient, right time, right route, and right drug. Steps to ensure safety include medication reconciliation, high-risk drug warnings, bar-coding for medication administration, computerized physician order entry, proactive medication review by pharmacists, use of smart pumps, and constant vigilance on the part of physicians and the nursing staff. A useful resource is http://www.ismp.org/.

Pharmacogenomics

Table 1.2 summarizes the potential to find genetic markers for more effective drug dosing and monitoring for adverse effects. It is assumed (and proven in certain circumstances) that underlying genetic factors are associated with variable drug responses (7,13–16). Pharmacogenomics is an emerging field and could have major implications for the drugs used in critically ill neurologic patients (17). Clinical pharmacists will be a reliable source of information for choosing medications and doses, as well as providing the right monitoring, as this field expands.

Neuropharmacology and Critical Care Pharmacology

Within a short period, neurocritical patients may become a living drug encyclopedia. It remains a major responsibility for the clinician, in conjunction with the ICU pharmacist, to tailor drug administration to the individual patient. Daily rounds must include a conscious effort to review medication lists and to promote drug reconciliation. Some drugs cannot be stopped without consequences (Table 1.3). Drug–drug interactions should be considered, antibiotic drug levels should be ordered regularly, and stop dates are needed to avoid prolonged use. The use of multiple antihypertensive agents is common,

Table 1.2 Pharmacogenomics

Genetic Marker	Relevant in	Most common in
CYP2C19 variant is responsible for the metabolism of 10–15% of drugs in practice.	Phenytoin, diazepam, lorazepam, omeprazole, clopidogrel	Asians
CYP2C9 variant	Warfarin, phenytoin	Blacks
VKORC1 deficiency	Warfarin	
CYP2D6 variant is responsible for the metabolism of about 25% of the drugs in practice.	Many psychoactive and cardiovascular medications	Caucasians
ABCB1 variant	Antiepileptic drugs	
HLA-B*1502 hypersensitivity reactions (Stevens-Johnson syndrome/toxic epidermal necrolysis)	Carbamazepine, phenytoin	Asians

Table 1.3 Problems with Inadvertently Holding Maintenance (Home) Medications

Drug Class	Rationale for Holding	Consequences
Beta-blockers	Permissive hypertension after ischemic stroke	Rebound hypertension, tachycardia
Antiepileptic medications	Decreased consciousness	Seizures
Diuretics	Permissive hypertension after ischemic stroke	Worsening heart failure
Serotonergic medications (e.g., selective serotonin reuptake inhibitors, tricyclic antidepressants)	Decreased consciousness, prolonged QT interval on electrocardiogram	Worsening depression, withdrawal (seizures), discontinuation syndrome (nausea/vomiting, sleep disturbances, arrhythmia, psychological symptoms)
Baclofen	Decreased consciousness	Withdrawal (hyperpyrexia, muscle rigidity, rhabdomyolysis)
Parkinson's medications (e.g., carbidopa/levodopa, amantadine, dopamine agonists)	Dyskinesias, orthostatic hypotension, hallucinations	Acute rigidity and hyperthermia, agitation, delirium
Benzodiazepines	Decreased consciousness	Tremors, anxiety, dysphoria, psychosis, seizures
Opioids	Decreased consciousness	Dysphoria, nausea/vomiting/diarrhea, muscle aches, pupillary dilation, lacrimation
Alpha-agonists (e.g., clonidine)	Decreased consciousness, hypotension	Rebound hypertension (sympathetic overdrive)

and they should be closely titrated and adjusted. Hypotension can be expected and severe when the recovered patient is mobilized. Antiepileptic drugs are frequently administered prophylactically, and evidence for long-term use is not sufficient. Critical review of all administered drugs helps the patient. Equally important is to regularly calculate creatinine clearance for renally cleared drugs and to make dose adjustments as indicated. Serum creatinine does not reflect clearance and can be normal with abnormal clearance.

Key Pointers

1. Intravenous drug administration in patients with acute brain injury is often necessary.
2. Nasogastric tube placement for enteral nutrition changes the absorption of drugs.
3. Antiepileptic drugs and sedatives are often associated with drug–drug interactions.

4. Certain drugs require central venous access.
5. Renal and hepatic disease, obesity, advanced age, and hypothermia have an impact on drug effects.

References

1. Smith, B.S., et al., *Introduction to drug pharmacokinetics in the critically ill patient*. Chest, 2012. **141**: 1327–1336.
2. Roberts, D.J. and Hall, R.I. *Drug absorption, distribution, metabolism and excretion considerations in critically ill adults*. Expert Opin Drug Metab Toxicol, 2013. **9**: 1067–1084.
3. Kasinathan, N., et al., *Strategies for drug delivery to the central nervous system by systemic route*. Drug Deliv, 2015. **22**: 243–257.
4. Kulkarni, A.D., et al., *Brain-blood ratio: implications in brain drug delivery*. Expert Opin Drug Deliv, 2016. **13**: 85–92.
5. Bennett, B., et al., *Medication management in patients with dysphagia: a service evaluation*. Nurs Stand, 2013. **27**: 41–48.
6. Carnaby-Mann, G. and Crary, M. *Pill swallowing by adults with dysphagia*. Arch Otolaryngol Head Neck Surg, 2005. **131**: 970–975.
7. Kelly, J., Wright, D. and Wood, J. *Medicine administration errors in patients with dysphagia in secondary care: a multi-centre observational study*. J Adv Nurs, 2011. **67**: 2615–2627.
8. Kelly, J., Wright, D. and Wood, J. *Medication errors in patients with dysphagia*. Nurs Times, 2012. **108**: 12–14.
9. Floroff, C.K., et al., *Potentially inappropriate medication use is associated with clinical outcomes in critically ill elderly patients with neurological injury*. Neurocrit Care, 2014. **21**: 526–533.
10. Keers, R.N., et al., *Causes of medication administration errors in hospitals: a systematic review of quantitative and qualitative evidence*. Drug Saf, 2013. **36**: 1045–1067.
11. Macdonald, M., *Patient safety: examining the adequacy of the 5 rights of medication administration*. Clin Nurse Spec, 2010. **24**: 196–201.
12. Marengoni, A., et al., *Understanding adverse drug reactions in older adults through drug-drug interactions*. Eur J Intern Med, 2014. **25**: 843–846.
13. Caudle, K.E., et al., *Clinical pharmacogenetics implementation consortium guidelines for CYP2C9 and HLA-B genotypes and phenytoin dosing*. Clin Pharmacol Ther, 2014. **96**: 542–548.
14. Chan, A., Pirmohamed, M. and Comabella, M. *Pharmacogenomics in neurology: current state and future steps*. Ann Neurol, 2011. **70**: 684–697.
15. Kasperaviciute, D. and Sisodiya, S.M. *Epilepsy pharmacogenetics*. Pharmacogenomics, 2009. **10**: 817–836.
16. Tate, S.K. and Sisodiya, S.M. *Multidrug resistance in epilepsy: a pharmacogenomic update*. Expert Opin Pharmacother, 2007. **8**: 1441–1449.
17. MacKenzie, M. and Hall, R. *Pharmacogenomics and pharmacogenetics for the intensive care unit: a narrative review*. Can J Anaesth, 2017. **64**: 45–64.

Chapter 2

Analgosedation and Neuromuscular Blockers

It is ostensibly a paradox, but many patients with acute brain injury receive sedation (1,2,9). Neurologic examination is rendered virtually impossible, and rapid neuroimaging may be the only option to assess the situation. These scenarios of emergent intubation and use of large amounts of anesthetic drugs are all too common in deteriorating patients with traumatic head injury, status epilepticus, or cerebral hemorrhage. In neurointervention suites, sedation is often used; starting as conscious sedation but then converted to general anesthesia in restless uncommunicative (aphasic) patients (2).

In the general intensive care unit (ICU) population, less or no sedation is associated with a better outcome (3), and daily sedation interruption is beneficial to the patient (4). Similar concerns apply to the use of neuromuscular blockers (NMBs), but now are used sparingly and mostly when there is a hard indication such as inability to ventilate properly in acute lung injury.

Deciding on Sedation

It remains a clinical judgment, but sedation is unnecessary when patients are not agitated or delirious, tolerate the endotracheal tube, or have a decreased responsiveness as a result of acute brain injury. Not every restless patient requires sedation. In fact, restlessness is often a good sign; transitioning from restlessness to stupor often is not. Indications for sedation are severe agitation resulting in possible harm to the patient, ventilator asynchrony, and poor gas exchange. We think that sedation is overused, for the wrong indications and at doses that are too high. Analgosedation is common in the general ICU but a controversial approach in acute brain injury. Some centers do routinely sedate patients after a severe acute brain injury, others are more reluctant knowing that there are misunderstandings about what sedation can do (Box 2.1). Analgosedation and often paralysis are considered in patients with refractory increased intracranial pressure, in situations that require targeted temperature management (e.g., post-cardiopulmonary resuscitation coma) or when control of extreme agitation is warranted (e.g., autoimmune encephalitis). Once sedated, interruption for a neurologic examination is needed but we have little understanding of what interruption of sedation (wake-up test) 'can do' to the patient physiologically with a damaged brain under pressure (16).

Box 2.1 Sedation in Critical Neurologic Patients—Hard Truths

- Sedation does not treat ICP effectively.
- Sedation does not always effectively suppress seizures.
- Sedation does not treat autonomic storming.
- Sedation does not improve cerebral metabolism.
- Sedation does not prevent self-extubation or catheter removal.

Sedative Drugs

The drugs most commonly used for sedation are propofol and midazolam. Dexmedetomidine is a good alternative and is often also a first choice. In the neurosciences ICU, physicians often switch between dexmedetomidine and propofol. Benzodiazepines are frequently administered in the neurosciences ICU and are used in combination with other sedatives to provide amnesia but are generally discouraged due to alleged increased rates of delirium and longer duration of mechanical ventilation. Sedation can be monitored with nursing scales such as the Richmond Agitation Sedation Scale (RASS), but reliance on these scales likely does not surpass close clinical observation focusing on patient comfort (5). As a rule, light sedation is better than deep sedation. Current consensus calls for a RASS score between 0 and -2.

Dexmedetomidine IV

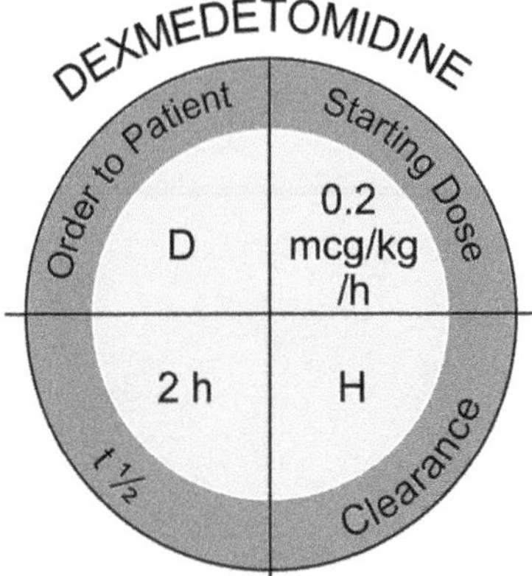

Pharmacologic Characteristics

- Selective alpha-2 agonist
- Effects are threefold: sedation, analgesia, and anxiolysis
- Peak effect in 15 minutes

- Reduces hypertension and tachycardia (reduces sympathetic drive)
- No significant effect on respiratory drive and can be used in non-ventilated patients
- Can decrease opioid, benzodiazepine, and propofol needs
- Shorter mechanical ventilation and increased patient communication to health care providers compared to propofol and midazolam, when used for sedation (18)

Dosing and Administration

- Loading dose: 1 mcg/kg over 10-minute intravenous (IV) infusion
- Continuous infusion: starting at 0.2 up to 0. 7 mcg/kg per hour
- Continuous infusion: up to 1.5 mcg/kg per hour IV allowed for duration of more than 24 hours

Monitoring

- Narrow therapeutic spectrum—side effects common with overshooting

Side Effects

- Hypotension when administered as a loading dose or at high infusion rates. Stop infusion—but can be restarted without a bolus and halved infusion rate
- Bradycardia
  - Bradyarrythmias have been associated with cardiac arrest
  - More common in hemodynamically unstable patients, the elderly, and patients with chronic hypertension
  - Discontinue immediately. Do not restart
- Agitation
- Seizures (rare)
- Nausea/vomiting

Propofol IV

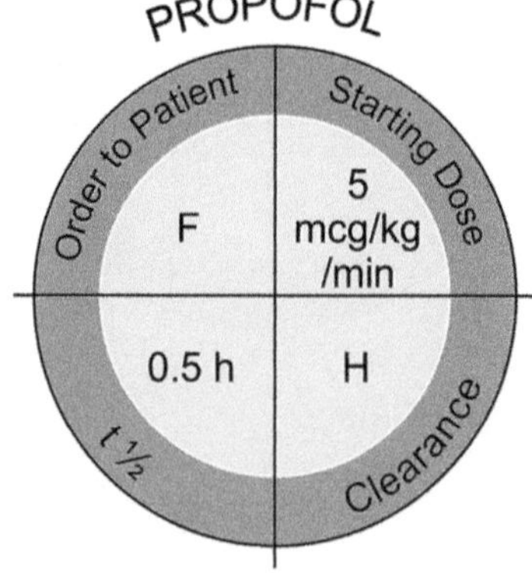

Pharmacologic Characteristics

- Pivotal sedative in any ICU
- Onset 10 to 50 seconds; duration 3 to10 minutes
- Preferred sedative because of rapid awakening when stopped (6–8)
- Reduces intracranial pressure only in very high doses and is ill advised for that indication
- Lower mortality in low doses than IV midazolam with earlier ICU discharge and fewer ventilator days

Dosing and Administration

- Dosing for procedural sedation: 1 mg/kg IV load, with 0.5 mg/kg IV repeated
- Infusion starting at 5 mcg/kg per minute, up to 80 mcg/kg per minute

Monitoring

- Clearance not significantly altered with renal or hepatic disease, but reduced clearance in critical illness due to decreased hepatic blood flow
- Prior alcohol use disorder may require higher doses
- Provides 1.1 kcal/ml from fat; calories should be counted toward daily nutrition allotments
- Frequent arterial blood gas (metabolic acidosis) and triglyceride levels (rising)—for anticipating propofol related infusion syndrome (These laboratory tests, however, are far from predictive)

Side Effects

- Hypotension common (vasodilatory response), especially with bolus administration or in patients with marginal volume status
- Propofol related infusion syndrome (rare)—acute-onset bradycardia or other dysrhythmia, metabolic acidosis, rhabdomyolysis or myoglobinuria, myocardial failure, followed by hypotension and circulatory collapse. Patient may be salvaged by extracorporeal membrane oxygenation (ECMO)
- Propofol related infusion syndrome more common with high doses (>80 mcg/kg per minute for >48 hours), in acute brain and spinal cord injury, in sepsis and with ketogenic diet
- Propofol may be associated with significant neuroexcitation while emerging from the drug with wild, agitated, bizarre behavior mimicking functional behavior, often in young individuals ("propofol frenzy"). Symptoms are self-limiting, may last hours, may repeat but only supportive care is required (17)

Midazolam IV

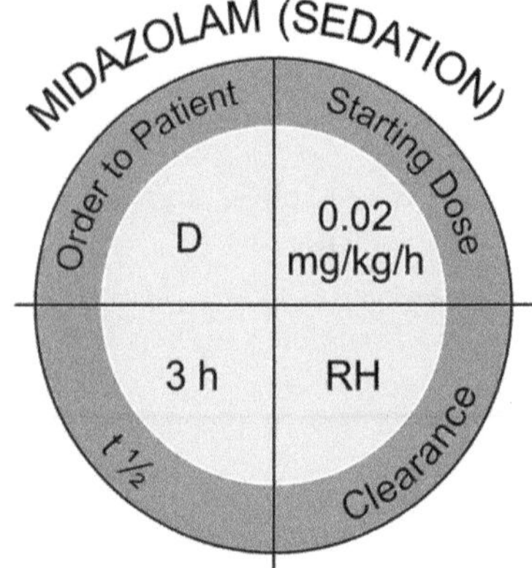

Pharmacologic Characteristics

- Gamma-aminobutyric acid (GABA)-A agonist
- Short-acting (30–90 seconds), rapid onset (1–2.5 minutes)
- Widely distributed into the cerebrospinal fluid (lipophilic drug)
- Half-life prolonged in cirrhosis, obesity, renal failure and with advanced age
- Extensively metabolized by the liver to active metabolite
- Induces anterograde—not retrograde—amnesia
- Opioid-sparing effect due to modulation of pain response

Dosing and Administration

- Bolus dose: 0.01 to 0.05 mg/kg, slow IV push over several minutes
- Starting dose: 0.02 mg/kg per hour and up to 0.1 mg/kg per hour continuous infusion, adjusted up by 25% to 50% to achieve level of sedation

Monitoring

- No reliable drug assays
- Active metabolites that accumulate in renal and hepatic dysfunction affect elimination half-life
- Metabolite (1-hydromidazolam glucuronide) has central nervous system depressant effects and can accumulate in renal failure
- Prolonged sedative effects in obese patients or those with reduced albumin levels (i.e., high lipophilicity and protein binding)

Side Effects

- Hypotension due to major cardiodepressant effect
- Respiratory depression and respiratory arrest
- Laryngospasm
- Tachyphylaxis (overstimulation of benzodiazepine receptors)

Lorazepam IV

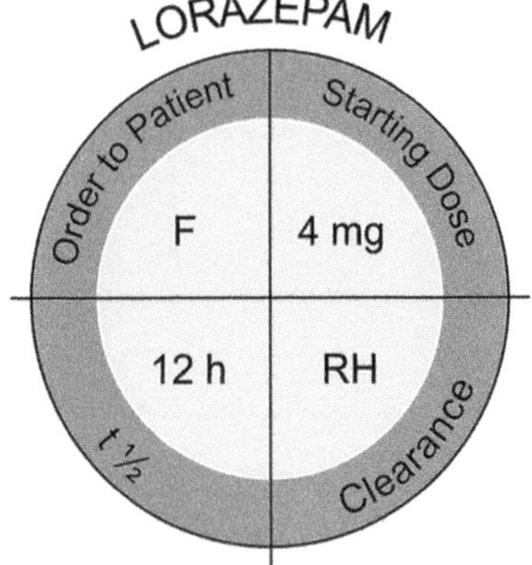

Pharmacologic Characteristics

- GABA-A agonist
- Slower onset than midazolam (2–3 minutes)
- Longer half-life than midazolam (12 hours), prolonged in end-stage renal disease (18 hours)
- Metabolized by hepatic conjugation to inactive metabolite

Dosing and Administration

- Continuous infusion: 0.01–0.1 mg/kg per hour (not commonly used)
- Intermittent dosing: 0.02–0.06 mg/kg

Monitoring

- Propylene glycol component in parenteral formulation and higher concentration may lead to toxicity (kidney injury, metabolic acidosis)
- 2 mg/hr = 20 g of propylene glycol (>10 times the WHO-recommended daily intake for 70-kg person)
- Screen for toxicity with doses of 50 mg/day or 1 mg/kg per day lorazepam using serum osmolar gap (toxicity ≥ 12)

Side Effects

- Propylene glycol toxicity and higher risk in pregnant patients, patients with renal or hepatic impairment, patients younger than 4 years, and patients receiving treatment with metronidazole. Hemodialysis will remove propylene glycol and correct the hyperosmolar gap.

Etomidate IV

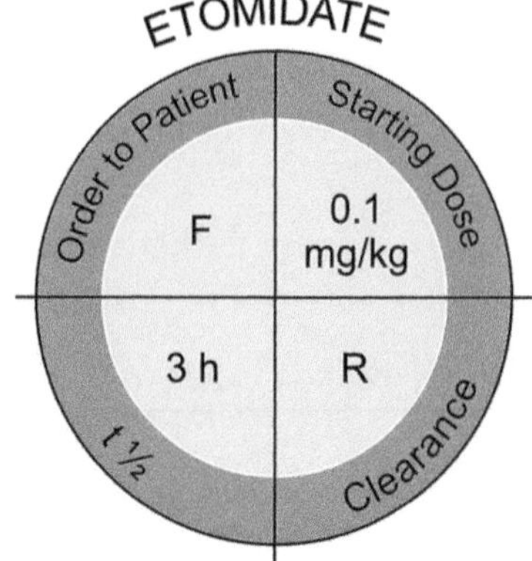

Pharmacologic Characteristics

- Ultra-short-acting non-barbiturate anesthetic agent
- Typically used in short procedures (e.g., endotracheal intubation)
- Preferred in hemodynamically unstable, agitated patients
- Rapid brain penetration and rapid elimination
- Short-term use only
- No known drug–drug interactions
- Produces electroencephalogram burst suppression at high doses
- Onset: 10–20 seconds; duration: 4–10 minutes

Dosing and Administration

- Sedation: 0.1–0.2 mg/kg; anesthesia: 0.3 mg/kg over 30 seconds

Monitoring

- Risk of toxicity in patients with renal impairment
- Free level increased in patients with hepatic cirrhosis or renal failure (75% protein-bound)
- Cardiac monitoring

Side Effects

- May induce cardiac depression in elderly patients with hypertension, who may need lower doses
- Increased mortality with continuous infusions
- Blocks 11-B hydroxylase (enzyme for adrenal steroid production). A single dose blocks adrenal cortisol production for 6–8 hours, up to 24 hours in elderly or debilitated patients
- Consider corticosteroids in severe stress

Analgesics

As a rule, opioids are avoided and are prescribed only when pain is obvious or unresponsive to simple analgesics. Opioid use leads to systemic effects such as bradycardia or hypotension. Opioids are used in combination with other sedatives for analgesia and have the potential to reduce the need of hypnotics when used in combination. Most nurses titrate the agent based on the use of arbitrary pain scales (verbal/nonverbal) or physiologic endpoints (Chapter 4). Opioids have significant side effects, most notably sedation, constipation, and vomiting. Dependency on opioids first prescribed in hospital settings (often after neurosurgical procedures) may be greater than appreciated.

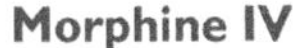

Morphine IV

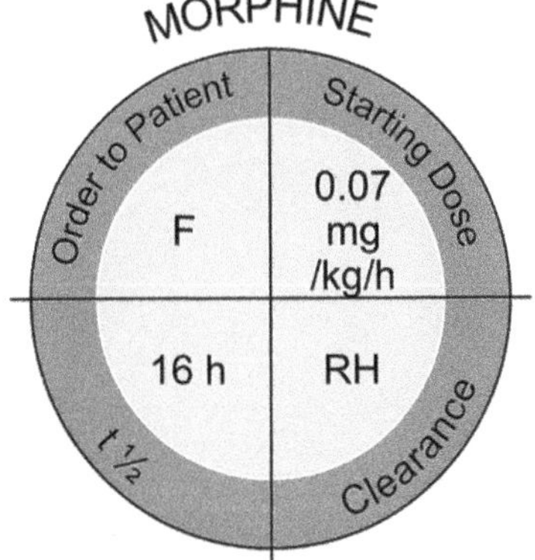

Pharmacologic Characteristics

- Binding to central opioid receptors in sensory pathways
- Onset: 5 minutes for analgesia
- Patients with altered P450 CYP2D6 enzyme activity may have no response to morphine or experience toxicity, depending on their metabolism
- Greater histamine release compared to fentanyl or hydromorphone

Dosing and Administration

- Continuous infusion: 0.07–0.5 mg/kg per hour for ventilated patients
- Intermittent dosing: 0.01–0.15 mg/kg every 1–2 hours
- Initiate at lower doses for renal failure; there is a decreased clearance because 90% of drug is renally excreted
- Initiate at lower doses for liver cirrhosis; elimination half-life is prolonged. Increase dosing interval 1.5 to 2 times of normal dosing regimen
- Active metabolite—accumulates several-fold in renal disease (morphine-6-glucuronide)
- Hydrophilic and low volume of distribution, and this leads to higher plasma concentrations

Monitoring

- Respiratory drive
- Gastrointestinal function

Side Effects

- Marked respiratory depression
- Constipation
- Gastrointestinal intolerance
- Hypotension, urticaria, pruritus, flushing, bronchospasm (from histamine release)
- Serotonin syndrome (Chapter 16) if used together with selective serotonin reuptake inhibitors (SSRIs)
- Adrenal suppression

Fentanyl IV

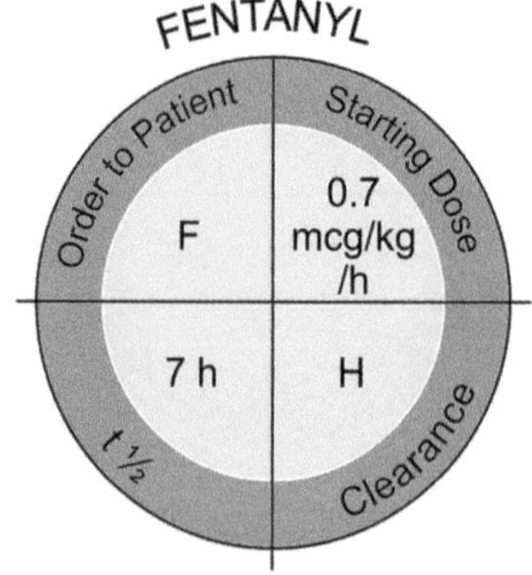

Pharmacologic Characteristics

- Binding to central mu-opioid receptors in sensory pathways
- Onset: almost immediate; duration: 1–2 hours
- Highly lipophilic thus fast onset (faster than morphine or hydromorphone)
- Comparative study with fentanyl versus propofol showed no difference in ICU length of stay or duration of ventilation, but there was a difference in the need for rescue opioids in those on propofol (10)
- Metabolized by the liver to inactive metabolites
- Half-life is prolonged with continuous infusions

Dosing and Administration

- Continuous infusion: 0.7–10 mcg/kg per hour or 25–200 mcg/hr
- Intermittent: 0.35–1.5 mcg/kg every hour for ventilated patients
- Conscious sedation: 0.5–1.5 mg/kg every 3 minutes, repeated if needed
- For mild renal failure, reduce to 75% of dose; severe failure, reduce to 50% of dose
- Hepatic blood flow affects fentanyl disposition

Monitoring

- Prolonged duration or effect after repeated doses (tissue accumulation in adipose tissues), especially in obese patients
- Significant accumulation with renal or hepatic disease
- Drug interactions: prolonged sedation/effects when used concomitantly with CYP3A4 inhibitors

Side Effects

- Marked respiratory depression
- Histamine release (less than morphine)
- Associated with serotonin syndrome if used with selective serotonin reuptake inhibitors (SSRIs)
- Adrenal suppression

Remifentanil IV

Pharmacologic Characteristics

- mu-receptor opioid agonist
- Rapid onset (1–3 minutes) and peak response (3–5 minutes); duration 3–10 minutes
- 500–1,000 times more potent than morphine

Dosing and Administration

- 0.025–2 mcg/kg per minute (when used with propofol or midazolam)
- 0.5–1 mcg/kg boluses every 2–5 minutes as needed
- Dosed based on ideal body weight in obesity

Monitoring

- Accumulation with renal failure
- Dialyzable: metabolite is 30% removed by hemodialysis

Side Effects

- Marked respiratory depression
- Histamine release (less than morphine)
- Associated with serotonin syndrome if used with selective serotonin reuptake inhibitors (SSRIs)
- Adrenal suppression
- Gastrointestinal intolerance

Hydromorphone IV

Pharmacologic Characteristics

- Binds to central opioid receptors in sensory pathways
- Onset: 5 minutes; duration: 3–4 hours
- Ideal agent for end-stage renal disease

Dosing and Administration

- Continuous infusion: 0.5–3 mg/hr
- Intermittent dosing: 0.2–1 mg every 2–3 hours

Monitoring

- Extensive hepatic metabolism to metabolites with unknown pharmacologic activity

Side Effects

- Marked respiratory depression
- Histamine release
- Associated with serotonin syndrome if used with selective serotonin reuptake inhibitors (SSRIs)
- Adrenal suppression

Ketamine IV

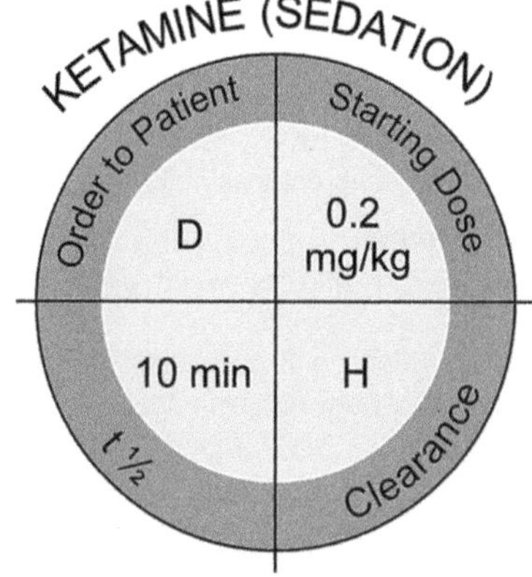

Pharmacologic Characteristics

- Noncompetitive NMDA receptor antagonist (excitatory neurotransmitter glutamate)
- Dissociative effect
- Deep analgesia and onset 30 seconds, duration 5–10 minutes
- May increase heart rate and blood pressure (useful in hypotensive patients)
- Contraindicated with myocardial ischemia (increases heart rate and cardiac output)
- Contraindicated in porphyria

Dosing and Administration

- Bolus: 0.5 mg/kg
- Profound rapid sedation: 0.2–2 mg/kg IV (maximal 4.5 mg/kg)
- 2 mcg/kg per minute continuous infusion for postoperative opioid-sparing effect

Monitoring

- Closely monitor for increased intracranial pressure
- Monitor for hypertension
- Monitor for tachycardia

Side Effects

- Hallucinations
- "K-hole" (derealization with visual and auditory hallucinations)
- Emergency reactions
- Risk of laryngospasm

Neuromuscular Blockers

Neuromuscular blockers (NMBs) are divided into depolarizing (e.g., succinylcholine) and nondepolarizing (e.g., vecuronium, rocuronium, atracurium, cisatracurium, pancuronium) classes (11). Depolarizing NMBs bind to receptors, depolarize the muscle membrane and open the calcium channels. Nondepolarizing NMBs bind to receptors but without channel opening, allowing rapid reversal (Fig. 2.1).

There are few neurologic reasons to use NMBs other than emergent intubation for airway control such as management of mechanical ventilation in patients with severe neurogenic pulmonary edema, targeted temperature management after cardiac resuscitation for prevention of shivering, and in some instances control of refractory intracranial pressure (ICP). There have been varying effects on ICP control with different agents based on systematic review, but administration for more than 12 hours resulted in longer ICU stays, higher occurrence of pneumonia, and a higher proportion of severely disabled survivors (12,13). Ultimately, the clinician must determine the risk/benefit ratio (11,14,15).

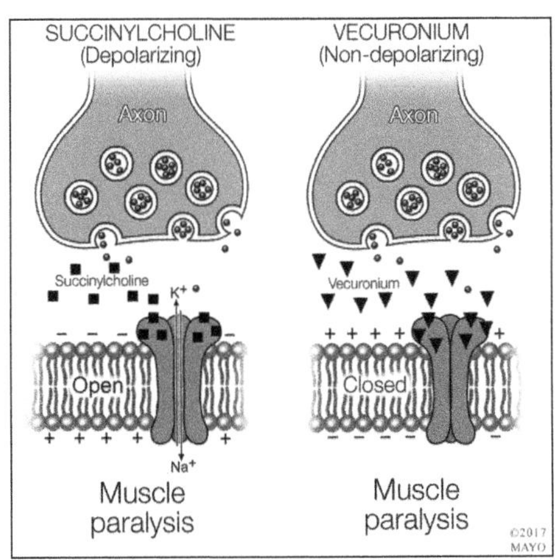

Figure 2.1 Mechanisms of depolarizing and nondepolarizing NMBs

Use of NMBs has decreased in the past years due to better awareness of the risks. Most importantly, neurologic examination is lost (except for pupil reaction to light) and seizures cannot be recognized clinically. Other substantial risks are prolonged ICU-acquired weakness, risk of patient awareness during paralysis, risk for deep venous thrombosis, anaphylaxis (IgE-mediated from ammonium ion), and corneal abrasions. Ultimately, many patients who have been paralyzed develop prolonged, flaccid limb weakness, caused by critical illness polyneuropathy, disturbances in microcirculation, protein malnutrition, systemic inflammation, and prolonged immobility. Adverse events caused by NMBs include hypersensitivity reactions (i.e., anaphylaxis), malignant hyperthermia, hypertension or hypotension, hyperkalemia, prolonged respiratory depression, rhabdomyolysis, myalgia, skeletal muscle weakness, and cardiac arrest. Train-of-four monitoring using a peripheral nerve stimulator should be used on all patients undergoing prolonged periods of NMB in order to determine the minimum drug dosage required to obtain a train-of-four of 2/4. It is important to obtain a baseline train-of-four assesment prior to initiating long term paralysis (19).

Neuromuscular Blockers in ICU Practice

NMBs are classified by their mode of action (depolarizing vs. nondepolarizing) and duration of action (short, intermediate, and long). Succinylcholine is often used for endotracheal intubation because of its short duration of action. Other NMBs are used to paralyze the patient for more prolonged periods.

Pharmacologic Characteristics of NMBs

Succinylcholine IV

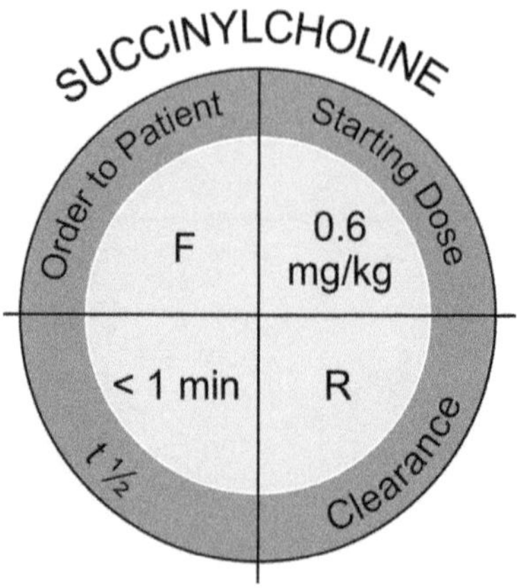

SUCCINYLCHOLINE

Order to Patient: F

Starting Dose: 0.6 mg/kg

t ½: < 1 min

Clearance: R

- 0.6 mg/kg (range 0.3–1.1 mg/kg) IV
- Onset 30–60 seconds; duration 6–10 minutes
- Slight ICP increase

- Drug of choice for rapid sequence intubation
- Hyperkalemia risk; use with caution in patients with preexisting hyperkalemia

Pancuronium IV

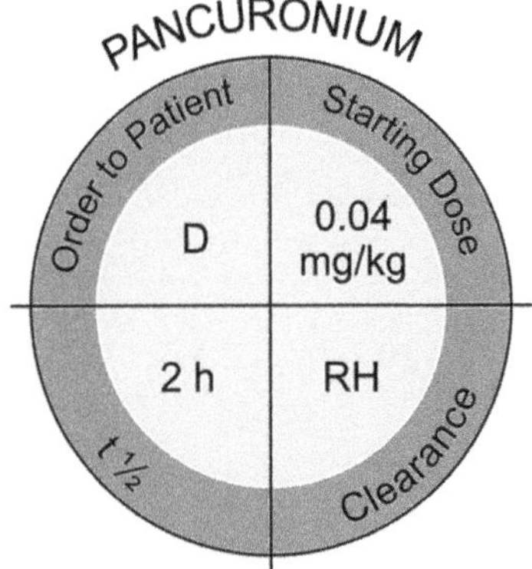

- 0.04–0.1 mg/kg IV
- Onset 120–180 seconds; duration 45–60 minutes
- Increases heart rate, blood pressure, and cardiac output
- Rarely used due to variable effects in renal dysfunction
- Prolonged effect in patients with myasthenia gravis and Lambert–Eaton myasthenic syndrome

Vecuronium IV

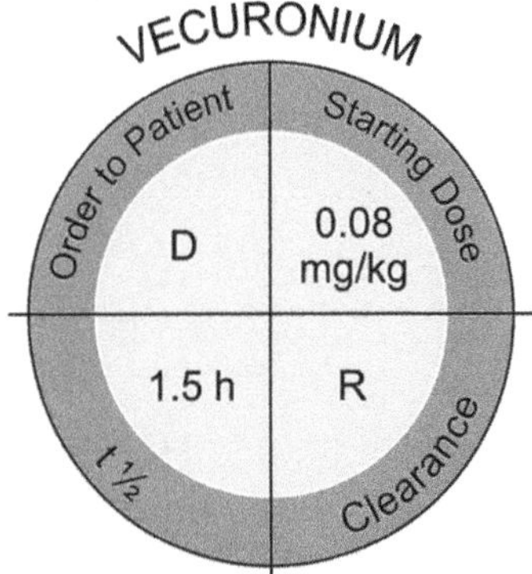

- 0.08–0.1 mg/kg IV
- Onset 2–4 minutes; duration 30–40 minutes

- No cardiovascular effect or ICP effect
- Rate of elimination decreased in patients with renal dysfunction

Cisatracurium IV

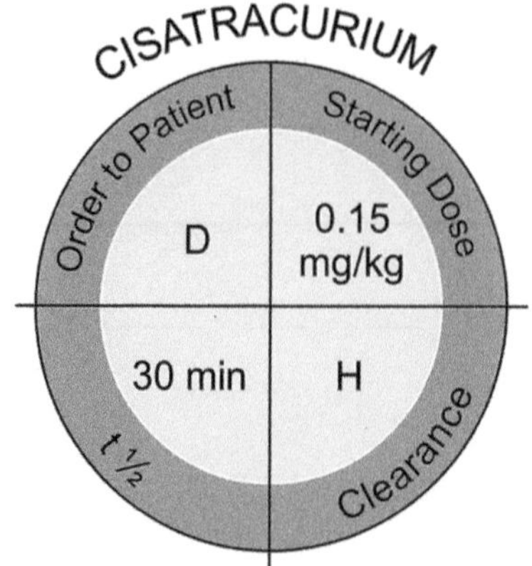

- 0.15–0.2 mg/kg IV
- Onset 90–120 seconds (2–3 minutes); duration 45–75 minutes
- Half-life prolonged in elderly patients
- More potent than atracurium
- Slower onset in patients with renal dysfunction
- Hofmann elimination (independent of liver, kidney, or enzymatic processes but metabolite hepatically cleared)

Rocuronium IV

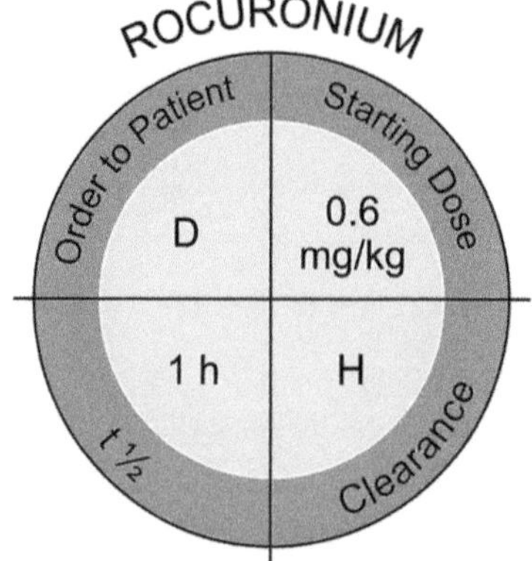

- 0.6–1.2 mg/kg
- Onset 60–90 seconds; duration 30 minutes
- Half-life prolonged in patients with renal disease
- Less potent than vecuronium
- Liver elimination, prolonged effect and elimination in patients with liver dysfunction
- Requires refrigeration

Atracurium IV

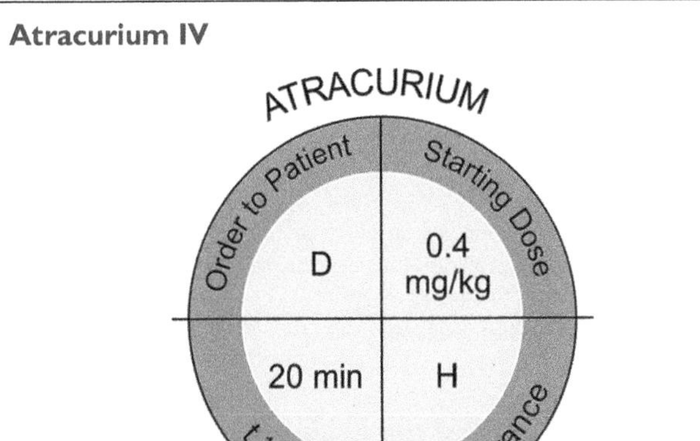

- 0.4–0.5 mg/kg
- Onset 2–5 minutes; duration 60–70 minutes
- Hypotension caused by histamine release
- Hofmann elimination (independent of liver, kidney, or enzymatic processes but metabolite hepatically cleared)

Monitoring of NMBs and Side Effects

- Train-of-four using a peripheral nerve stimulator; goal 2/4 twitches
- Important pharmacokinetic and pharmacodynamic changes in critically ill patients
  - Age—decrease in total body water, lean body mass, and serum albumin. May lead to decreased volume of distribution for NMBs, leading to increased drug effect and a decrease in drug elimination
  - Hypothermia—may prolong duration of action of NMBs due to altered sensitivity of neuromuscular junction, decreased acetylcholine, decreased muscle contraction, and reduced renal or hepatic clearance
  - Hypokalemia—may augment blockage by nondepolarizing agents and may reduce ability of neostigmine to reverse blockade

- Hypermagnesemia—prolongs the duration of blockade by inhibiting calcium
- Hypercalcemia—calcium triggers acetylcholine release; may reduce sensitivity to NMBs and decrease the duration of effect. Calcium may antagonize the potentiating effects of magnesium with NMBs
- Acidosis may enhance blockade effects of nondepolarizing agents
- Organ dysfunction: pancuronium half-life is increased in patients with liver failure; vecuronium and pancuronium have prolonged action as a result of metabolite accumulation in patients with renal disease
- Drug–drug interactions
  - Phenytoin, carbamazepine, other antiepileptic drugs may cause resistance to NMBs
  - Administration of succinylcholine after the administration of a nondepolarizing agent will cause a prolonged effect of succinylcholine
  - Cyclosporine may inhibit NMB metabolism and prolong effect
  - Uncertain effect of cardiac drugs
  - Uncertain effects of antibiotics

Reversal of Neuromuscular Blockers

- Neostigmine
  - Dose: 0.04–0.07 mg/kg IV
  - Reversal within 1 minute with a peak effect for 9 minutes
  - Increases the amount of acetylcholine in the neuromuscular junction
- Antimuscarinics needed to counteract side effects of acetylcholinesterases such as bradycardia, bradyarrhythmias, increased secretions, and bronchoconstriction
  - Atropine 0.01–0.02 mg/kg IV with neostigmine 0.04 mg/kg IV
  - Edrophonium 10 mg IV over 30–45 seconds
  - Glycopyrrolate 0.2 mg IV for every 1 mg neostigmine
- Sugammadex (steroidal muscle relaxant encapsulator) for urgent rocuronium reversal. Sugammadex forms a complex with the NMJ blocker to prevent binding to the nicotinic receptor in the NMJ. This results in the NMJ blockade reversal.
  - For immediate clinical need: 16 mg/kg IV for 1.2 mg/kg single rocuronium administration
  - Reversal in less than 3 minutes
  - Dosing based on actual body weight
  - For routine reversal: 4 mg/kg IV bolus (actual body weight)
- If tendon reflexes are intact, reversal mostly complete

Key Pointers

1. Light sedation is preferred to deep sedation. Sedation is overused and is used for longer than necessary, for the wrong reasons, and at doses that are too high.
2. The agent used for sedation often switches between dexmedetomidine, propofol and midazolam.
3. Propofol related infusion syndrome is more common with high doses for more than 48 hours and manifests comparatively more often in patients with acute neurocritical illness.
4. Opioids are used in combination with other sedatives and may reduce hypnotics (i.e., analgosedation).
5. Phenytoin, carbamazepine, and other antiepileptic drugs increase resistance to NMBs.

References

1. Devabhakthuni, S., et al., *Analgosedation: a paradigm shift in intensive care unit sedation practice*. Ann Pharmacother, 2012. **46**: 530–540.
2. Devlin, J.W. and Roberts, R.J. *Pharmacology of commonly used analgesics and sedatives in the ICU: benzodiazepines, propofol, and opioids*. Anesthesiol Clin, 2011. **29**: 567–585.
3. Jackson, D.L., et al., *A systematic review of the impact of sedation practice in the ICU on resource use, costs and patient safety*. Crit Care, 2010. **14**: R59.
4. Mehta, S., et al., *Daily sedation interruption in mechanically ventilated critically ill patients cared for with a sedation protocol: a randomized controlled trial*. JAMA, 2012. **308**: 1985–1992.
5. Riker, R.R., et al., *Clinical monitoring scales in acute brain injury: assessment of coma, pain, agitation, and delirium*. Neurocrit Care, 2014. **21 Suppl 2**: S27–37.
6. Angelini, G., Ketzler, J.T. and Coursin, D.B. *Use of propofol and other nonbenzodiazepine sedatives in the intensive care unit*. Crit Care Clin, 2001. **17**: 863–880.
7. Flower, O. and Hellings, S. *Sedation in traumatic brain injury*. Emerg Med Int, 2012. **2012**: 637171.
8. Lonardo, N.W., et al., *Propofol is associated with favorable outcomes compared with benzodiazepines in ventilated intensive care unit patients*. Am J Respir Crit Care Med, 2014. **189**: 1383–1394.
9. Oddo, M., Crippa, I.A., Mehta, S., Menon, D., Payen, J.F., Taccone, F.S. and Citerio, G. *Optimizing sedation in patients with acute brain injury*. Crit Care, 2016. **20**(1): Review.
10. Tedders, K.M., McNorton, K.N. and Edwin, S.B. *Efficacy and safety of analgosedation with fentanyl compared with traditional sedation with propofol*. Pharmacotherapy, 2014. **34**: 643–647.
11. Greenberg, S.B. and Vender, J. *The use of neuromuscular blocking agents in the ICU: where are we now?* Crit Care Med, 2013. **41**: 1332–1344.
12. Sanfilippo, F., et al., *The role of neuromuscular blockade in patients with traumatic brain injury: a systematic review*. Neurocrit Care, 2015. **22**: 325–334.

13. deBacker, J., Hart, N. and Fan, E. *Neuromuscular blockade in the 21st Century Management of the Critically Ill Patient.* Chest, 2017. **151**: 697–706.
14. Murray, M.J., et al., *Clinical practice guidelines for sustained neuromuscular blockade in the adult critically ill patient.* Crit Care Med, 2002. **30**: 142–156.
15. Schepens, T. and Cammu, G. *Neuromuscular blockade: what was, is and will be.* Acta Anaesthesiol Belg, 2014. **65**: 151–159.
16. Marklund, N. *The Neurological Wake-up Test-A Role in Neurocritical Care Monitoring of Traumatic Brain Injury Patients?* Front Neurol, 2017. **8**: 540.
17. Carvalho, D.Z., Townley, R.A., Burkle, C.M., Rabinstein, A.A. and Wijdicks, E.F.M. *Propofol Frenzy: Clinical Spectrum in 3 Patients.* Mayo Clin Proc, 2017. **92**: 1682–1687.
18. Jakob, S.M., Ruokonen, E., Grounds, R.M. et al. *Dexmedetomidine vs midazolam or propofol for sedation during prolonged mechanical ventilation: two randomized controlled trials.* JAMA, 2012. **307**: 1151–1160.
19. Murray, M.J., DeBlock, H., Erstad, B. et al. *Clinical Practice Guidelines for Sustained Neuromuscular Blockade in the Adult Critically Ill Patient.* Crit Care Med, 2016. **44**: 2079–2103.

Chapter 3

Agitation and Delirium

Agitation is common, particularly in patients with acute right hemispheric or frontal lobe lesions (1–3). In general intensive care units (ICUs), agitation and delirium occur in the sickest patients, those undergoing major surgery, those with multiple-organ failure, and those with a history of alcohol or drug abuse (4–6) (Chapter 18). There is a high likelihood that delirium in the elderly is more common in those with previously unrecognized or known dementia. Older age and frailty remain the most robust risk factors for delirium in surgical and medical ICUs, and thus, are confounding co-variables.

Delirium involves abnormalities in perception and, often, the inability to maintain attention and failure of the observer to correct behavior. There is a current tendency to divide delirium into *hypoactive* and *hyperactive* delirium, with the former characterized by less attention and paucity of movement. Most neurologists agree that patients are typically restless. A hypoactive delirium is very difficult to diagnose reliably and only, perhaps, after a comprehensive evaluation for other neurologic (e.g., posterior reversible encephalopathy syndrome, drug neurotoxicity, diencephalic or cortical lesions) and medical disorders (e.g., metabolic derangements) has been performed. The diagnosis subsyndromal delirium is even more controversial, and there is no standard definition or interobserver studies. When used to diagnose patients there is a—not unexpectedly—very high incidence in critical illness (1). For all of these manifestations, consensus definitions are wanting and the diagnosis are difficult to make due to its subjectivity.

The current view is to recognize delirium (often first observed by the nursing staff) and to avoid administering medications associated with higher risks of delirium (7,8). Yet, drugs should also be used cautiously and not in everyone who teeters at the brink of delirium. (As a corollary, physicians have learned a lesson with overprescribing opioids when pain became a high priority vital sign.)

Causes of Delirium

Contributing factors for delirium consistently found in large hospital series include advanced age (defined as > 65 years old), alcoholism, prior cognitive impairment or depression, a prior history of delirium, advanced respiratory disease, hypertension, and a number of drugs (Box 3.1). Polypharmacy used at home may be a major factor. Withdrawal of alcohol or drugs of abuse remains an underappreciated cause of delirium, and often family members provide a much different history than what is volunteered by the patient.

Box 3.1 Drugs Contributing to Delirium

- Sedative-hypnotics
- Narcotics
- Anticholinergics
- Benzodiazepines
- Corticosteroids
- Antimicrobials
- Stimulants
- H2 blockers

Once in the hospital, use of opioids in elderly patients, particularly meperidine, can cause significant agitation and behavioral changes. Similar effects can occur with high-dose corticosteroids, such as intravenous (IV) methylprednisolone. Benzodiazepine infusions (in high daily doses) are a major risk factor (2,4,9). Other predisposing factors are acute hospital-acquired infections, fever, a new appearance of hypoxemia or hypercapnia, and disturbance of sleep—an unavoidable problem in many ICUs.

Delirium may be prevented by simple measures in low-risk patients (Box 3.2). For high-risk patients (and those rapidly scoring positive on the Clinical Institute Withdrawal Assessment for Alcohol [CIWA] protocol), pharmacotherapy is needed.

A special group of patients are those admitted with an autoimmune encephalitis and refractory agitation, which is comparatively difficult to treat. Patients may show disinhibition, self-injurious behaviors, hallucinations and delusions. The broad psychiatric clinical spectrum may include catatonic symptoms such as mutism, rigidity, posturing, stupor, staring, and gegenhalten alternating with combativeness (11). The NMDA hypofunction model of psychosis suggests that drugs such as olanzapine, clozapine, and lamotrigine can arrest the acute neurotoxic process. Mood stabilizers such as lithium and valproic acid have been used to treat manic symptoms. Benzodiazepines are the first choice to treat the catatonic symptoms, and electroconvulsive therapy

Box 3.2 Prevention of Delirium

- Early physical and occupational therapy
- Sleep enhancement (reduction of light and noise)
- Music therapy
- Improved daylight exposure
- Single-room ICU
- Minimize disruptions to sleep
- Hearing and vision aids for those with impairments
- Pain control
- Avoid physical restraints when able
- Reorientation to environment
- Risperidone or low-dose haloperidol in very high-risk patients (10)

(ECT) may be warranted in patients with life-threatening malignant catatonia or catatonia refractory to other treatments (12,13). Multiple medication trials, including sertraline, ziprasidone, quetiapine, olanzapine, and valproic acid, have generally been unsuccessful, and some patients are better protected with endotracheal intubation, mechanical ventilation, and midazolam infusion while undergoing plasma exchange and corticosteroid treatment.

Clinical Features of Delirium

Generally when in a delirium, patients fidget or thrash and may yell, hallucinate, grab nursing staff, or try to leave. Hallucinations of animals (e.g., seeing rodents) are common in alcohol-withdrawal delirium. Autonomic overdrive (i.e., tachycardia, sweating, and hypertension) is common and may lead to cardiac arrhythmias, electrocardiographic (EKG) changes, and increased creatine phosphokinase (CPK) values. Screening tools have been developed and validated (14,15). Tables 3.1 and 3.2 show the delirium detection and Confusion Assessment Method for the Intensive Care Unit (CAM-ICU) scores used by nursing staff to alert physicians and to administer medications when certain thresholds are reached.

Table 3.1 Delirium Detection Score

Symptoms	Points
1 Orientation	
Orientated to time, place, and personal identity; able to concentrate	☐ 0
Not sure about time and/or place, not able to concentrate	☐ 1
Not orientated to time and/or place	☐ 4
Not orientated to time, place, and personal identity	☐ 7
2 Hallucinations	
None	☐ 0
Mild hallucinations at times	☐ 1
Permanent mild-to-moderate hallucinations	☐ 4
Permanent severe hallucinations	☐ 7
3 Agitation	
Normal activity	☐ 0
Slightly higher activity	☐ 1
Moderate restlessness	☐ 4
Severe restlessness	☐ 7
4 Anxiety	
No anxiety when resting	☐ 0
Slight anxiety	☐ 1
Moderate anxiety at times	☐ 4
Acute panic attacks	☐ 7

(continued)

Table 3.1 (Continued)

Symptoms	Points
5 Myoclonus/Convulsions	
None	□ 0
Myoclonus	□ 1
Convulsions	□ 7
6 Paroxysmal Sweating	
No sweating	□ 0
Almost undetectable, only palms	□ 1
Beads of perspiration on the forehead	□ 4
Heavy sweating	□ 7
7 Altered Sleep-Waking Cycle	
None	□ 0
Mild, patient complaints about problems to sleep	□ 1
Patient sleeps only with high dose of medication	□ 4
Patient does not sleep despite medication at night, tired at day time	□ 7
8 Tremor	□ 1
None	□ 4
Not visible, but can be felt	□ 7
Moderate tremor (arms stretched out)	□
Severe tremor (without stretching arms)	□
Delirium	≥8
No delirium	<8

Table 3.2 Confusion Assessment Method for the Intensive Care Unit (CAM-ICU)

Feature 1: Acute Onset or Fluctuating Course: Positive if you answer "yes" to either 1A or 1B.	Positive	Negative
1A: Is the patient different from his/her baseline mental status?	Yes	No
1B: Has the patient had any fluctuation in mental status in the past 24 hrs as evidenced by fluctuation on a sedation scale (e.g., RASS), GCS, or previous delirium assessment?		
Feature 2: Inattention: Positive if either score for 2A or 2B is <8. Attempt the ASE letters first. If patient is able to perform this test and the score is clear, record this score and move to Feature 3. If patient is unable to perform this test or the score is unclear, then perform the ASE Pictures. If you perform both tests, use the ASE Pictures' results to score the Feature.	Positive	Negative

(continued)

Table 3.2 (Continued)		
2A: ASE Letters: Record score (enter NT for not tested). Directions: Say to the patient, *"I am going to read you a series of 10 letters. Whenever you hear the letter 'A', indicate by squeezing my hand."* Read letters from the following letter list in a normal tone. S A V E A H A A R T Scoring: Errors are counted when patient fails to squeeze on the letter "A" and when the patient squeezes on any letter other than "A."	Score (out of 10): ______	
2B: ASE Pictures: Record score (enter NT for not tested). Directions are included on the picture packets.	Score (out of 10): ______	
Feature 3: Disorganized Thinking. Positive if the combined score is <4.	Positive	Negative
3A: Yes/No Questions (Use either Set A or Set B, alternate on consecutive days if necessary): Set A / Set B 1. Will a stone float on water? / 1. Will a leaf float on water? 2. Are there fish in the sea? / 2. Are there elephants in the sea? 3. Does one pound weigh more than two pounds? / 3. Do two pounds weigh more than one pound? 4. Can you use a hammer to pound a nail? / 4. Can you use a hammer to cut wood? Score ____ (Patient earns 1 point for each correct answer out of 4)	Combined Score (3A + 3B): ______ (out of 5)	
3B: Command: Say to patient: *"Hold up this many fingers."* (Examiner holds two fingers in front of patient.) *"Now do the same thing with the other hand."* (Not repeating the number of fingers.) *If patient is unable to move both arms, for the second part of the command, ask patient, *"Add one more finger."* Score ____ (Patient earns 1 point if able to successfully complete the entire command.)		
Feature 4: Altered Level of Consciousness: Positive if the Actual RASS score is anything other than "0" (zero).	Positive	Negative
Overall CAM-ICU: (Features 1 and 2 and either Feature 3 or 4).	Positive	Negative

Pharmacologic Treatment of Agitation

Several drugs can aggravate or cause agitation or delirium, and our current understanding points to upregulation of neurotransmitters, mostly GABA receptors. Anticholinergic medications can also cause delirium, suggesting cholinergic deficiency as a potential mechanism.

The consensus is to avoid benzodiazepines unless there is an alcohol-withdrawal delirium or withdrawal from benzodiazepines. The evidence that benzodiazepines are a risk factor for delirium is comparatively strong. Antipsychotics also raise a concern, because these drugs increase the risk of a prolonged QT interval on the electrocardiogram, and thus the risk of ventricular tachycardia or torsades de pointes. Caution should be used when administering opioid medications and other central nervous system depressants.

In the neurosciences ICU, there is no compelling reason to start drugs to help prevent a possible delirium, and there has been no convincing study to support such an approach. (This is different with the use of dexmedetomidine to prevent postoperative delirium, for which there is evidence of an effect in clinical trials.)

A reasonable start is quetiapine 12.5 to 25 mg orally at bedtime in incremental doses if sedation or seizures are not a major concern. If oral administration is a problem, the next approach can be haloperidol 1 mg given intravenously (IV). The dose can be repeated every 30 minutes if agitation persists and eventually settling on a maintenance dose. Dexmedetomidine remains a rescue drug of choice when haloperidol fails. If agitation is extreme, as is seen in patients with autoimmune encephalitis, patients may simply have to be intubated using high-dose intravenous midazolam, propofol or a combination (16,17). Prescribers should use the lowest, most effective dose and for a limited duration.

Neuroleptics

Haloperidol IV

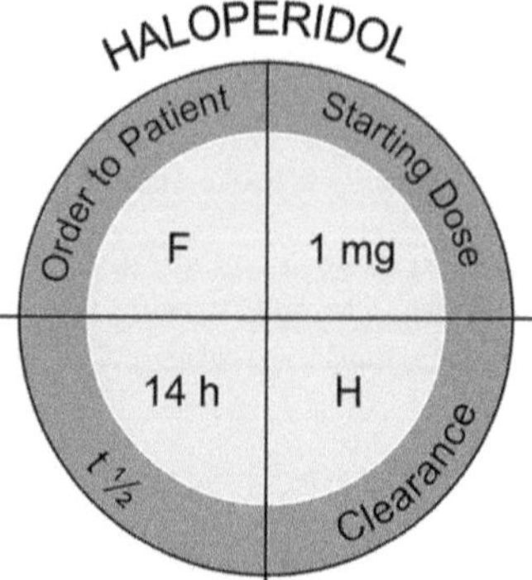

Pharmacologic Characteristics

- Potent dopamine receptor antagonist
- Best clinical experience and often first-line therapy for delirium
- Clearance: 50–60% cleared by liver via CYP3A4 with active metabolites
- Lipophilic and freely crosses the blood–brain barrier

- Concentration in cerebrospinal fluid can be 10 times more than in serum after intramuscular (IM) administration (10,18,19)
- Onset of action is 30 minutes with IV route (injection product is not approved by the U.S. Food and Drug Administration [FDA] for IV use, but it is frequently used clinically)

Dosing and Administration

- 0.5–1 mg IV
- Repeat dose every 30 minutes (usually half of initial dose)
- Maintenance 2 mg every 6 hours IV
- Maximum dose 5–10 mg IV

Monitoring

- EKG for QT interval prolongation
- CAM-ICU scores

Side Effects

- Greater risk of QT prolongation and torsades de pointes with IV administration and with higher doses
- Acute dystonic reactions (i.e., oculogyric crisis, torticollis)
- Akathisia (less acute)
- Worsening of Parkinson's symptoms
- Hypotension, cardiac arrhythmia

Quetiapine PO

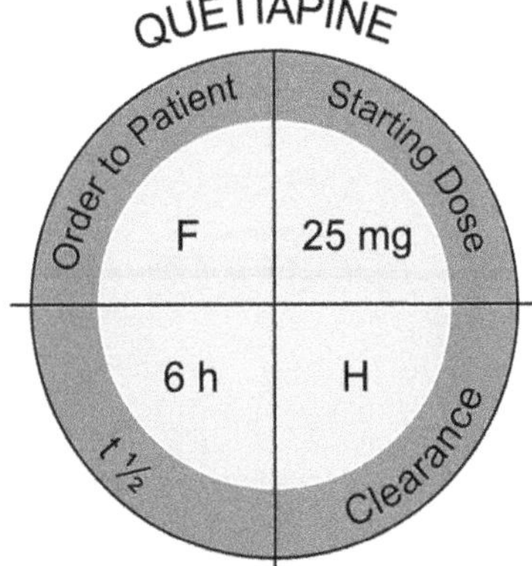

Pharmacologic Characteristics

- Antagonist of 5HT1 and 5HT2 (serotonin) receptors, dopamine D1 and D2 receptors, histamine-1 and alpha-1 and alpha-2 receptors centrally
- Generally greater sedative H1 effect at lower doses, greater neuroleptic D2 effect at higher doses (20)

- Useful in many moderately agitated patients, but sedation may be a limiting factor
- Preferred neuroleptic for treating delirium in Parkinson's disease
- Extensive first-pass metabolism, 83% protein-bound
- Primarily metabolized in the liver via CYP3A4 to active and inactive metabolites
- Time to peak: 1.5 hours

Dosing and Administration

- Initiate at 25 mg nightly; titrate to response
- 25–200 mg orally every 12 hours, maximum 10 days and until improved

Monitoring

- Anticholinergic effects (e.g., constipation, urinary retention)
- Lower risk of QT prolongation compared with haloperidol but more than olanzapine
- Cholesterol (with long term use)
- Weight, gain (with long term use)
- Extrapyramidal symptoms

Side Effects

- Sedation (high incidence and often unexpected with low dose)
- Orthostatic hypotension
- Hyperglycemia
- Hyponatremia (rare)
- Seizures (rare, more common with prior dementia)

Olanzapine PO

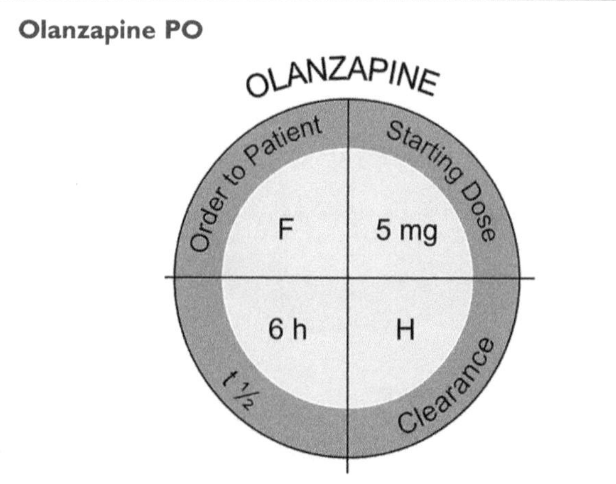

Pharmacologic Characteristics

- Dopamine and 5HT receptor antagonist, with histamine, alpha-adrenergic, and muscarinic receptor affinity
- Dopamine blockade increases with increasing doses
- Peak effect: 6 hours (orally); 15–45 minutes (IM)
- Extensive first-pass metabolism
- Increased urinary drug clearance in smokers

Dosing and Administration

- 5 mg orally nightly for up to 5 days or until improved
- 2.5 mg/day starting dose in elderly
- Available as oral dissolving tablet for rapid absorption
- IM for severe agitation, when spitting or refusing oral route
- Not for IV administration
- Do not administer within 1 hour of parenteral benzodiazepine

Monitoring

- QT prolongation (less than haloperidol, but more than quetiapine)
- Extrapyramidal symptoms (less than haloperidol)
- Weight, gain (long-term use)

Side Effects

- Orthostatic hypotension
- Abnormal liver function test results
- Anticholinergic effects
- Blood dyscrasias
- Seizures (rare, more common with prior dementia)
- Increase in serum prolactin

Dexmedetomidine IV

Pharmacologic Characteristics

- Dexmedetomidine is a selective alpha-2 agonist
- Effects are threefold: sedation, analgesia, and anxiolysis
- Decreases blood pressure and heart rate (reduces sympathetic drive)
- No significant effect on respiratory drive and can be used in non-ventilated patients
- Ability to use lower doses of opioids, benzodiazepines, and propofol concurrently
- Shorter ICU stay compared to propofol, when used for sedation, and less ICU delirium compared to propofol
- Time to peak 15 minutes

Dosing and Administration

- Loading dose: 1 mcg/kg over 10-minute IV infusion
- Continuous infusion: starting at 0.2–0.7 mcg/kg per hour
- Continuous infusion: up to 1.5 mg/kg per hour IV allowed for duration >24 hours
- Titrate infusion no faster than every 30 minutes to avoid hypotension

Monitoring

- Narrow therapeutic spectrum—overshoots common
- Blood pressure and heart rate
- Level of sedation (i.e., RASS)

Side Effects

- Hypotension is common, when administered as a loading dose or at high infusion rates. Can be restarted without a bolus and at half previous infusion rate
- Bradycardia
  - Bradyarrhythmias have been associated with cardiac arrest
  - More common in hemodynamically unstable patients, elderly patients, and patients with chronic hypertension
  - Discontinue immediately; do not restart
- Agitation
- Seizures
- Nausea and vomiting

Benzodiazepines

These drugs are useful in severely agitated patients and those experiencing alcohol withdrawal symptoms. Benzodiazepine use otherwise is not recommended for the management of delirium.

Midazolam IV

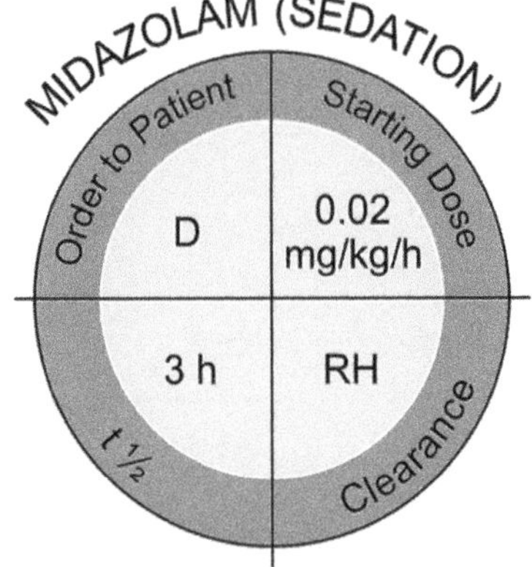

Pharmacologic Characteristics

- Gamma-Aminobutyric acid (GABA) agonist
- Short-acting (30–90 seconds), rapid onset (1–2.5 minutes)
- Induces anterograde—not retrograde—amnesia
- Opioid-sparing effect due to modulation of pain response
- Extensively metabolized by the liver

Dosing and Administration

- Bolus dose: 0.01–0.05 mg/kg, slow IV push over several minutes
- Starting dose: 0.02 mg/kg per hour and up to 0.1 mg/kg per hour continuous infusion, increased by 25–50% to achieve level of sedation

Monitoring

- No reliable drug assays
- Active metabolites that accumulate in renal and hepatic dysfunction have an impact on half-life
- Metabolite (1-hydromidazolam glucuronide) has central nervous system depressant effects and can accumulate in renal failure
- Prolonged sedative effects in obese patients or those with reduced albumin levels because of lipophilicity and protein binding

Side Effects

- Hypotension due to major cardiodepressant effect
- Respiratory depression and respiratory arrest
- Laryngospasm, hiccups

Lorazepam IV

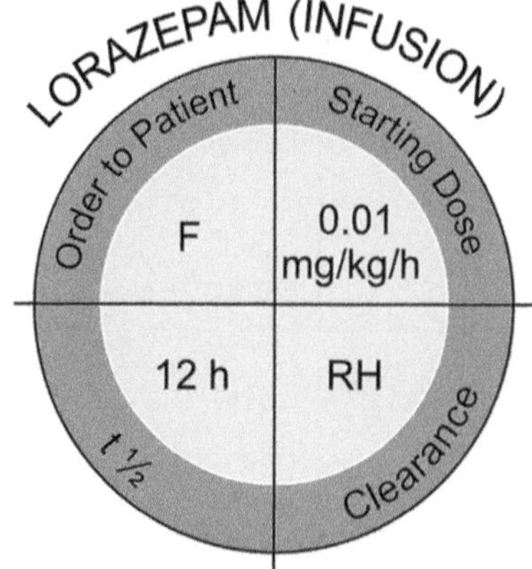

Pharmacologic Characteristics

- GABA agonist
- Slower onset than midazolam (within 2 minutes)
- Longer half-life than midazolam (about 14 hours), prolonged in renal dysfunction
- Metabolized extensively by the liver to inactive metabolite, highly protein-bound (~90%)

Dosing and Administration

- Continuous infusion: 0.01–0.1 mg/kg per hour
- Intermittent dosing: 0.02–0.06 mg/kg
- Dilute IV product 1:1 with saline prior to intermittent dose administration

Monitoring

- Propylene glycol component in parenteral formulation and higher concentration may lead to toxicity (e.g., kidney injury, metabolic acidosis)
- 2 mg per hour = ~20 g of propylene glycol (> 10 times the WHO-recommended daily intake for a 70-kg person)
- Screen for toxicity with doses of 50 mg/day or 1 mg/kg per day lorazepam using serum osmolar gap
- Respiratory and cardiac function

Side Effects

- Propylene glycol toxicity and higher risk in pregnant patients, patients with renal or hepatic impairment, children age < 4 years, patients being treated with metronidazole
- Hemodialysis will remove propylene glycol and correct hyperosmolar gap
- Extrapyramidal reactions

Preventive Drugs

These agents are considered for use in high-risk patients and not for treatment of florid delirium.

Donepezil PO

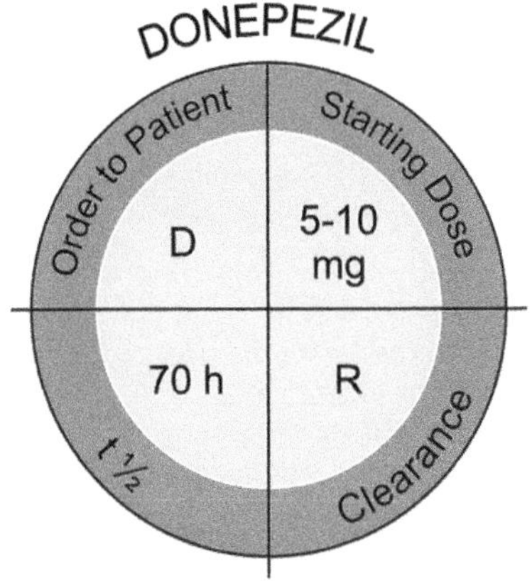

Pharmacologic Characteristics

- Centrally acting acetylcholinesterase inhibitor (increases acetylcholine concentration presynaptically) (16)
- Used in high-risk patients but clinical trials have not shown a markedly decreased incidence of delirium

Dosing and Administration

- 5 mg orally once daily at bedtime
- Up to 23 mg orally daily for multi-infarct dementia
- No established maximum dose in agitation (off-label use)

Monitoring

- Improved sleep pattern

Side Effects

- Hypotension
- Can cause dream disturbances (dose in the morning if problematic)
- Greater number of side effects than alternatives
- Cholinergic effects (e.g., nausea, diarrhea)

Melatonin PO

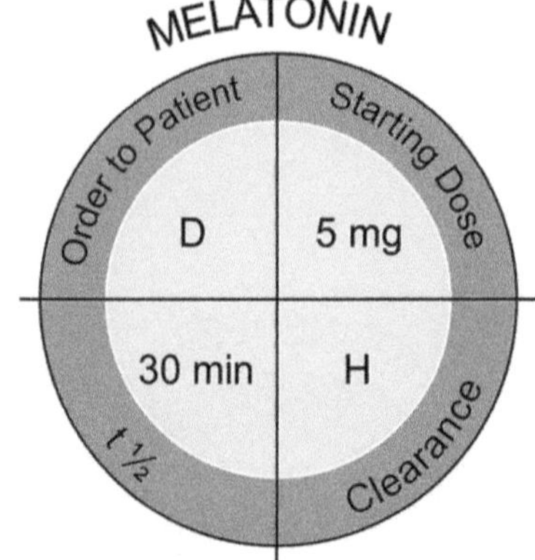

Pharmacologic Characteristics

- Secreted by the pineal gland from the amino acid tryptophan; decreased secretion in delirium
- Helps regulate circadian rhythm (21)
- Optimal role in treating ICU delirium unknown
- Extensively cleared by the liver, half-life prolonged in cirrhosis
- Onset: 2 hours, administer before intended hour of sleep
- Peak effect: 90 minutes

Dosing and Administration

- Starting dose: 5 mg nightly, may be doubled

Monitoring

- Improved sleep pattern
- Liver function tests

Side Effects

- Daytime sleepiness
- Headaches
- Dizziness

Key Pointers

1. Delirium is best prevented, and if mild, treated first with non-pharmacologic measures.
2. Atypical antipsychotics are the first-line treatment for delirium.
3. Haloperidol is a potent and effective drug, but its use is limited due to QT prolongation.
4. Dexmedetomidine is a rescue drug for patients with severe agitation.
5. Benzodiazepines should be avoided in non-withdrawal delirium.

References

1. Brummel, N.E., Boehm, L.M., Girard, T.D. et al., *Subsyndromal delirium and institutionalization among patients with critical illness.* Am J Crit Care, 2017. **26**: 447–455.
2. Pandharipande, P., et al., *Prevalence and risk factors for development of delirium in surgical and trauma intensive care unit patients.* J Trauma, 2008. **65**: 34–41.
3. Pandharipande, P.P., et al., *Effect of dexmedetomidine versus lorazepam on outcome in patients with sepsis: an* a priori*-designed analysis of the MENDS randomized controlled trial.* Crit Care, 2010. **14**: R38.
4. Dubois, M.J., et al., *Delirium in an intensive care unit: a study of risk factors.* Intensive Care Med, 2001. **27**: 1297–1304.
5. Ebersoldt, M., Sharshar, T. and Annane, D. *Sepsis-associated delirium.* Intensive Care Med, 2007. **33**: 941–950.
6. Shehabi, Y., et al., *Delirium duration and mortality in lightly sedated, mechanically ventilated intensive care patients.* Crit Care Med, 2010. **38**: 2311–2318.
7. Garrett, K.M., *Best practices for managing pain, sedation, and delirium in the mechanically ventilated patient.* Crit Care Nurs Clin North Am, 2016. **28**: 437–450.
8. Fick, D.M., Auerbach, A.D., Avidan, M.S. et al.; NIDUS Delirium Network, *Network for Investigation of Delirium across the U.S.: Advancing the Field of Delirium with a New Interdisciplinary Research Network.* J Am Geriatr Soc, 2017. **65**: 2158–2160.
9. Zaal, I.J., et al., *Benzodiazepine-associated delirium in critically ill adults.* Intensive Care Med, 2015. **41**: 2130–2137.
10. Wang, W., et al., *Haloperidol prophylaxis decreases delirium incidence in elderly patients after noncardiac surgery: a randomized controlled trial.* Crit Care Med, 2012. **40**: 731–739.
11. Kuppuswamy, P.S., Takala, C.R. and Sola, C.L. *Management of psychiatric symptoms in anti-NMDAR encephalitis: a case series, literature review and future directions.* Gen Hosp Psychiatry, 2014. **36**: 388–391.
12. Braakman, H.M., et al., *Pearls & Oysters: electroconvulsive therapy in anti-NMDA receptor encephalitis.* Neurology, 2010. **75**: e44–46.
13. Chapman, M.R. and Vause, H.E. *Anti-NMDA receptor encephalitis: diagnosis, psychiatric presentation, and treatment.* Am J Psychiatry, 2011. **168**: 245–251.
14. Ely, E.W., et al., *Evaluation of delirium in critically ill patients: validation of the Confusion Assessment Method for the Intensive Care Unit (CAM-ICU).* Crit Care Med, 2001. **29**: 1370–1379.
15. Neto, A.S., et al., *Delirium screening in critically ill patients: a systematic review and meta-analysis.* Crit Care Med, 2012. **40**: 1946–1951.
16. Al-Qadheeb, N.S., et al., *Preventing ICU subsyndromal delirium conversion to delirium with low-dose IV haloperidol: a double-blind, placebo-controlled pilot study.* Crit Care Med, 2016. **44**: 583–591.
17. Barr, J. and Pandharipande, P.P. *The pain, agitation, and delirium care bundle: synergistic benefits of implementing the 2013 Pain, Agitation, and Delirium Guidelines in an integrated and interdisciplinary fashion.* Crit Care Med, 2013. **41**: S99–115.
18. Fok, M.C., et al., *Do antipsychotics prevent postoperative delirium? A systematic review and meta-analysis.* Int J Geriatr Psychiatry, 2015. **30**: 333–344.

19. Turunen, H., et al., *Dexmedetomidine versus standard care sedation with propofol or midazolam in intensive care: an economic evaluation.* Crit Care, 2015. **19**: 67.

20. Devlin, J.W., et al., *Efficacy and safety of quetiapine in critically ill patients with delirium: a prospective, multicenter, randomized, double-blind, placebo-controlled pilot study.* Crit Care Med, 2010. **38**: 419–427.

21. Al-Aama, T., et al., *Melatonin decreases delirium in elderly patients: a randomized, placebo-controlled trial.* Int J Geriatr Psychiatry, 2011. **26**: 687–694.

Chapter 4

Pain Management

Many central (brain and spinal cord) and peripheral (nerve roots and peripheral nerve) neurologic disorders are demonstrably painful. Pain control is important, and pain has been arguably considered by the Joint Commission a vital sign next to blood pressure, heart rate, temperature, airway and breathing. Adequate pain control has a high priority, but pain control does not manage major other discomforts (4). Moreover, overprescribing with opioids may be common resulting in the American Medical Association to re-emphasize that pain is a symptom and not a vital sign.

The pharmacopeia of pain management in hospital setting is growing and changing, and several trends have been noted. Tricyclic antidepressants, selective serotonin and norepinephrine reuptake inhibitors, and antiepileptic drugs found their way in pain treatment.

Grading Pain

Patients in the intensive care unit (ICU) who are communicative can be asked to rate the pain on a visual analog scale of 0 to 10 (0, no pain; 10, excruciating and unbearable pain). The numeric pain-rating scale using faces has been validated (Fig. 4.1) (1–3). In less responsive patients, pain is signaled by moaning, grimacing, and extreme restlessness, but these remain very subjective measures and could lead to overtreatment.

0-10 Numeric Pain Intensity Scale (NPIS)

0 1 2 3 4 5 6 7 8 9 10

No pain — Moderate pain — Worst possible pain

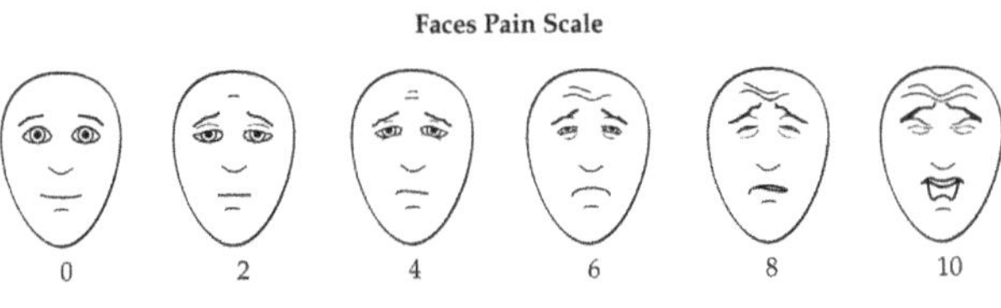

Figure 4.1 Numerical Pain Rating Scale

Table 4.1 Critical-Care Pain Observation Tool (CPOT)

Indicator	Description	Score	
Facial expression	No muscular tension observed	Relaxed, neutral	0
	Presence of frowning, brow lowering, orbit tightening, and levator contraction	Tense	1
	All of the above facial movements plus eyelid tightly closed	Grimacing	2
Body movements	No movement at all (may not mean absence of pain)	Absence of movements	0
	Slow, cautious movements, touching or rubbing the pain site, seeking attention through movements	Protection	1
	Pulling tube, attempting to sit up, moving limbs/thrashing, not following commands, striking at staff, trying to climb out of bed	Restlessness	2
Muscle tension	No resistance to passive movements	Relaxed	0
	Resistance to passive movements	Tense, rigid	1
	Strong resistance to passive movements, inability to complete them	Very tense or rigid	2
Ventilator Compliance	Alarms not activated	Tolerating ventilator or movement	0
OR	Alarms stop spontaneously	Coughing but tolerating ventilator	1
	Asynchrony: blocking ventilation, alarms frequently activated	Fighting ventilator	2
Vocalization	Normal conversational tone or no sound		0
	Sighing, moaning		1
	Crying out, sobbing		2
Total, range			**0–8**

Tables 4.1 and 4.2 show commonly used nursing scales, and high scores are triggers to give pain medication. The Critical-Care Pain Observation Tool (CPOT) (Table 4.1) and the Behavioral Pain Scale (BPS) (Table 4.2) are validated and useful in most ICU patients, including those with acute brain and spine injury. The critical care pain observation tool identifies several domains: facial expression, movements, muscle tension, and how well the ventilator is tolerated. In non-intubated patients, sounds and moaning are graded. Inadequate pain control leads to disturbed sleep, fighting the ventilator, rapidly escalating anxiety and restlessness but also endocrine changes, delayed gastric emptying (and vomiting), as well as very obvious tachycardia, hypertension, and dyspnea. It is just as important to grade pain at rest or during turning. Wide pupils have been used as indirect markers of pain but are not very useful in neurologic patients.

Table 4.2 Behavioral Pain Scale

Categories	0	1 Rare	2 Occasional	3 Frequent	4 Constant
FACE (Expression)	Relaxed, no particular expression or smile	Grimacing, frowning, or wrinkled forehead		Grimacing, tearing, frowning, or wrinkled forehead	
ACTIVITY (Movement)	Lying quietly, normal position, no guarding	Uneasiness, splinting areas of the body, tenseness, or slow, cautious movement		Restlessness, excessive movement of arms or legs, withdrawal reflexes, rigidness, or stiffness	
VITAL SIGN CHANGE*	**0**	**1**		**2**	
	Stable or no change in past 4 hours:	**Change over past 4 hours greater than:**		**Change over past 4 hours greater than:**	
	SpO_2	Decreased SpO_2 5		Decreased SpO_2 10	
	RR	Increased RR 10		Increased RR 20	
	HR	Increased HR 20		Increased HR 25	
	SBP	Increased SBP 20		Increased SBP 30	

*** Vital Sign Change = change in 1 or more vital signs:** SpO_2 = pulse oximetry, RR = respiratory rate, HR = heart rate, SBP = systolic blood pressure

In 2013 the American College of Critical Care Medicine published a comprehensive update on pain and delirium management (5). Pain is underreported in the ICU and should be treated when indicated. Opioids are considered the main analgesic of choice in critically ill patients with non-neuropathic pain, and non-opioid drugs are recommended to reduce the dose of opioid drugs. Gabapentin or carbamazepine is considered a first-line choice for patients with neuropathic pain. So called "bundle strategies" (comprehensive order sets) are encouraged.

Types of Pain in the Neurosciences ICU

Conditions in the neurosciences ICU associated with headache are hemorrhagic stroke (often with a rapid decline in consciousness), cerebellar infarcts, meningitis, and cerebrospinal fluid hypotension headache (with upright position). Excruciating pain associated with a ruptured cerebral aneurysm has not subsided in patients who have been admitted to the neurosciences ICU, and often there is a severe lingering, holocephalic pain causing nausea and vomiting. Typically we see a curled-up, immobilized patient trying to find any relief.

The headache associated with a ruptured aneurysm starts as a split-second excruciating head pain moving quickly into the neck. A "thunderclap" headache refers to a split-second, extremely intense ("10 out of 10"), totally unexpected headache. The sudden onset can often be recognized by the patient if the examiner demonstrates a handclap or finger snap. The headache with an arteriovenous malformation is much less explosive and may have migrainous characteristics.

Box 4.1 Worsening Headache

- Recurrent subarachnoid hemorrhage
- Enlarging hematoma
- New hematoma
- Raised intracranial pressure
- Nosocomial meningitis
- Hypertensive urgency

Pain is generated from meningeal vessels containing pain-sensing fibers as the result of an inflammatory response and subsequent meningeal irritation. Less severe pain is seen after a craniotomy, but it is still often severe enough to warrant strong analgesics. Because it associated with vomiting, oral medication is not always effective or appropriate. Pain is associated with increased intracranial pressure and often proven with resolution after reduction of pressure (e.g., ventriculostomy). Conversely, low-pressure headache (i.e., spontaneous intracranial hypovolemia syndrome) causes headache in a sitting position. In any event, a worsening headache may signal a new problem (Box 4.1) (6,7).

Another category is patients with an acute spinal cord injury or acute poly-radiculoneuropathy. Pain can be defined as allodynia (pain with a stimulus not usually causing pain) or hyperalgesia (exaggerated pain with a painful stimulus), but also pain can be absent in areas that should be normally painful (analgesia). Pain in acute polyneuropathy may appear in several forms, including hyperalgesia, sciatica, muscle pain and cramps, and joint stiffness. Patients may complain of tingling or burning, prickling, tightness, or shooting (lancinating) pain. Typical is the nocturnal aggravation of pain that keeps patients from rest and sleep. Neuropathic pain may be electric and shock-like (8–13). Pain associated with avulsion of nerves can cause excruciating deafferentation pain, and the best-known is avulsion of the brachial plexus, but this usually occurs much later. These types of pain can be continuous, often a burning or throbbing pain (assumed to be due to thalamic neuroplasticity), or shooting paroxysms (assumed to be due to dorsal horn hyperactivity).

Drugs for Pain

Acetaminophen should be the first agent used in pain management. Next are weak narcotic analgesics (e.g., codeine and tramadol), which could have less severe side effects than stronger opioid analgesics. They must be reserved for patients who cannot tolerate acetaminophen or who have mild to moderate pain. They must be used preferentially in patients with acute brain injury in whom sedation is unacceptable. If opioids are the only option, oral codeine is the agent of choice for relief of severe pain in acute central nervous system disorders. Intravenous (IV) medication is

Box 4.2 Management of Pain with Subarachnoid Hemorrhage

- Acetaminophen oral, rectal or IV 500-1000 mg (may be repeated)
- Tramadol, oral 400 mg/day (divided doses)
- Gabapentin, oral 300 mg every 8 hours
- Codeine, oral 30 mg every 6 hours as needed
- Dexamethasone, oral 2 mg every 6 hours

generally preferred in the critically ill patient because of varying degrees of gastrointestinal dysfunction in this population. There is evidence of serious underuse of analgesics when neurosciences ICUs are surveyed (14). Suggestions for pain treatment in subarachnoid hemorrhage are shown in Box 4.2, and pain treatment for post-neurosurgical patients is covered in Box 4.3.

Several drug options are available (15,16). First-choice headache drugs are acetaminophen, codeine, tramadol, and, recently, gabapentin (17). Intravenous acetaminophen is expensive but is currently explored as an option in craniotomy to reduce the need for opioids (18). Ketamine is emerging as a possible alternative to opioids in acute pain management (19).

Control of Specific Headaches

Posttraumatic Headache

Valproic Acid

- 1,000–1,500 mg orally once daily
- Best avoided in patients with unstable brain contusions
- Do not use in pregnancy or in patients with liver disease
- Major side effects include hyperammonemia, hepatitis, pancreatitis and thrombocytopenia
- Assess baseline liver function test results and pancreatic enzymes if there is a strong suspicion of dysfunction
- Multiple drug formulations are available; extended-release formulation is marketed for headache prevention

Propranolol

- Nonselective beta-blocker
- 80 mg orally daily in divided doses initially; titrate to maximum (tolerated) dose of 240 mg/day in divided doses
- Major side effects: hypotension, bradycardia
- Use caution in patients with airway disease due to risk of bronchospasm
- Do not discontinue use abruptly, but taper off slowly
- Extensive first-pass liver metabolism, higher drug exposure noted in liver dysfunction

Box 4.3 Management of Post-Neurosurgical Patients

- Acetaminophen 1000 mg orally four times daily
- Codeine 30 mg per dose orally, maximum 360 mg/day
- Morphine, 2 mg IV hourly as needed
- Morphine patient-controlled analgesia

Reversible Cerebral Vasoconstriction Syndrome

Nimodipine

- Dihydropyridine calcium-channel blocker, with greater central-acting than peripheral-acting effects (on blood pressure)
- 60 mg orally every 4 hours; reduce dose to 30 mg every 4 hours in patients with cirrhosis
- Administer on an empty stomach 1 hour before or 2 hours after food
- Large, solution-filled capsules; patients with dysphagia may have difficulty swallowing. Could puncture capsules and withdraw solution with a needle
- Major side effect: hypotension
- Avoid use with strong CYP3A4 inhibitors

Verapamil

- Non-dihydropyridine calcium-channel blocker. Decreases calcium efflux into smooth muscle and reduces vasodilation and vasoconstriction of blood vessels
- 360 mg orally daily, in three divided doses
- Common side effects: constipation, hypotension, bradycardia, peripheral edema

Cerebrospinal Fluid Hypotension Syndrome

Dexamethasone

- 4 mg orally once daily for 4 days
- Long-acting corticosteroid with very few mineralocorticoid properties
- Common side effects: gastrointestinal irritation, hyperglycemia, insomnia

Caffeine

- Causes cerebral vasoconstriction; stimulates cerebrospinal fluid production by stimulating Na/K ATPase pumps
- 300 mg orally as needed (every 4 hours)
- 500 mg IV in 1 L saline infused over 1 hour
- Major side effects: insomnia, agitation, restlessness

Acetaminophen PO

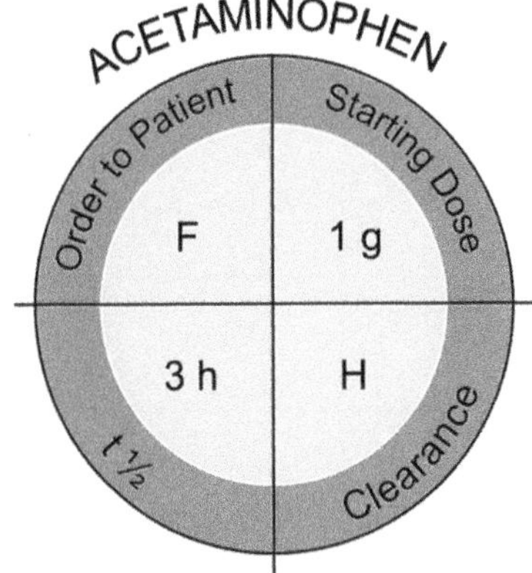

Pharmacologic Characteristics

- Analgesic and antipyretic
- Inhibits prostaglandin synthesis in the central nervous system
- Effect in <1 hour orally
- Effect in 5–10 min for IV (peak analgesic effect IV in 1 hour)
- Effect lasts 4–6 hours (both IV and orally)
- Half-life may be doubled with severe renal failure (glomerular filtration rate [GFR] <30 ml/min)

Dosing and Administration

- 1,000 mg orally or enterally (maximal 4000 mg in 24 hours)
- IV given as infusion over 15 minutes (not "pushed")
- IV only if no oral route (IV is no more effective than oral and is more costly)
- IV use is contraindicated in hepatic disease

Monitoring

- Pain response
- Regular liver and kidney function tests
- Stop use if liver function test results are abnormal
- Increase administration interval with kidney failure (GFR ≤10–50 ml/min)

Side Effects

- Hypotension (decrease of >15%) with IV administration
- Nausea and vomiting with IV infusion
- Caution with 6GPD deficiency (accumulation of toxic metabolite)

Codeine PO

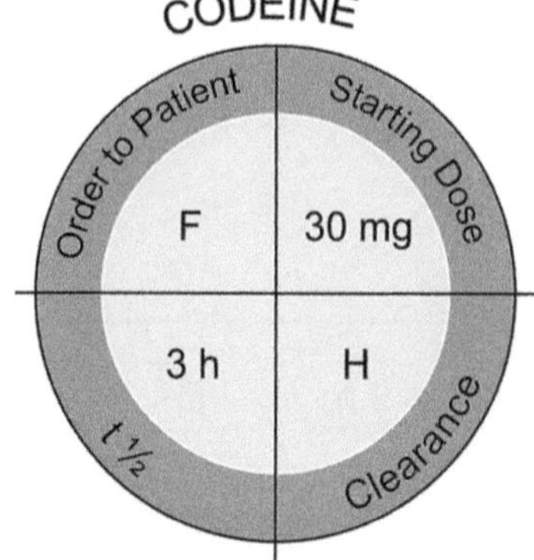

Pharmacologic Characteristics

- Mu-receptor agonist
- Metabolized rapidly by CYP2D6 to morphine. If patient is a poor metabolizer, will not achieve adequate patient response; if patient is an ultra-rapid metabolizer, will potentially "overdose" on analgesia
- Use with strong CYP2D6 inhibitors may prevent codeine conversion to morphine (decreased analgesia response)
- Duration: 4–6 hours
- Onset: 30–60 minutes

Dosing and Administration

- 30–60 mg orally every 4 hours as needed
- Maximum 360 mg/24 hours

Monitoring

- Pain response
- Degree of sedation
- Respiratory rate

Side Effects

- Nausea and vomiting
- Constipation (i.e., reduced bowel sounds, abdominal distention)
- Respiratory depression

Morphine IV

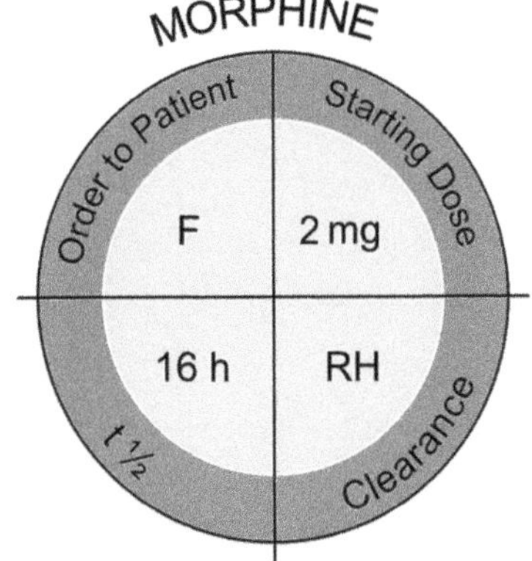

Dosing and Administration

- 2–4 mg IV every 3–4 hours, over slow IV push (4–5 minutes)
- Continuous infusion: 2–30 mg/hr (0.07–0.5 mg/kg per hour)
  Peak: 30 minutes for oral, 5–10 minutes for IV
- Decrease doses in patients with renal dysfunction
- Onset: 5 minutes, duration 4 hours

Monitoring

- Renal function tests
- Pain control
- Respiratory rate
- Heart rate and blood pressure

Side Effects

- Nausea and vomiting
- Respiratory depression
- Hypotension
- Bronchospasm
- Bradycardia
- Constipation, ileus
- Urinary retention
- Seizures (rare)

Fentanyl IV

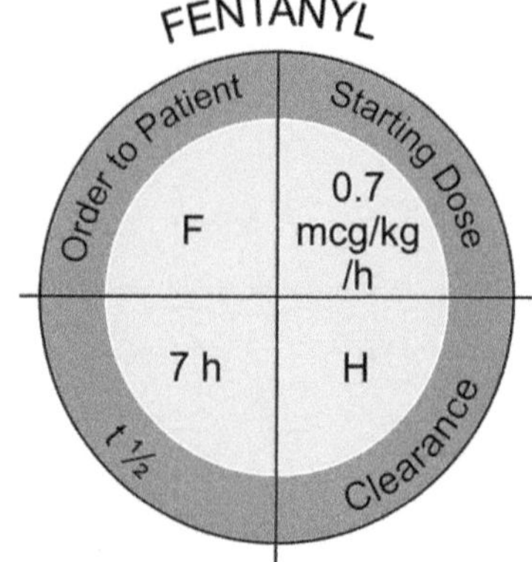

Pharmacologic Characteristics

- 50–100 times more potent than morphine
- Synthetic derivative of morphine
- Short half-life with intermittent doses (2–4 hours)
- Long half-life with infusion (9–16 hours)
- Highly lipophilic, fast onset; may accumulate in adipose tissue, causing prolonged sedation when discontinued

Dosing and Administration

- Slow IV push 25–35 mcg every 30 minutes (0.5 mcg/kg)
- Continuous infusion: 0.7–10 mcg/kg per hour
- Patient-controlled analgesia
  - <50 mcg/hr basal rate
  - 10–20 mcg demand dose

Monitoring

- Respiratory rate
- Heart rate and blood pressure
- Pain response

Side Effects

- Respiratory depression
- Hypotension
- Bronchospasm
- Bradycardia
- Impaired gastrointestinal motility, constipation, ileus
- Seizures (rare)
- Nausea and vomiting
- Urinary retention

Oxycodone PO

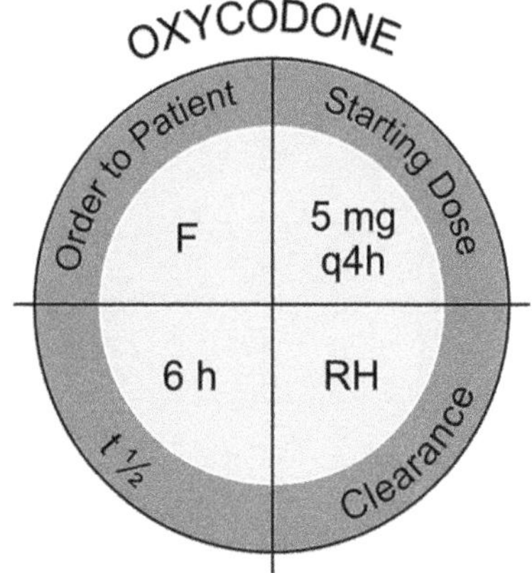

Pharmacologic Characteristics

- Semisynthetic derivative of morphine
- Onset: 10–15 minutes
- Peak effect: 0.5–1 hour

Dosing and Administration

- Dosing: 5–15 mg orally every 4–6 hours
- Decrease initial dose by 33–50% in patients with renal dysfunction

Monitoring

- Pain response
- Respiratory rate
- Heart rate and blood pressure

Side Effects

- Respiratory depression
- Hypotension
- Bronchospasm
- Bradycardia
- Impaired gastrointestinal motility, constipation, ileus
- Seizures (rare)
- Nausea and vomiting
- Urinary retention

Tramadol PO

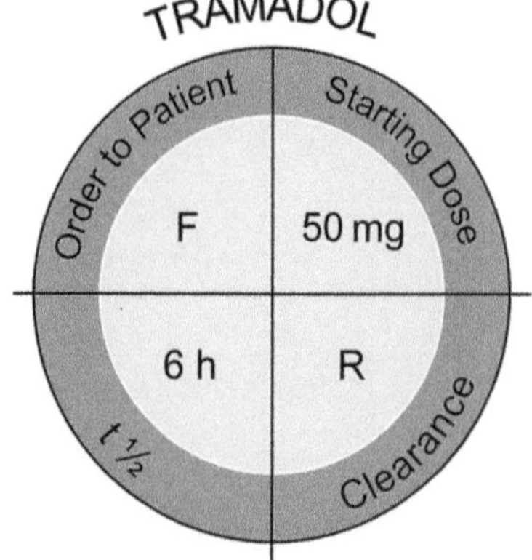

Pharmacologic Characteristics

- Indirect binding of mu-opioid receptors and inhibition of norepinephrine and serotonin reuptake
- Used as pain management when pain is severe enough to require daily opioids ("opioid-sparing" drug)
- Effect within 1 hour, peak 2–3 hours

Dosing and Administration

- 50–100 mg every 4 hours
- Maximum 400 mg/day with normal renal function
- Renally cleared, dose reduced in diminished renal function (maximum 200 mg/day when creatinine clearance [CrCl] <30 ml/min), extend interval to every 12 hours
- Removed by hemodialysis

Monitoring

- Respiratory rate
- Liver function tests
- Renal function tests

Side Effects

- Potential for seizures
- Respiratory depression
- Constipation
- Bradycardia in high doses
- Sedation
- Do not use within 14 days of monoamine oxidase inhibitors

Ketorolac IM

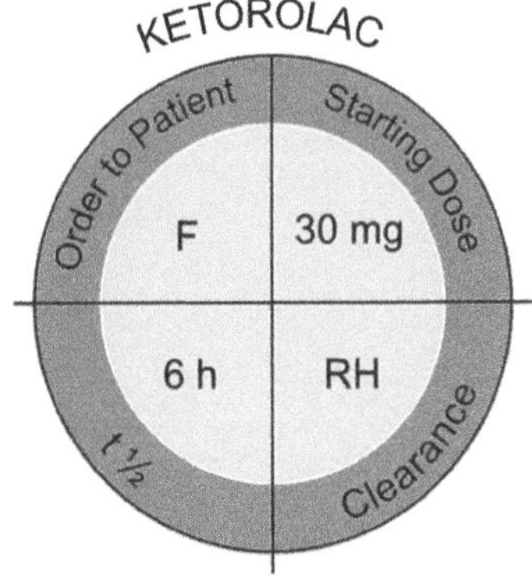

Pharmacologic Characteristics

- Fast onset of analgesia: 30 minutes for injection (intramuscular [IM] or IV)
- Less sedation than opioids
- Nonselective nonsteroidal anti-inflammatory (NSAID; blocks both cyclooxygenase [COX]-1 and COX-2 enzymes), resulting in decreased prostaglandin precursors; has antipyretic, analgesic, and anti-inflammatory properties
- Useful in patients with postoperative pain
- Half-life is doubled in patients with renal failure

Dosing and Administration

- Single dose 30 mg IM, slowly and deeply into muscle tissue
- IV administration over 15 seconds
- Adjust dose for weight <50 kg and age >65 years (maximum 15 mg per dose, 60 mg/day); there is an increased risk of adverse events in these patients

Monitoring

- Pain response
- Laboratory or clinical signs of gastrointestinal bleeding
- Renal function tests

Side Effects

- Risk of renal injury; use is contraindicated in patients with advanced renal disease
- Limited to 5 days of consecutive use due to risk of serious gastro-intestinal adverse events (bleeding)
- Renal dysfunction

Celecoxib PO

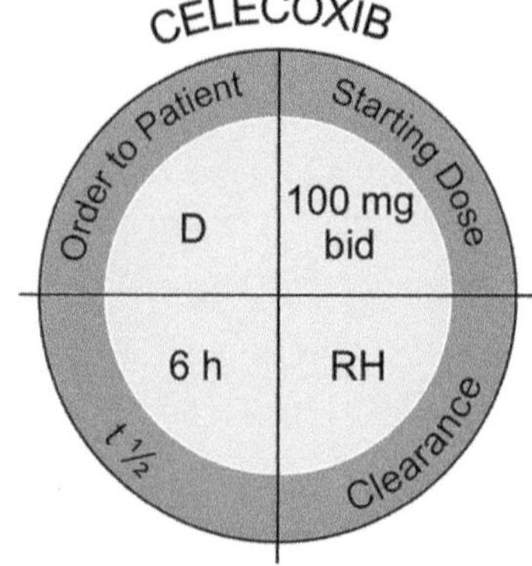

Pharmacologic Characteristics

- Selective inhibitor of COX-2 non-opioid NSAID, resulting in decreased prostaglandin precursors; has analgesic, anti-inflammatory, and antipyretic properties

Dosing and Administration

- Dose: 100–200 mg orally, twice a day
- Reduce dose by 50% in patients with hepatic dysfunction

Monitoring

- Pain response
- Laboratory or clinical signs of gastrointestinal bleeding
- Avoid in patients with severe renal disease
- Avoid in patients with sulfa allergy

Side Effects

- NSAIDs carry the risk of increased cardiovascular adverse events, including fatal myocardial infarction and stroke
- Increased risk of gastrointestinal adverse events, including bleeding, ulceration, or perforation

Gabapentin PO

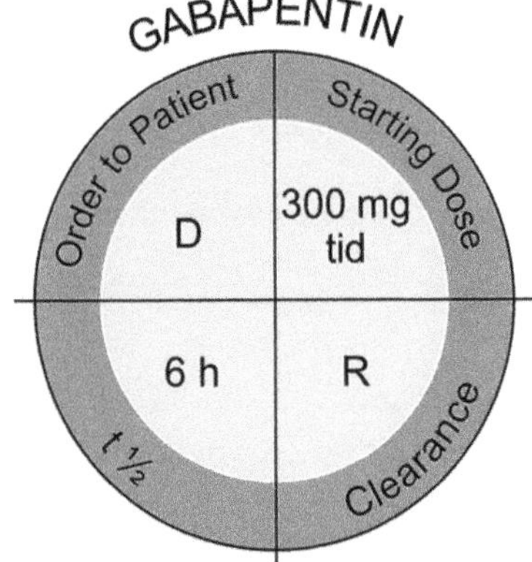

Pharmacologic Characteristics

- Structurally related to GABA but does not bind to GABA-A or GABA-B receptors. Binds to voltage-gated Ca channels in the central nervous system (alpha-2-delta-1 subunit) to modulate release of excitatory neurotransmitters (effecting pain response).
- Bioavailability is inversely related to dose administered (i.e., higher absorption with lower doses).

Dosing and Administration

- Initial dosing: 100 mg three times daily maintenance 300–1,200 mg/day, rapid titration (with normal renal function) (17)
- Postoperative pain: 300–1,200 mg the night prior to surgery, and 1–2 hours before surgery or immediately following surgery (17)
- Neuralgic pain (up to 3,600 mg/day, in divided doses [i.e., 1,200 mg three times a day]), with normal renal function (17)
- Renally cleared; reduce dose in patients with renal dysfunction

Monitoring

- Space antacids and other cation medications (e.g., calcium, magnesium, iron) at least 2 hours before gabapentin administration
- Level of alertness
- Pain response
- Renal function

Side Effects

- Dizziness
- Ataxia

Carbamazepine PO

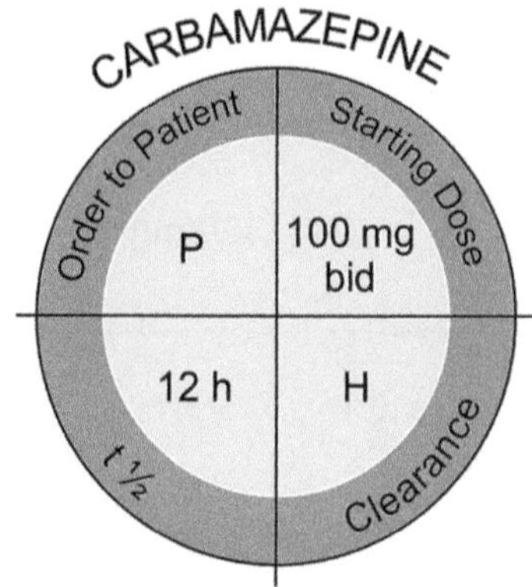

Pharmacologic Characteristics

- Anticholinergic, antineuralgic, muscle relaxant, and antidepressant properties
- Chemically related to tricyclic antidepressants; decreased neural impulse transmission by blocking sodium impulse through membranes

Dosing and Administration

- Oral: 50–100 mg twice daily
- Maintenance 100–200 mg every 4–6 hours; maximum 1,200 mg/day (in divided doses)
- Reduce dose in patients with renal dysfunction; give 75% of normal dose
- Often combined with IV opioids

Monitoring

- Complete blood count
- Renal function tests
- Liver function tests
- Serum sodium
- Dermatologic reactions

Side Effects

- Dizziness
- Drowsiness
- Ataxia
- Nausea and vomiting
- Hyponatremia, Syndrome of inappropriate antidiuretic hormone secretion (SIADH)
- Agranulocytosis (rare) and anemia
- Hepatotoxicity
- Hypersensitivity reactions (i.e., Stevens-Johnson syndrome, toxic epidermal necrosis)

Ketamine IV

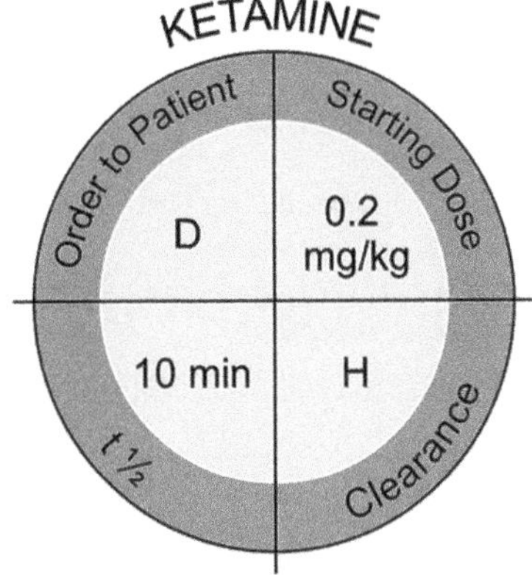

Pharmacologic Characteristics

- NMDA receptor antagonist, blocks glutamine release by binding to opioid receptors
- Adjunctive or opioid-sparing agent
- Used with opioids to help manage tolerance, withdrawal, hyperalgesia, and neuropathic pain

Dosing and Administration

- Bolus: 0.2–0.5 mg/kg
- Infusion: 0.05–0.4 mg/kg per hour

Monitoring

- Pain control
- Level of sedation
- Heart rate and blood pressure

Side Effects

- Hypertension
- Tachycardia
- Theoretical increase in intracranial pressure
- Emergence reactions after discontinuation

Patient-Controlled Analgesia

Commonly used in patients with longstanding, refractory pain, this treatment is a last resort and requires patient cooperation. Mistakes can be made in programming the pump, and oversedation seen at the end of a lockout period can cause respiratory depression. Monitoring of the patient involves specific attention in five areas: (1) at least 4 hours at stable dose, (2) patient's pain level is rated 4 or less (on a traditional 1-to-10 scale),

Box 4.4 Patient-Controlled Analgesia

- Patient should be able to self-administer medication (i.e., push the button)
- Appropriate for rapid drug titration
- Oral medication inappropriate or inadequate response from oral medication
- Provides pain relief much more quickly than with traditional nurse and pharmacy preparations
- Often hydromorphone (0.1–0.3 mg) is administered with a 10 minutes lock out and 0.6 mg one hour limit
- Initiation of dose by family members has been observed and should be avoided

(3) oxygen saturations are greater than 90%, (4) respirations are more than 10 per minute, and (5) level of sedation is a Richmond Agitation Sedation Scale (RASS) score of 0/1 (Box 4.4).

Key Pointers

1. Pain has many distinguishing features, and they need to be recognized and treated.
2. Pain in alert patients may be underrated, and use of nursing pain scales may be helpful.
3. Acetaminophen and codeine are preferred drugs for mild to moderate pain.
4. Patient-controlled analgesia can be used in patients with refractory pain but is discouraged in the neurosciences ICU.
5. Ketamine can be used as an opioid-sparing agent (19).

References

1. Ferreira-Valente, M.A., J.L. Pais-Ribeiro, and Jensen, M.P. *Validity of four pain intensity rating scales*. Pain, 2011. **152**: 2399–2404.
2. Breivik, H., et al., *Assessment of pain*. Br J Anaesth, 2008. **101**: 17–24.
3. Stites, M., *Observational pain scales in critically ill adults*. Crit Care Nurse, 2013. **33**: 68–78.
4. Berntzen, H., Bjork, I.T. and Woien, H. *"Pain relieved, but still struggling"—critically ill patients' experiences of pain and other discomforts during analgosedation*. J Clin Nurs, 2017. **1–2**: e223–e234.
5. Barr, J., et al., *Clinical practice guidelines for the management of pain, agitation, and delirium in adult patients in the intensive care unit*. Crit Care Med, 2013. **41**: 263–306.
6. Lew, H.L., et al., *Characteristics and treatment of headache after traumatic brain injury: a focused review*. Am J Phys Med Rehabil, 2006. **85**: 619–627.

7. Petzold, A. and Girbes, A. *Pain management in neurocritical care*. Neurocrit Care, 2013. **19**: 232–256.

8. Chanques, G., et al., *The measurement of pain in intensive care unit: comparison of 5 self-report intensity scales*. Pain, 2010. **151**: 711–721.

9. Erstad, B.L., et al., *Pain management principles in the critically ill*. Chest, 2009. **135**: 1075–1086.

10. Gelinas, C., *Pain assessment in the critically ill adult: Recent evidence and new trends*. Intensive Crit Care Nurs, 2016. **34**: 1–11.

11. Gelinas, C., et al., *Validation of the critical-care pain observation tool in adult patients*. Am J Crit Care, 2006. **15**: 420–427.

12. Gelinas, C., et al., *Pain assessment and management in critically ill intubated patients: a retrospective study*. Am J Crit Care, 2004. **13**: 126–135.

13. Olsen, B.F., et al., *Development of a pain management algorithm for intensive care units*. Heart Lung, 2015. **44**: 521–527.

14. Zeiler, F.A., et al., *Analgesia in Neurocritical Care: An International Survey and Practice Audit*. Crit Care Med, 2016. **44**: 973–980.

15. Dhakal, L.P., et al., *Headache and Its Approach in Today's NeuroIntensive Care Unit*. Neurocrit Care, 2016. **25**: 320–334.

16. Goddeau, R.P. and Alhazzani, A. *Headache in stroke: a review*. Headache, 2013. **53**: 1019–1022.

17. Chang, C.Y., et al., *Gabapentin in acute postoperative pain management*. Biomed Res Int, 2014. **2014**: 631756.

18. Greenberg, S., Murphy, G.S., and Avram, M.J. *Postoperative intravenous acetaminophen for craniotomy patients: a randomized controlled trial*. World Neurosurg, World Neurosurg, 2018. **109**: e554–e562.

19. Gottlieb, M., Ryan, K.W., and Binkley, C. *Is Low-Dose Ketamine an Effective Alternative to Opioids for the Treatment of Acute Pain in the Emergency Department?* Ann Emerg Med, 2017. Dec 8.

Chapter 5

Osmotic Therapy

Using any concentrated solution, fluids can be drawn from tissue through osmosis. These osmotic fluids can act as therapeutic agents, and sugar and salt solutions are used by physicians caring for acute brain swelling with mass effect.

Mannitol and hypertonic saline are readily available in emergency departments and intensive care units but are used often without knowing the true intracranial pressure (ICP) and after interpreting computed tomography scans and clinical findings. These osmotic fluids change fluid compartments and cannot be used indiscriminately. If administered regularly, close monitoring is needed and target goals should be set.

The Constants of Brain Volume

Because more than 75% of the brain parenchyma consists of water, mostly intracellular, the intracranial compartment is, in essence, a fluid-filled space. Fluids are physically largely incompressible; thus, a change (increase or decrease) in one compartment should be followed by a change (increase or decrease) in the other compartments. This relationship can be depicted as a pressure–volume curve that is hyperbolic. Therefore, after the knee of the curve is passed, even a small volume increase leads to a much higher increase in pressure. Realistically, up to 10% of new volume can be tolerated, but this depends on the volume of the brain parenchyma—there is more accommodation with atrophy and much less in younger brains (Fig. 5.1). Two situations that also hamper the tolerance of a new mass are (1) when the cerebrospinal fluid fails to egress to the spinal canal and (2) when vasodilatation is sustained with hypercapnia, hyperthermia, or hypoxemia. Intracranial crowding eventually leads to increased ICP. A new intracranial mass for which no accommodation can be made displaces and compresses the central thalamus–brainstem structure and impairs its function; the result is coma and later loss of brainstem function. One can expect tissues to move after a rapid increase of more than 20% in volume, and this is reflected by a change in the pupil size and response to light. A Cushing reflex (bradycardia, hypertension, and apnea) appears typically after the pupils become fixed and dilated.

Increased ICP reduces cerebral perfusion pressure. When ICP increases to a certain threshold—mostly in the range of 40 mmHg—cerebral perfusion pressure closes down and global ischemia occurs.

There are several causes of increased ICP (Box 5.1). Common triggers for the use of hyperosmotic agents are shown in Box 5.2.

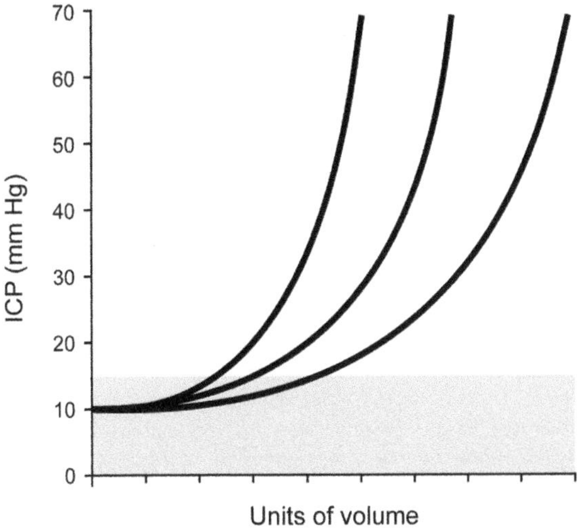

Figure 5.1 Pressure–volume curves. Different curves for age: sharper break ("knee") and steep curve in young, gradually ascending curve in the elderly.

Box 5.1 Causes of Increased ICP

- Cerebral edema
- Mass lesion with shift
- Acute cerebrospinal fluid flow obstruction causing hydrocephalus
- Cerebral vasodilatation (hypercapnia, hypoxemia)
- Cerebral venous thrombosis
- Bucking the ventilator, causing increased intrathoracic pressure
- Febrile state or hyperthermia
- Status epilepticus

Box 5.2 Triggers for the Use of Osmotic Agents

- Assumed increased ICP (swelling on computed tomography scan)
- Documented increased ICP (by monitor)
- New fixed and dilated pupil
- New decorticate or decerebrate posturing
- New decline in level of consciousness with more mass effect, shift, or cerebral edema

Hyperosmolar Fluids

If there is swelling and crowding, hyperosmolar fluids create more space after shrinking the unaffected parts of the brain. Osmotic fluids (also known as hyperosmolar agents) increase the intravascular osmolality, draw water from the brain, reduce or temporize shift, and reduce globally increased ICP from any cause (1–4). There is evidence that osmotic diuretics flatten the shape of the pressure–volume curve and make the brain more tolerant of additional volume. The blood–brain barrier is semi-permeable when intact. Although solutes such as mannitol and hypertonic sodium move through the barrier, water does not (5).

Since their introduction as a neurosurgical therapy, after being used by nephrologists as diuretics (6,7), neurosurgeons have used osmotic agents in craniotomies to reduce brain bulk. When mannitol was introduced into perioperative neurosurgical practice, it replaced (more toxic) urea (8). Mannitol (20%) is inert and nontoxic and still is used most commonly, although hypertonic saline is popular in some neurocritical care practices.

The infusates currently used are 20% and 25% mannitol solution and several concentrates of hypertonic saline (e.g., 3% NaCl, 7.5% NaCl, 14.6% NaCl, and 23.4% NaCl). The osmolarity of these fluids is shown in Table 5.1. There is little evidence that these concentrated solutions differ much in efficacy if used in equimolar dose—the mechanism by which they are effective (5,9–14).

The main mechanism of action is to create a new intravascular osmotic pressure to induce distribution of fluids to the intravascular compartment; an intact blood–brain barrier is needed. Another mechanism is that osmotic agents increase plasma volume and decrease blood viscosity. This leads to immediate cerebral vasoconstriction and reduced cerebral blood volume in intact autoregulated areas. One crucial difference is that mannitol depletes and hypertonic saline expands the volume status. Mannitol will decrease sodium as a result of dilution; hypertonic saline will increase sodium, but it will remain

Table 5.1 Osmotic Fluids and Osmolarity

20%	Mannitol	1100 mOsm/L
25%	Mannitol	1375 mOsm/L
3%	Hypertonic saline	1027 mOsm/L
7.5%	Hypertonic saline	2566 mOsm/L
14.6%	Hypertonic saline	5370 mOsm/L
23.4%	Hypertonic saline	8008 mOsm/L

somewhat diluted by water influx. Mannitol causes diuresis, and hypertonic saline does not (15,16).

The blood–brain barrier osmotic gradient can be used as a metric and is estimated as follows:

Osmolar gap = calculated – measured osmolality.

Serum osmolality is calculated as

Osmolality = 2 Na + glucose/18 + blood urea nitrogen/2.8.

An acute osmotic gradient of 10 mOsm is most effective, and this value can be used to guide the need for an additional bolus of mannitol. An additional dose of mannitol is warranted if clinically indicated and the osmolar gap is less than 10 or the serum osmolality is less than 320 mOsm.

In urgent situations, it is common practice to continue to administer mannitol infusions until the serum sodium level is between 145 and 150 mmol/L or an osmolality of 320 mOsm/kg is reached (17). With hypertonic saline, the target sodium level is similar but less than 160 mmol/L. Both osmotic fluids have a rapid (within an hour) effect, with duration varying from 2 to 6 hours. We usually also switch to 1.5% NaCl maintenance infusion but carefully monitor the serum sodium level. Usually either mannitol or hypertonic saline is used when prolonged treatment is needed (e.g., gradually worsening massive ischemic cytotoxic swelling).

These osmotic agents are administered using a peripheral vein (mannitol) or central access (hypertonic saline). With no intravenous access these fluids can be hyperacutely administered through the interosseous route or femoral vein cannulation when reliably identified with ultrasound.

Mannitol IV

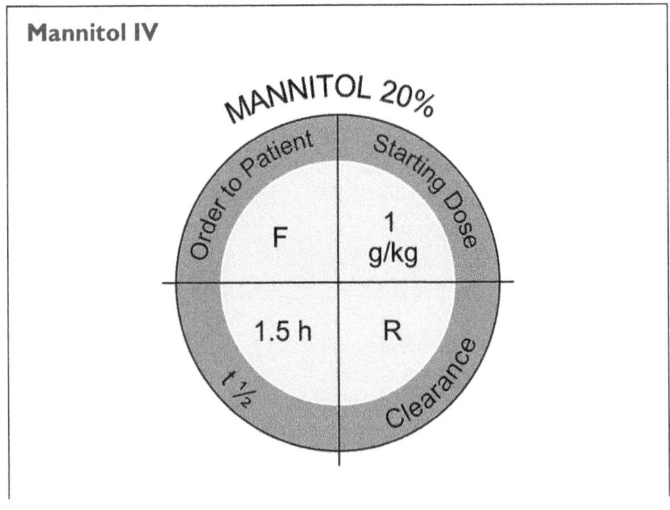

Pharmacologic Characteristics

- Volume expansion results in cerebral vasoconstriction but requires intact autoregulation. This action reduces cerebral blood volume and ICP
- Potent osmotic diuretic (and aquaretic) with expected diuresis volume five times greater than volume administered (Fig. 5.2)

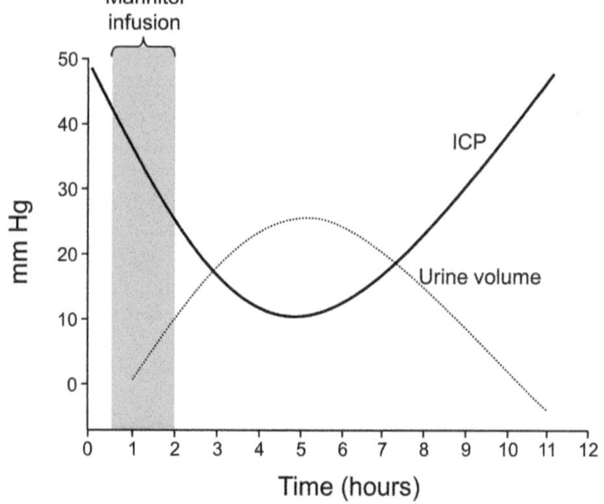

Figure 5.2 Mannitol's effect on ICP and concomitant diuresis

- Greater response in lowering ICP for those with higher ICP
- Decrease in ICP may vary proportionally to dose used
- Some transport over the blood–brain barrier despite near-perfect reflection coefficient, but generally does not pass
- Renal excretion 1% per minute after loading dose with little metabolized
- Duration: 1–4 hours and affected by glomerular filtration
- Reduction in ICP from onset is 15–30 minutes

Dosing and Administration

- 0.5–1 g/kg IV (maximum 2 g/kg)
- Doses <0.5 g/kg not effective; doses >2 g/kg may lead to renal failure
- Infusion over 15–30 minutes (with filter)
- Administration every 4–6 hours
- If some of the mannitol is crystallized, heating dissolves it quickly
- Mannitol cannot be combined with blood transfusion

Monitoring

- Renal function indices (creatinine, glomerular filtration rate)
- Electrolytes and fluid status
- Rapid administration (30 minutes) results in peak increase in serum osmolality up to 20 mOsm/kg and reduces ICP by 30% to 60%
- Repeat dose of mannitol with an osmolar gap <10 mOsm/kg
- Hold mannitol with an osmolar gap ≥10–20 mOsm/kg
- Hold mannitol with a serum osmolality of 320 mOsm/kg
- "Rebound" ICP with sudden discontinuation

Side Effects

- Hypotension with <15-minute infusion
- Renal failure ("osmotic nephrosis") usually with high osmolar gap
- Renal failure may be mannitol-induced vasoconstriction (usually high dose)
- Renal failure reversible with hemodialysis
- Hypochloremia
- Hypernatremia (from excessive free water loss)
- Hyponatremia (high doses)
- Hypophosphatemia (high doses)
- Hyperkalemia (high doses)
- Diastolic cardiac failure with pulmonary edema
- Tissue extravasation

Hypertonic Saline IV

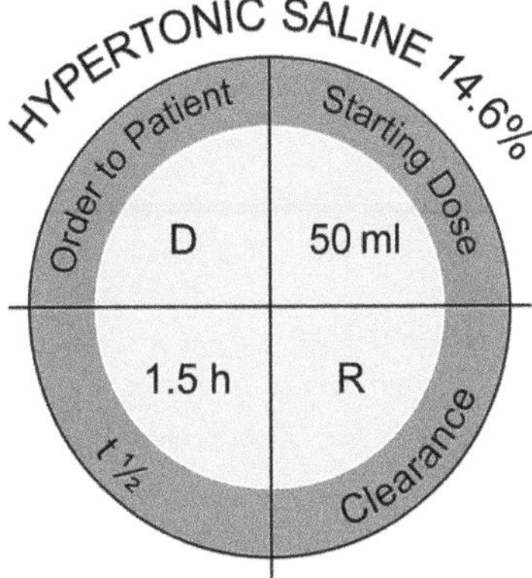

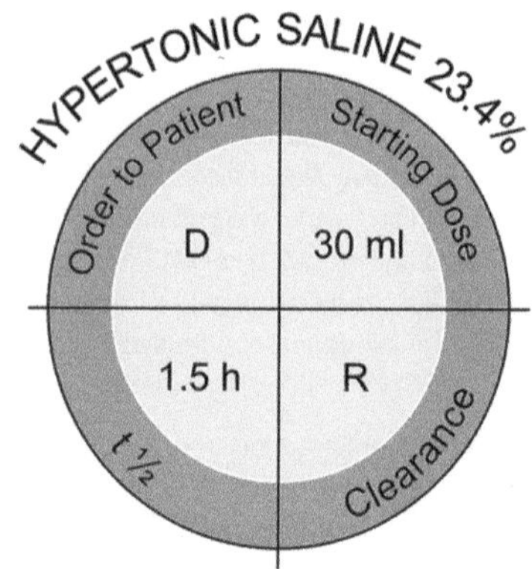

Pharmacologic Characteristics

- Several concentrations with significant sodium content
- Volume expander and no diuretic action
- Volume expansion results in cerebral vasoconstriction with intact autoregulation and reduces cerebral blood volume and ICP
- At least as effective as mannitol in lowering ICP but some extra benefits:
  - May increase cerebral perfusion pressure
  - Decreases leukocyte adhesion (18)
  - Reduces extracellular glutamate (19)
  - Improves brain tissue oxygen tension
  - No concern for crossing blood–brain barrier compared with mannitol due to perfect reflection coefficient

Dosing and Administration

- Bolus preferred over infusion (slow IV administration over 15 minutes)
- Commonly used preparations: hypertonic saline 14.6% NaCl, or 23.4% NaCl
- Hypertonic saline is preferred in polytrauma with hypotension
- Hypertonic saline 3% NaCl infusion may be effective if serum sodium level is kept between 145 and 155 mmol/L
- "Rebound" ICP (as with mannitol, but less so)

Monitoring

- Bronchospasm (responds to short-acting beta agonist)
- Chloride, electrolytes
- Renal indices

Side Effects

- Hypotension with rapid bolus administration
- Renal failure (chloride in the renal tubules activates tubuloglomerular feedback resulting in afferent arteriole vasoconstriction), less in chloride-restricted hypertonic saline
- Hyperchloremia and acidosis with repeated dosing (switch to equimolar sodium acetate when Cl is >110 mmol/L)

- Hypokalemia (transient)
- Cardiac failure (worsening from preexistent) and pulmonary edema
- Marked, prolonged hypernatremia
- Infusion phlebitis more common with infusions (>3% NaCl) than with bolus
- Extravasation
- No evidence of osmotic demyelination, but risk may be increased in malnourished alcoholics

Osmotic Agents in Clinical Practice

Osmotic agents should be seen as part of a comprehensive therapeutic plan. The first measure to take, therefore, is elevating the head to 30 degrees while avoiding any jugular venous obstruction. Patients should have excellent oxygen saturation with SPO_2 of more than 97%, and the $PaCO_2$ should be normal or low normal. The mode of mechanical ventilation does not significantly influence ICP. High levels of positive end-expiratory pressure (PEEP; 15–20 cm H_2O) do not markedly influence cerebral venous return. Reduction of pulmonary compliance in patients with acute respiratory distress syndrome—the typical situation in which PEEP is indicated—does not modulate ICP, but PEEP may interfere with systemic arterial pressure by causing arteriolar vasodilatation.

The first measure is to start hyperventilation that reduces the $PaCO_2$ to the low 30s. Acute hyperventilation causes a rapid acute alkalosis in cerebrospinal fluid, and cerebral vasoconstriction reduces intracranial blood volume.

The next step to consider is temperature management. Core temperature should be reduced to 37°C and cooling devices are effective.

Most practices in the emergency department and in intensive care units will start with mannitol first because of its easy and immediate accessibility. Mannitol 20% must be administered in a substantial dose of at least 1 g/kg. This will allow assessment of a response if there is any. There is no need to initially administer 2 g/kg, which may produce a very brisk—sometimes unexpectedly profound—diuresis.

The ICP goal must be less than 15 mmHg, and this cutoff value seems reasonable. However, ICPs moving into the double digits in a clinically deteriorating patient are just as significant, and then lower single digits are better goals. Moreover, in most situations, ICP values may not be available, and clinical and computed tomography scan changes must provide guidance. Once osmotic agents have been administered, there is often improvement of pupil size and light reflex, but improvement with mannitol infusion may involve resolution of hemispheric signs such as aphasia and hemiparesis. Once there is a clear clinical effect, mannitol can be repeated, but other measures may still be needed to control ICP (e.g., neurosurgical intervention).

After a mannitol bolus, it is common practice to continue mannitol every 4 hours using a lower dose (0.25–0.5 g/kg). If diuresis is significant, the maintenance fluid can be switched to 1.5% NaCl starting at 60 ml/hr. The plasma osmolality or plasma sodium level should be closely monitored, but the risk of renal failure with mannitol—previously known as "osmotic nephrosis" and possibly due to arterial vasoconstriction—is low in patients who have normal prior renal function and to whom no other potentially nephrotoxic agents are being administered.

When to make the transition to hypertonic saline is not well defined, and practice varies widely. The use of hypertonic saline is mostly limited by the presence of a central catheter. For safe administration, use is restricted to a smart pump or by a provider trained in slow drug administration through a large vessel. Normally, 50 ml of 14.6% or 30 ml of 23.4% NaCl, followed by a repeated dose every 4 hours, may be sufficient to treat increased ICP. The aim is to cause a hypernatremia with values between 150 and 155 mmol/L. Continuous infusion of 1.5% hypertonic saline (as opposed to repeated bolus) has been considered as an alternative to bolus administration, but its osmotic effect is not sufficient. Infusion of 3% NaCl may reduce ICP, but it also causes significant fluid retention and pulmonary edema in susceptible patients. Hypertonic saline may have a theoretical benefit over mannitol when treating traumatic brain injury with elevated ICP in a patient who also is hypovolemic. Hypertonic saline has also been proven more effective than isotonic fluids in patients with traumatic brain injury and polytrauma during fluid resuscitation.

It is important to continuously consider the equimolar doses of osmotic agents, which are summarized in Table 5.2. As a comparison, 200 ml of 20% mannitol is about equivalent to giving 30 ml of 23.4% NaCl.

Some ICP control may be achieved with adequate sedation (Chapter 2). However, this may lead to a loss of findings on the neurologic examination, which is a tradeoff. Adequate sedation often can be started with intravenous propofol but typically without a bolus to avoid the expected hypotension. Maintenance with a propofol dosage of between 5 and 50 mcg/kg per minute (0.3–3 mg/kg per hour) is usually very successful in sedating the patient. Adding an analgesic agent (e.g., intravenous fentanyl) should be completely avoided. Most patients who need sedation for increasing ICP are comatose and will have reduced pain sensation. Intravenous opioids such as fentanyl will make a neurologic examination quite difficult and may even raise ICP. However, transient increases in ICP may occur concomitant with a decrease in blood pressure and thus may be due to the autoregulatory decrease in cerebrovascular resistance triggered by systemic hypotension. The use of intravenous fentanyl is indicated only if the patient is bucking

Table 5.2 Equimolar Doses of Osmotic Agents

23.4%	Hypertonic saline	30 ml
14.6%	Hypertonic saline	50 ml
7.5%	Hypertonic saline	100 ml
3%	Hypertonic saline	250 ml
20%	Mannitol	225 ml
25%	Mannitol	175 ml

the ventilator or if there is significant tachypnea or mechanical ventilator dyssynchrony (see chapter 2 for analgosedation concerns).

Once ICP is under control and the inciting factors are removed, gradual weaning of osmotic agents is recommended, taking 2 to 3 days until discontinuation. Few clinicians use barbiturates because of significant myocardiac depression, resulting in significant systemic hypotension with incremental use of vasopressors or inotropes, and the long elimination half-life (up to 2 days in certain circumstances). Refractory ICP can be effectively treated only by a decompressive craniectomy or evacuation of a mass.

Key Pointers

1. Mannitol is a potent diuretic.
2. Hypertonic saline is a volume expander.
3. Repeated doses are necessary to control ICP.
4. Monitor effect with either serum sodium levels or serum osmolality.
5. Osmotic diuretics are effective only if used with other measures.

References

1. Diringer, M.N., *New trends in hyperosmolar therapy?* Curr Opin Crit Care, 2013. **19**: 77–82.
2. Li, M., et al., *Comparison of equimolar doses of mannitol and hypertonic saline for the treatment of elevated intracranial pressure after traumatic brain injury: a systematic review and meta-analysis.* Medicine, 2015. **94**: e736.
3. Czosnyka, M., Pickard, J.D., and Steiner, L.A., *Principles of intracranial pressure monitoring and treatment.* Handb Clin Neurol, 2017. **140**: 67–89.
4. Todd, M.M., *Hyperosmolar therapy and the brain: a hundred years of hard-earned lessons.* Anesthesiology, 2013. **118**: 777–779.
5. Francony, G., et al., *Equimolar doses of mannitol and hypertonic saline in the treatment of increased intracranial pressure.* Crit Care Med, 2008. **36**: 795–800.
6. Wise, B.L. and Chater, N. *Effect of mannitol on cerebrospinal fluid pressure. The actions of hypertonic mannitol solutions and of urea compared.* Arch Neurol, 1961. **4**: 200–202.
7. Wise, B.L. and Chater, N. *Use of hypertonic mannitol solutions to lower cerebrospinal fluid pressure and decrease brain bulk in man.* Surg Forum, 1961. **12**: 398–399.
8. Langfitt, T.W., *Possible mechanisms of action of hypertonic urea in reducing intracranial pressure.* Neurology, 1961. **11**: 196–209.
9. Battison, C., et al., *Randomized, controlled trial on the effect of a 20% mannitol solution and a 7.5% saline/6% dextran solution on increased intracranial pressure after brain injury.* Crit Care Med, 2005. **33**: 196–202.
10. Burgess, S., et al., *A systematic review of randomized controlled trials comparing hypertonic sodium solutions and mannitol for traumatic brain injury: implications for emergency department management.* Ann Pharmacother, 2016. **50**: 291–300.
11. Cottenceau, V., et al., *Comparison of effects of equiosmolar doses of mannitol and hypertonic saline on cerebral blood flow and metabolism in traumatic brain injury.* J Neurotrauma, 2011. **28**: 2003–2012.

12. Carter, C. and Human, T. Efficacy, *safety, and timing of 5% sodium chloride compared with 23.4% sodium chloride for osmotic therapy.* Ann Pharmacother, 2017. **51**: 625–629.
13. Jagannatha, A.T., et al., *An equiosmolar study on early intracranial physiology and long-term outcome in severe traumatic brain injury comparing mannitol and hypertonic saline.* J Clin Neurosci, 2016. **27**: 68–73.
14. Witherspoon, B. and Ashby, N.E. *The use of mannitol and hypertonic saline therapies in patients with elevated intracranial pressure: a review of the evidence.* Nurs Clin North Am, 2017. **52**: 249–260.
15. Thenuwara, K., Todd, M.M. and Brian, Jr., J.E. *Effect of mannitol and furosemide on plasma osmolality and brain water.* Anesthesiology, 2002. **96**: 416–421.
16. Todd, M.M., Cutkomp, J. and Brian, J.E. *Influence of mannitol and furosemide, alone and in combination, on brain water content after fluid percussion injury.* Anesthesiology, 2006. **105**: 1176–1181.
17. Ropper, A.H., *Hyperosmolar therapy for raised intracranial pressure.* N Engl J Med, 2012. **367**: 746–752.
18. Boone, M.D., et al., *Mannitol or hypertonic saline in the setting of traumatic brain injury: What have we learned?* Surg Neurol Int, 2015. **6**: 177.
19. Shackford, S.R., Schmoker, J.D. and Zhuang, J. *The effect of hypertonic resuscitation on pial arteriolar tone after brain injury and shock.* J Trauma, 1994. **37**: 899–908.

Chapter 6

Antiepileptic Drugs

Seizures are typically self-limiting, and few return straight away so in most instances treatment is not critically urgent. However, this changes with any recurrence and if there is a major precipitating factor such as acute brain injury (1,2). In this chapter, we will discuss antiepileptic drugs (AED) used for the management of seizures in the acute setting, but we exclude drugs used for outpatient management of complex epilepsy syndromes. (A clinicians' manual on AEDs in this series of books has been published by Oxford University Press (3).)

Status epilepticus is basically one seizure after another——overt or covert, focal or generalized, convulsive or non-convulsive. The management of convulsive status epilepticus has a number of critical challenges. There is a delay in diagnosis, inadequate dosing of AEDs, and no unequivocal consensus on how best to escalate intravenous drugs with ongoing seizures (4–6).

Seizures in the ICU

In the neurosciences intensive care unit (NICU), the causes of recurrent seizures include brain tumors or metastasis, meningitis or encephalitis, acute subdural hematoma or traumatic contusions, and (less likely) acute stroke. Drug toxicity or alcohol withdrawal remains a major risk factor for seizures (Chapter 18). Abruptly withdrawn AEDs are common causes for seizures, and these seizures are not always effectively managed by simply restarting the drug. Additionally, with no evidence of a new structural lesion, one of the first questions is whether a seizure is provoked by a certain drug at toxic levels or in predisposed patients (Table 6.1) or by acute, potentially correctable metabolic derangements (e.g., severe hyponatremia, hypoglycemia).

Treatment Protocols

The choice of which AED to administer depends on the pharmacologic characteristics of the drug, the patient's past medical history and particular end organ function, and the type of seizure. Continuous electroencephalogram (EEG) is an important guide in monitoring treatment effect and must be available. In most patients and in many practices, a single seizure (focal or generalized) will lead to treatment with 1,000 mg of levetiracetam followed by 750 mg twice a day as maintenance but with adjustment for renal failure. The decision to prevent seizures in high-risk patients (e.g., traumatic brain

Table 6.1 Drug-Associated Seizures

Drug	Circumstance
Tricyclic antidepressants	At toxic doses
Lithium	At toxic doses
Anticholinergics	At toxic doses
Carbapenem	Renal dysfunction
Cephalosporins (highest with fourth generation)	Renal dysfunction at toxic doses
Tramadol	In high-risk patients
Clozapine	In high-risk patients
Bupropion	In high-risk patients
Venlafaxine, selective serotonin reuptake inhibitors (SSRIs), monoamine oxidase (MAO) inhibitors	In high-risk patients
Phenothiazines	In high-risk patients
Quinolone antibiotics	In high-risk patients
Immunosuppressants	With escalating doses

injury, brain tumor) also often leads to use of levetiracetam but without a loading dose and starting at 500–750 mg twice a day.

The choices are far more urgent and different when the patient is in status epilepticus. There is a sense that when adequate doses of an intravenous (IV) benzodiazepine and first-line anticonvulsant are given, status epilepticus can often be terminated.

There are no recent head-to-head large-scale hospital-based clinical trials currently available to guide treatment. To address the lack of evidence regarding second-line treatment agents, the Established Status Epilepticus Treatment Trial will compare fosphenytoin, valproic acid, and levetiracetam loading doses for the treatment of benzodiazepine-refractory status.

For now there has been a consensus to be formulaic in managing status epilepticus. In most practices, a combination of lorazepam with fosphenytoin, valproic acid, or levetiracetam is used. Some patients may already have received intramuscular or intranasal midazolam or rectal diazepam before transport to the emergency department, and this may have already ended status epilepticus in some patients.

A protocol with a timeline is shown in Figure 6.1, and quick decisions on moving to the next drug in the event of failed responses are imperative. Status epilepticus should be under control within an hour of presentation because a longer wait may lead to early neuronal injury and possible seizure perpetuation and more difficulty with treatment over time. Refractoriness is due to pharmacoresistance and alteration in the GABA-receptor sensitivity and, thus, the inability of agonists, such as benzodiazepines and other first-line AEDs, to work. At its extreme, super-refractory status epilepticus develops; this is defined as status

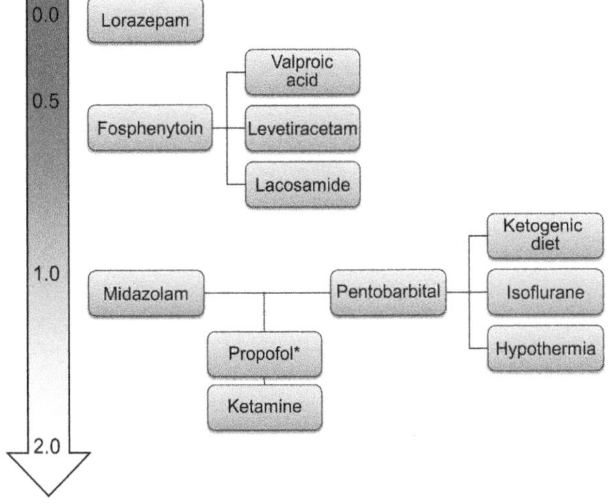

Figure 6.1 Treatment algorithm for status epilepticus. First choices are listed in the first column and additional AEDs are given in other columns. The time bar shows how quickly time passes before seizures are under control. *There are serious concerns with using long-term high-dose propofol infusions.

epilepticus that continues or recurs 24 hours or more after the onset of anesthetic therapy. The poor outcome for patients with such refractory status epilepticus can be as high as 60%. In our practice and that of others (7,8), the diagnosis of refractory generalized status epilepticus is already evident if we have to start a continuous infusion of an anesthetic agent. This decision requires endotracheal intubation for airway protection and continuous EEG monitoring. Among the many anesthetic agents, IV midazolam is preferred because of its comparatively favorable pharmacokinetic properties. IV midazolam infusions can be effective in aborting status epilepticus, but high doses are usually needed. The infusion rate is rapidly increased until seizures are suppressed; doses as high as 3 mg/kg per hour have been required in the most refractory cases.

Use of an algorithm for decision making is common in the management of refractory status epilepticus, but the drug priority constantly changes (9–12). Our approach remains the administration of IV midazolam—combined, if necessary, with IV ketamine—before resorting to pentobarbital infusion (Box 6.1). We have largely eliminated propofol for treatment after a series of patients developed propofol related infusion syndrome. We may consider administering IV propofol in low doses as a bridge to midazolam and ketamine, knowing that preparation of these drugs may take some time.

Box 6.1 Stepwise Treatment of Status Epilepticus

- Adequate dose of IV lorazepam
- Load IV (fos)phenytoin
- Add IV levetiracetam (or IV valproic acid)
- IV midazolam with intubation
- Combine IV midazolam with IV ketamine
- IV pentobarbital
- Consider adjunctive therapy with oral lacosamide, felbamate, topiramate

Antiepileptic Drugs Used in ICU Practice

Lorazepam IV

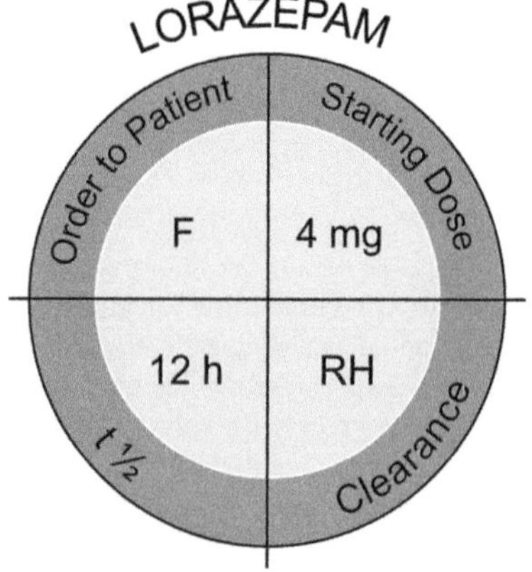

Pharmacologic Characteristics

- Direct binding to GABA-A benzodiazepine receptor complex
- Onset 10 minutes and peak at 2 hours
- 85–90% protein binding, higher percentage of free drug in elderly patients
- Highly lipophilic and remains in cerebrospinal fluid for a prolonged time (6–8 hours)
- Longer duration of action compared to other benzodiazepines

Dosing and Administration

- 4 mg IV and inject 2 mg/min
- 0.05 mg/kg IV repeat doses
- Maximum total dose: 8 mg
- Dilute IV dose with equal volume of normal saline

Monitoring

- Ongoing seizure activity
- Respiratory drive and presence of an open airway

Side Effects

- Hypotension (rapid IV administration)
- Metabolic acidosis, renal failure, osmolar gap with high doses as a result of propylene glycol in drug's vehicle
- Sedation, respiratory depression

Midazolam IV

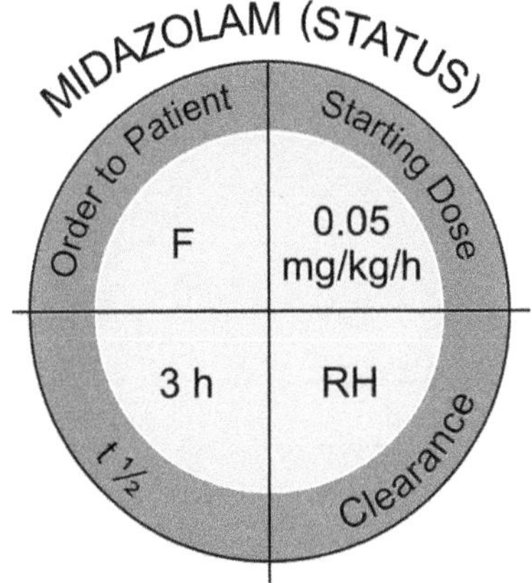

Pharmacologic Characteristics

- Binds to postsynaptic GABA-A receptors
- Onset: 3–5 minutes (IV), ~15 minutes (intramuscular [IM])
- Peak effect 30–60 minutes; duration <2 hours (IV), up to 6 hours (IM)
- Shorter duration of action than lorazepam (rapid redistribution and lower lipophilicity)

Dosing and Administration

- Prehospital setting: midazolam 10 mg IM
- 0.2 mg/kg IV bolus (maximum 10 mg) followed by 0.05 mg/kg per hour IV infusion, titrating up to no clinical or EEG seizures
- Doses can go as high as 3 mg/kg per hour
- Maintain infusion for 24–48 hours of EEG control before tapering

Monitoring

- Maintain continuous EEG showing burst suppression and no brief ictal rhythmic discharges (BIRDS)

- No dosage adjustment in patients with renal dysfunction, but drug accumulation and increased risk of side effects in renal dysfunction, such as prolonged sedation and hypotension
- Use with caution in patients with hepatic dysfunction

Side Effects

- Tachyphylaxis with prolonged administration as a result of decreased sensitivity to GABA-A receptors
- Hypotension
- Hypoventilation
- Prolonged sedation in patients with renal and hepatic failure

Fosphenytoin IV

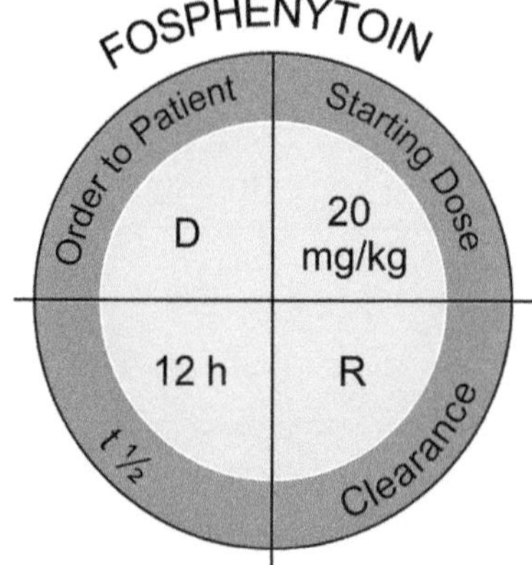

Pharmacologic Characteristics

- Fosphenytoin has largely replaced phenytoin in the United States but not elsewhere
- Fosphenytoin is a pro-drug of phenytoin and is converted in the body by plasma esterases to active moiety
- Increases influx and efflux of sodium ions to stabilize neuronal membranes
- 95–99% protein binding (higher free levels in malnourished, pregnant, and elderly patients and those with renal and liver dysfunction)
- Nonlinear pharmacokinetics with oral phenytoin administration
- Avoid if concern for concurrent tricyclic antidepressant toxicity due to additional risk of cardiac arrhythmias
- Use with caution in patients with bundle-branch block (class I b antiarrhythmic)
- Time to peak: 15 minutes

Dosing and Administration

- 18–20 mg phenytoin equivalents (PE)/kg IV

- IV push rate up to 150 mg PE/min (increased arrhythmias, hypotension with faster rates)
- Phenytoin has same dose, but the rate of administration is three times slower (e.g., 50 mg PE/min)
- With prior phenytoin use, calculated loading dose as 0.8 × weight × desired serum level – current serum level (= mg/kg dose)
- Maintenance: 5–6 mg/kg per day (IV or orally)
- Dilute manufacturer product 50 mg/ml (IM) 1:1 with saline prior to IV administration (25 mg/ml)
- Can be administered IM (undiluted product)
- No adjustment in patients with renal dysfunction but closer monitoring of free levels

Monitoring

- Serum drug levels 5 days after start: therapeutic range 10–20 mcg/ml (free 1–2 mcg/ml)
- Total serum level is sufficient for most patients
- Free level in patients with hypoalbuminemia and drug–drug interactions for protein binding, hepatic disease or pregnancy
- Steady state reached in 10–14 days of maintenance therapy

Side Effects

- Drug rash
- Bradycardia, hypotension (related to administration rate; electrocardiographic [EKG] monitoring required)
- Nystagmus, ataxia
- Drug reaction with eosinophilia and systemic symptoms (DRESS)
- "Purple glove" syndrome (e.g., edema, discoloration, pain at infusion site) with IV phenytoin use
- Rarely, increased liver function test results (<1%)

Levetiracetam IV

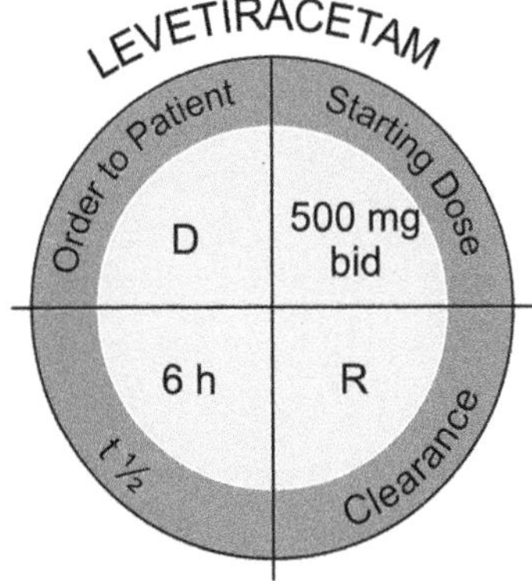

Pharmacologic Characteristics

- Mechanism of action largely unknown; interaction with SV2A receptor proposed
- Rapid absorption, peak concentration in 60 minutes

Dosing and Administration

- IV push loading dose over 5 minutes or infused over 15 minutes
- Usually loading 1,000–3,000 mg with acute seizures, not as adjunctive therapy; maximum 4,500 mg (or 60 mg/kg) loading dose
- Maintenance: 750 mg twice a day (IV or orally); maximum 1,500 mg twice daily
- Adjustment with abnormal creatinine clearance (CrCl):
  - CrCl <30 ml/min: change to 250–500 mg twice daily
  - CrCl 30–50 ml/min: change to 250–750 mg twice daily
  - Hemodialysis: 500–1,000 mg once daily
  - Continuous renal replacement therapy: 250–750 mg twice daily
  - Supplemental 250-500 mg dose needed after intermittent hemodialysis

Monitoring

- No interaction with other AEDs
- No adjustment in patients with hepatic dysfunction
- No cardiac monitoring needed
- Renal function

Side Effects

- Psychiatric behavior (e.g., aggression, agitation, depression, mood changes, hostility, paranoia)
- Acute renal failure

Valproate IV

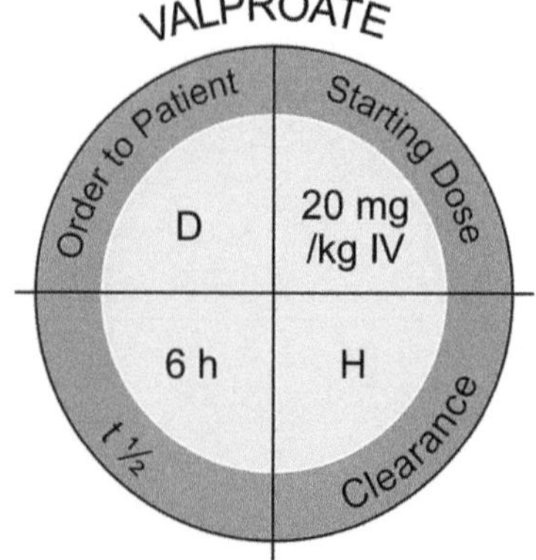

Pharmacologic Characteristics

- Increased availability of GABA to neurons, increased activity of GABA
- No adjustment in patients with renal impairment, but may see higher free drug levels due to decreased protein binding
- Do not use in pregnant women, unless there are no alternatives for use
- Do not use in patients with liver disease
- Do not use in patients with mitochondrial disease

Dosing and Administration

- 20–30 mg/kg IV load
- May administer another 20 mg/kg after 10 minutes
- Maximum 60 mg/kg per day in four divided doses
- Administration rate: 5–10 mg/kg per minute bolus, or infusion of no more than 20 mg/min

Monitoring

- Liver function tests
- Drug levels: 50–100 mcg/ml, free drug 5–15 mcg/ml
- aPTT, PT prior to surgical procedures (clinical relevance remains unclear)
- Does not require cardiac monitoring

Side Effects

- Hyperammonemia
- Hepatitis (higher risk in children <2 years)
- Pancreatitis
- Thrombocytopenia (mild)
- Leukopenia, neutropenia (rare)
- DRESS (rare)

Ketamine IV

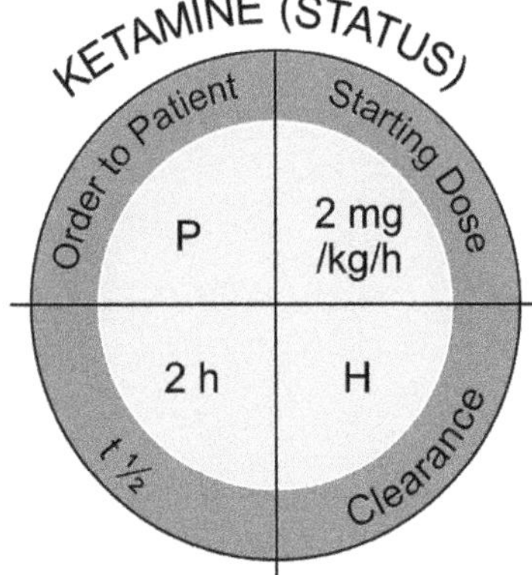

Pharmacologic Characteristics

- Glutamatergic NMDA antagonist, involvement with opioid receptors in central nervous system and spinal cord; interaction with norepinephrine, histamine, and muscarinic cholinergic receptors (16)
- Onset: immediate
- Usually used in refractory status epilepticus after multiple AEDs have been tried but early use in some practices.

Dosing and Administration

- Bolus: 1–2 mg/kg (maximum 5 mg/kg)
- Infusion: 2–10 mg/kg per hour

Monitoring

- Cardiac function (can be associated with hypertension and tachycardia with initial doses). Use with caution in patients with cardiac failure (increasing myocardial oxygen demand)
- EEG, seizure response

Side Effects

- Respiratory depression
- Hypertension
- Increase in intracranial pressure reported (evidence weak)
- Emergence reactions (e.g., vivid dreams, hallucinations, delirium): greater in patients >16 years, in females, or if infused too quickly. Pre-administration of a benzodiazepine mitigates response. May occur with bolus and after infusion irrespective of dose.
- Hypersalivation (atropine or scopolamine prophylactic use)
- Increased skeletal muscle tension—differentiate from seizure activity

Propofol IV

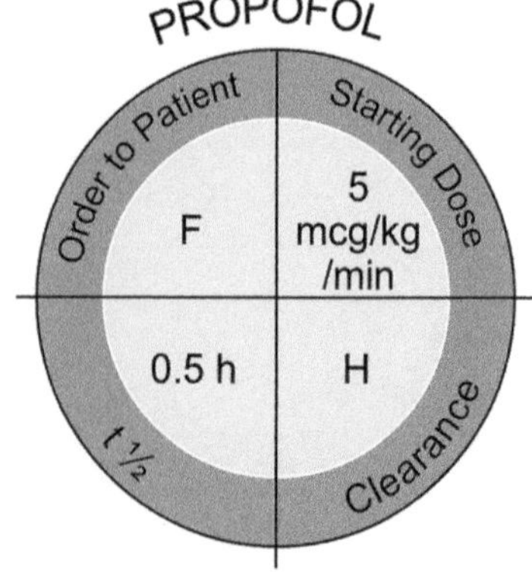

Pharmacologic Characteristics

- General anesthetic, global central nervous system depression with possible gamma-aminobutyric acid (GABA) agonist and N-Methyl-D-aspartate (NDMA) antagonist properties
- Onset: seconds (highly lipophilic)
- Duration: 3–10 minutes after single bolus dose
- Half-life prolonged with extended infusions

Dosing and Administration

- Bolus: 1–2 mg/kg
- Infusion: 5–200 mcg/kg per minute
- Avoid administering >80 mcg/kg per minute or 5 mg/kg per hour for >48 hours
- No dose adjustment in patients with renal or hepatic dysfunction

Monitoring

- EEG, achieve burst suppression prior to wean
- EKG, can prolong QTc interval
- Arterial blood gas (for metabolic acidosis)
- Potassium (may rise)
- Creatinine phosphokinase (may rise)
- Triglycerides (may rise but predictive value not strong)

Side Effects

- Hypotension
- Bradycardia
- Propofol related infusion syndrome—presents with acute metabolic acidosis and cardiovascular collapse. This is a serious concern when high doses are given for several days, but the exact threshold is not defined
- Hypoventilation to apnea
- Hypertriglyceridemia (10% fat emulsion)

Pentobarbital IV

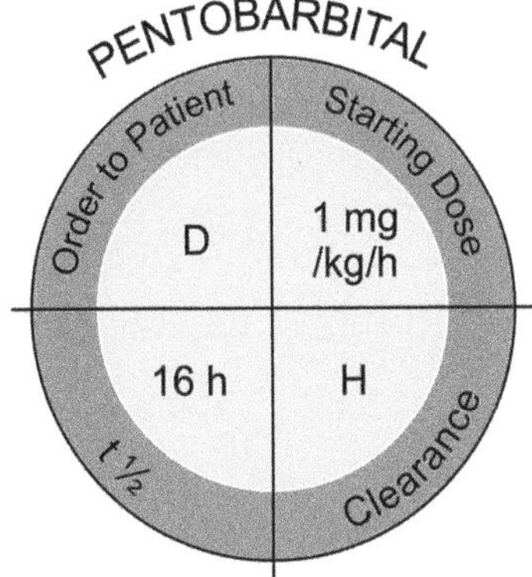

Pharmacologic Characteristics

- Barbiturate with sedative, hypnotic, and anticonvulsant activity
- Exhibits GABA-like effects
- Onset: immediate, 3–5 minutes
- Duration: 15–45 minutes after bolus
- Half life longer with higher doses

Dosing and Administration

- Bolus: 5–15 mg/kg over 10 minutes (maximum rate 50 mg/min)
- Continuous infusion: 1–5 mg/kg per hour titrated to burst suppression on EEG
- May give additional boluses of 5–10 mg/kg as needed

Monitoring

- Liver function tests
- Drug interactions (potent CYP P450 enzyme induction)
- EEG, maintain burst suppression for 48 hours prior to tapering trial
- Serum drug levels are not useful for monitoring seizures (1–5 mcg/ml sedation, 30–40 mcg/ml for coma)

Side Effects

- Hypotension requiring vasopressor support
- Respiratory depression
- Myocardial depression
- Infections
- Adynamic ileus
- Propylene glycol toxicity (e.g., hyperosmolality, lactic acidosis, respiratory depression, seizures)
- Extravasation risk (highly alkaline substance)
- Skin breakdown
- Macroglossus

Lacosamide IV

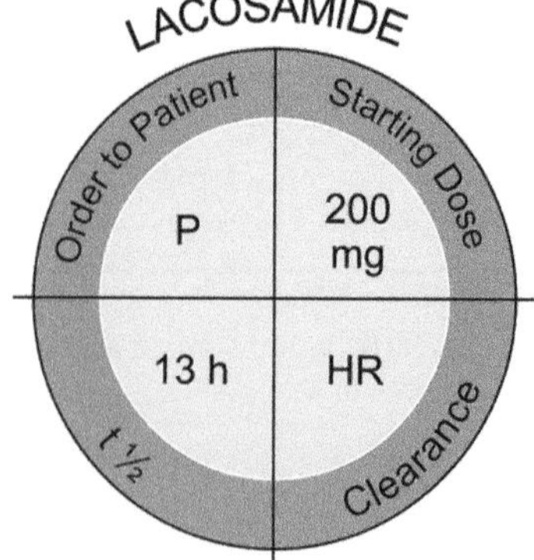

Pharmacologic Characteristics

- Exact mechanism of action unknown. Stabilizes excitable neuronal membranes by activating slow Na channels. Binds to CRMP-2 as part of signal transduction pathway (17)
- Avoid use in patients with severe liver failure. Adjust dose in patients with mild or moderate liver failure
- Product may contain phenylalanine or propylene glycol

Dosing and Administration

- Loading dose 200–400 mg IV, then maintenance dose 200–600 mg/day IV/PO
- Recommended IV infusion over 15 minutes, but can be given IV push
- Dosage adjustments in patients with renal dysfunction:
  - CrCl <30 ml/min: maximal dose 300 mg/day
  - With hemodialysis, supplement dose (50% of maintenance dose) after 4 hours

Monitoring

- Baseline EKG
- Complete blood count with differential

Side Effects

- Dose-dependent increase in PR interval
- First-degree atrioventricular block
- Drug reaction with eosinophilia and systemic symptoms (DRESS)

Topiramate PO

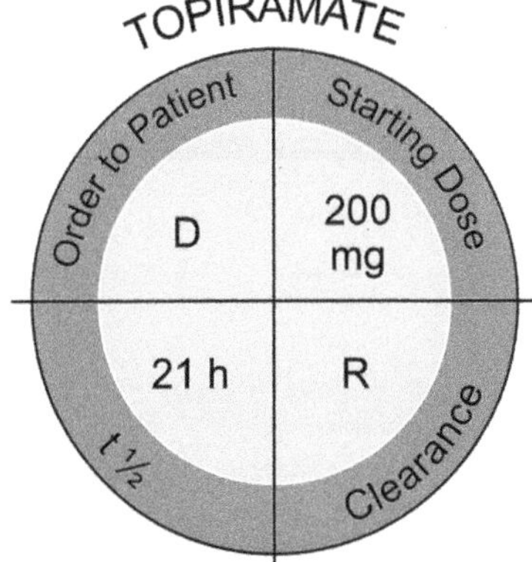

Pharmacologic Characteristics

- Mode of action is blocking of sodium channel activation, enhances GABA-A receptor activity, antagonizes AMPA/glutamate receptors, inhibits carbonic anhydrase
- Off-label use for refractory status epilepticus

Dosing and Administration

- Loading dose: 200–400 mg (oral), not available in IV form in the United States
- Maintenance: 300–1,600 mg/day in divided doses
- Supplemental dose in patients on hemodialysis

Monitoring

- Therapeutic drug level: 5–20 mcg/ml
- Renal function, serum bicarbonate
- Adequate hydration
- Body temperature (risk for hyperthermia)

Side Effects

- Anorexia, weight loss
- Renal calculi, nephrolithiasis
- Paresthesias
- Metabolic acidosis
- Memory impairment, confusion
- Increased intraocular pressure

Interactions and Adjustments

Most drugs can be started without preconditions, but there are two important caveats:

- AEDs interact with other AEDs (Table 6.2). This is largely unavoidable but should be kept in mind with escalating doses. Monitoring the patient's clinical status is all that is required. Serum drug concentrations, when available, can assist in addressing drug toxicity or subtherapeutic levels due to drug–drug interactions.
- Although this is a less common concern in the neurosciences ICU, dose adjustments of AEDs are needed in patients receiving intermittent dialysis, but not with continuous veno-venous hemodialysis (Fig. 6.2).

Table 6.2 AED–AED Interactions

AED	Inhibits its Metabolism
Carbamazepine	Felbamate, valproic acid (7)
Ethosuximide	Isoniazid, valproic acid
Lamotrigine	Valproic acid
Phenobarbital	Felbamate, valproic acid
Phenytoin	Felbamate, oxcarbazepine (high doses), topiramate (high doses), valproic acid (8)
Valproic acid	Felbamate, topiramate

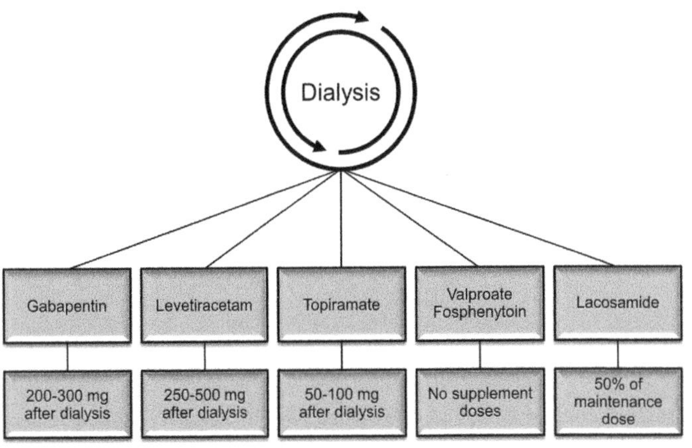

Figure 6.2 Supplemental AED dosing after dialysis

Key Pointers

1. Treatment of a single seizure in acute brain injury is best accomplished with levetiracetam.
2. The best drug to use for status epilepticus after adequate doses of lorazepam and fosphenytoin have been given has not been established, but IV midazolam is a popular choice (18).
3. Midazolam and ketamine can be combined and may effectively treat status epilepticus.
4. Alternatively, IV valproate (20-30 mg/kg) is considered. High dose IV valproate (40 mg/kg) is currently tested for efficacy and safety.
5. Significant AED–AED interactions occur, but clinical monitoring may be all that is necessary.

References

1. Olmes, D.G. and Hamer, H.M. *The debate: Treatment after the first seizure—The PRO*. Seizure, 2017. **49**: 90–91.
2. Steinhoff, B.J., *The debate: Treatment after the first seizure—The CONTRA*. Seizure, 2017. **49**: 92–94.
3. Asadi-Pooya, A.A. and Sperling, M.R. *Antiepileptic Drugs: A Clinician's Manual*. 2nd ed. 2016, New York: Oxford University Press.
4. Hill, C.E., et al., *Timing is everything: Where status epilepticus treatment fails*. Ann Neurol, 2017. **82**: 155–165.
5. Chen, H.Y., Albertson, T.E. and Olson, K.R. *Treatment of drug-induced seizures*. Br J Clin Pharmacol, 2016. **81**: 412–419.
6. Cock, H.R., *Drug-induced status epilepticus*. Epilepsy Behav, 2015. **49**: 76–82.
7. Falco-Walter, J.J. and Bleck, T. *Treatment of established status epilepticus*. J Clin Med, 2016. **5**. pii: E49.

8. Rossetti, A.O., *Are newer AEDs better than the classic ones in the treatment of status epilepticus?* J Clin Neurophysiol, 2016. **33**: 18–21.

9. Bleck, T., et al., *The established status epilepticus trial 2013*. Epilepsia, 2013. **54** Suppl 6: 89–92.

10. Glauser, T., et al., *Evidence-based guideline: treatment of convulsive status epilepticus in children and adults: report of the Guideline Committee of the American Epilepsy Society*. Epilepsy Curr, 2016. **16**: 48–61.

11. Trinka, E., et al., *A definition and classification of status epilepticus—Report of the ILAE Task Force on Classification of Status Epilepticus*. Epilepsia, 2015. **56**: 1515–1523.

12. Trinka, E., et al., *Pharmacologic treatment of status epilepticus*. Expert Opin Pharmacother, 2016. **17**: 513–534.

13. Brophy, G.M., et al., *Guidelines for the evaluation and management of status epilepticus*. Neurocrit Care, 2012. **17**: 3–23.

14. Claassen, J., et al., *Treatment of refractory status epilepticus with pentobarbital, propofol, or midazolam: a systematic review*. Epilepsia, 2002. **43**: 146–153.

15. Trinka, E., et al., *Efficacy and safety of intravenous valproate for status epilepticus: a systematic review*. CNS Drugs, 2014. **28**: 623–639.

16. Fang, Y. and Wang, X. *Ketamine for the treatment of refractory status epilepticus*. Seizure, 2015. **30**: 14–20.

17. Strzelczyk, A., et al., *Lacosamide in status epilepticus: systematic review of current evidence*. Epilepsia, 2017. **58**: 933–950.

18. Zaccara, G., Giannasi, G., Oggioni, R. et al., *Challenges in the treatment of convulsive status epilepticus*. Seizure, 2017. **47**: 17–24.

Chapter 7

Anticoagulation and Reversal Drugs

Management of anticoagulation—either initiation or reversal—is common ICU practice. Anticoagulation in the neurosciences ICU mostly involves subcutaneous unfractionated heparin (UFH) or low molecular weight heparin (LMWH). There are few strong indications for anticoagulation in ischemic stroke, and exceptions are discussed. Reversal of anticoagulation in cerebral hemorrhage has recently received significant attention mostly because it is inadequately done and the outcome could potentially improve with more aggressive action. Acute ischemic strokes due to cardiogenic emboli or an acute carotid or vertebral artery dissection may need treatment with full anticoagulation since early anticoagulation could prevent recurrence of a more devastating stroke. Unfractionated heparin infusion to bridge warfarin may be considered in patients whose stroke is due to atrial fibrillation or myocardial infarction. In cerebral venous sinus thrombosis, with or without hemorrhagic infarcts, immediate high-intensity heparinization with UFH (better factor Xa inhibition) is required, followed by LMWH. Concern for worsening cerebral hematoma becoming symptomatic with anticoagulation should be weighed against the risk of newly appearing hemorrhagic infarcts in a patient when anticoagulation is held. Generally, there has been a shifting trend toward the use of LMWH and diminishing use of UFH in treatment of an acute cerebral venous sinus thrombosis.

Approximately 10% to 15% of patients with intracranial hemorrhage have been on warfarin, often in a setting of atrial fibrillation or mechanical heart valves. With the increased use of warfarin, the risk of cerebral hemorrhage has markedly increased irrespective of the International Normalized Ratio (INR). Direct oral anticoagulants (DOACs) have reduced the risk of cerebral hemorrhage, and the outcome of DOAC-associated cerebral hemorrhage is not worse when compared with warfarin-associated cerebral hemorrhage (1). Reversal of warfarin must be considered an emergency intervention because without reversal, outcomes are worse and mortality is high. However, the reverse may not be true: Expansion of the hematoma is rapid, and urgent reversal may not reduce expansion or even have an impact on mortality or functional outcome.

Current reversal protocols require intravenous vitamin K, fresh-frozen plasma (FFP), and, more often, prothrombin complex concentrate (PCC). The long delay in reversal of INR with FFP is well known, so the use of PCC is preferred in warfarin reversal. While there remains only one DOAC-reversal agent on the market that has been approved by the U.S. Food and

Drug Administration (FDA), there are others undergoing phase III and phase IV studies. Individual reversal agents are discussed here (2–8).

Heparin and Warfarin

Heparin is a thrombin inhibitor due to its binding with antithrombin III. This binding enhances its inhibition properties, including thrombin and factor X, but also factors IX, XI, and XII. Heparin binds antithrombin III and causes a conformational change resulting in more than a 1,000-fold activation of antithrombin. The binding of factor Xa also reduces the conversion from prothrombin to thrombin, and thus it is partly a factor Xa inhibitor. This in return reduces the conversion from fibrinogen to fibrin clot and targets of available drugs are depicted in Figure 7.1. LMWHs are fragments of UFH but

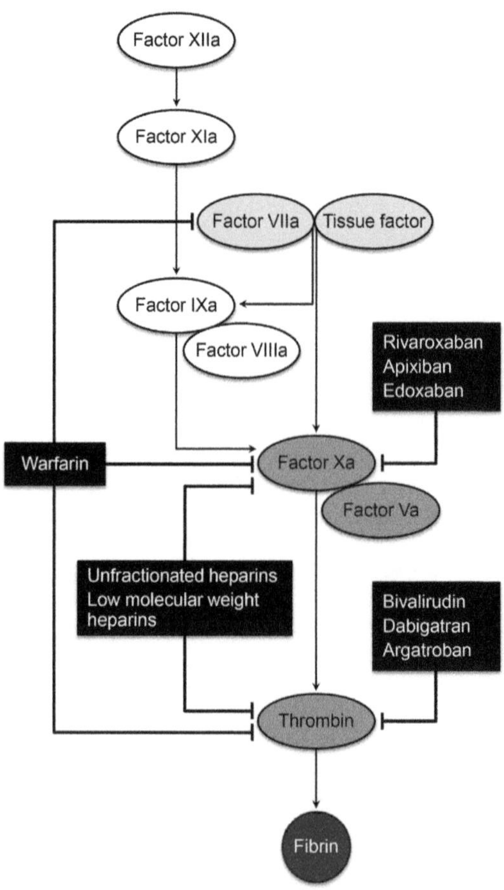

Figure 7.1 Targets of commonly used anticoagulants

have less inhibitory activity against thrombin than UFH and are much less responsive to reversal with protamine sulfate.

LMWHs have advantages over UFH because they have greater bioavailability, and the duration of anticoagulation effect is greater. LMWH is also much less likely to cause immune-mediated thrombocytopenia.

The most common monitoring tests are prothrombin time (PT), and INR, for warfarin and activated partial thromboplastin time (aPTT) and anti Xa for heparin. The PT/INR assesses the extrinsic clotting cascade, which consists of factor VIIa, tissue factor, and the common pathway of coagulation (factors II, Va, and Xa and fibrinogen). The aPTT assesses the intrinsic pathway of clotting, which consists of factors VIIIa, IXa, XIIa, and XIIIa and the common pathway. Modern monitoring now includes anti-factor Xa assays; these are used to measure the degree of anticoagulation for patients receiving heparin therapy and can be used as a quantitative marker. Anti-factor Xa reflects therapy more accurately because aPTT values and measurements can be influenced by a host of factors (e.g., reagents used). For patients with cerebral venous thrombosis, a high intensity level of anticoagulation with heparin is often employed; for all other neurologic indications, low-intensity nomograms are used (Tables 7.1 and 7.2).

Table 7.1 High-Intensity Heparin-Dosing Nomogram

Start 18 units/kg per hour				
Anti-Xa (units/ml)	***IV push loading dose***	**Infusion**	***IV rate change units/kg per hour***	**Repeat Anti-Xa**
<0.1	80 units/kg	Continue	Increase by 4 units/kg per hour	6 hours
0.1–0.2	40 units/kg	Continue	Increase by 2 units/kg per hour	6 hours
0.21–0.29	0	Continue	Increase by 2 units/kg per hour	6 hours
0.3–0.7	0	Continue	No change	If within first 24 hours of heparin, two consecutive therapeutic anti-Xa levels are required before defaulting to daily anti-Xa each morning.
0.71–0.99	0	Stop for 1 hour	Decrease by 2 units/kg per hour	6 hours after heparin resumed
1 or greater	0	Stop for 2 hours	Decrease by 4 units/kg per hour	6 hours after heparin resumed

Table 7.2 Low-Intensity Heparin-Dosing Nomogram

Start 12 units/kg per hour				
Anti-Xa (units/ml)	***IV push loading dose***	**Infusion**	***IV rate change units/kg per hour***	**Repeat Anti-Xa**
<0.1	0	Continue	Increase by 4 units/kg per hour	6 hours
0.1–0.19	0	Continue	Increase by 2 units/kg per hour	6 hours
0.2–0.5	0	Continue	No change	If within first 24 hours of heparin, two consecutive therapeutic anti-Xa levels are required before defaulting to daily anti-Xa each morning.
0.51–0.6	0	Continue	Decrease by 1 unit/kg per hour	6 hours after rate change
0.61–0.9	0	Stop for 1 hour	Decrease by 2 units/kg per hour	6 hours after heparin resumed
0.91 or greater	0	Stop for 2 hours	Decrease by 4 units/kg per hour	6 hours after heparin resumed

Heparin IV

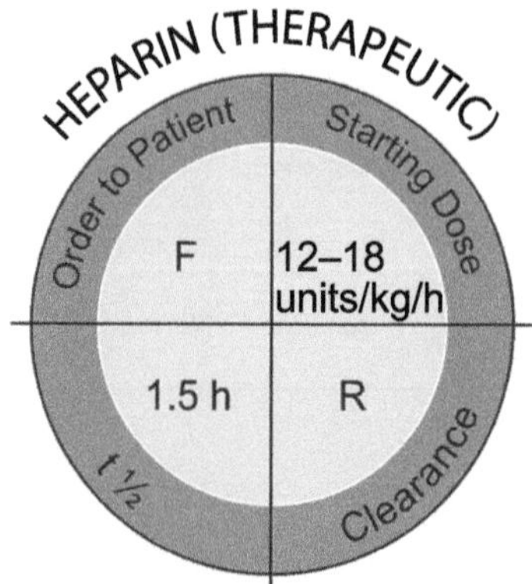

Pharmacologic Characteristics

- Thrombin inhibitor binds to antithrombin III and factor Xa
- Metabolized by the liver via reticuloendothelial system
- Half-life is related to age and is affected by body habitus
- Renal clearance, but at high doses, elimination occurs via non-renal methods

- Preferred injectable anticoagulant in renal disease (vs. LWMH or fondaparinux)
- High-risk drug with multiple concentrations commercially available

Dosing and Administration

- Onset immediate when administered intravenously (IV)
- Usually no bolus administered in neurologic indications but in other urgent anticoagulation indications, 60–80 units/kg IV push
- In cerebral venous thrombosis heparin infusion, give 18 units/kg per hour and adjust dosage to anti-Xa levels every 6 hours until anti-Xa level is within the therapeutic range for two consecutive results

Monitoring

- aPTT (1.5–2.5 x baseline)
- Anti-Xa levels (ideal range is 0.3–0.7)
- Platelet count
- Abnormal bleeding

Side Effects

- Heparin-induced thrombocytopenia (HIT)—antibody-mediated. The PF4-dependent P-selectin expression assay measures antibodies; if positive, need to replace with fondaparinux, argatroban, bivalirudin, or (Table 7.3)

Table 7.3 Treatment of Heparin Induced Thrombocytopenia

- **Fondaparinux** 5–10 mg and decrease dose to 1.5 mg subcutaneously once daily for CrCl 30–50 ml/min
- **Argatroban** (not with severe liver failure) 2 mcg/kg/minute starting dose with subsequent adjustments maintaining 1.5–2.5 times baseline aPTT
- **Bivalirudin** 0.2 mg/kg/hour (creatinine clearance >60 mL/minute) starting dose with subsequent adjustments maintaining 1.5–2.5 times baseline aPTT
  - 0.15 mg/kg/hour (creatinine clearance 30 to 60 mL/minute)
  - 0.075 mg/kg/hour (creatinine clearance 10 to 29 mL/minute)
  - 0.025 mg/kg/hour (creatine clearance <10 mL/minute)

- Mild, transient thrombocytopenia—not antibody-mediated
- Hyperkalemia (suppression of aldosterone synthesis)
- Minor bleeding: unexplained bruising, gingival hemorrhage
- Major bleeding: pulmonary hemorrhage, retroperitoneal hemorrhage
- Anaphylaxis resulting in skin necrosis
- Heparin resistance (possibly explained by increased heparin clearance, high dosing requirement to maintain therapeutic anticoagulation, increase in heparin binding proteins, elevations in factor VIII and fibrinogen)

Enoxaparin SQ

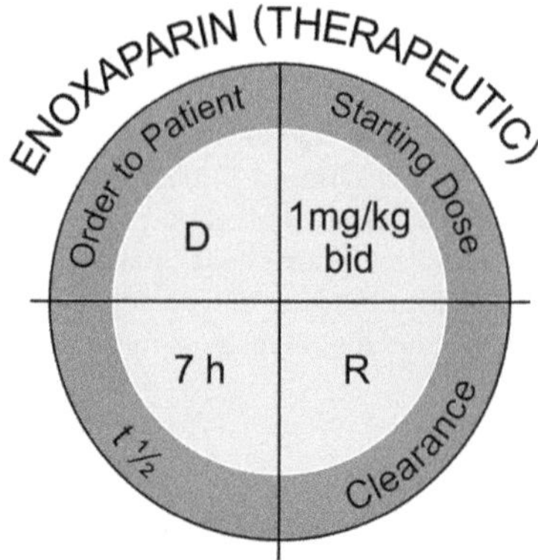

Pharmacologic Characteristics

- Derived from unfractionated heparin
- Low molecular weight: 4,000–5,000 Daltons (compared with UFH ~15,000 Daltons)
- Factor Xa inhibitor with some activity against antithrombin
- Therapeutic dose in deep venous thrombosis, cerebral venous thrombosis, pulmonary embolus, atrial thrombus (10)

Dosing and Administration

- Therapeutic dose (normal renal function): enoxaparin 1 mg/kg every 12 hours SQ
- Increasing the dose by 20-30% in patients with BMI > 40 kg/m^2 may be appropriate, but the ideal dose is not known in this patient demographic
- If creatinine clearance (CrCl) is <30 ml/min, reduce enoxaparin dose to 30 mg/day. Patients have significantly increased plasma levels and increased odds of bleeding
- When transitioning from UFH infusion, give dose of enoxaparin simultaneously after stopping the infusion

Monitoring

- Monitor activity with anti-Xa levels (especially in patients with renal disease, obesity). Measure anti-Xa level when drug is at steady state and 4 hours after the last dose was administered (for therapeutic dosing)
- Anti-Xa levels (ideal range is 0.3–1 and slightly higher than with UFH)

Side Effects

- Incidence of HIT: <1%
- Hypersensitivity angioedema, pruritus, urticaria, hyperkalemia (rare)
- Vesiculobullous rash and ischemic skin necrosis (rare)
- Major bleeding that cannot be adequately reversed with protamine (1%)
- Transient increase in liver function test results (4–10%)

Warfarin PO

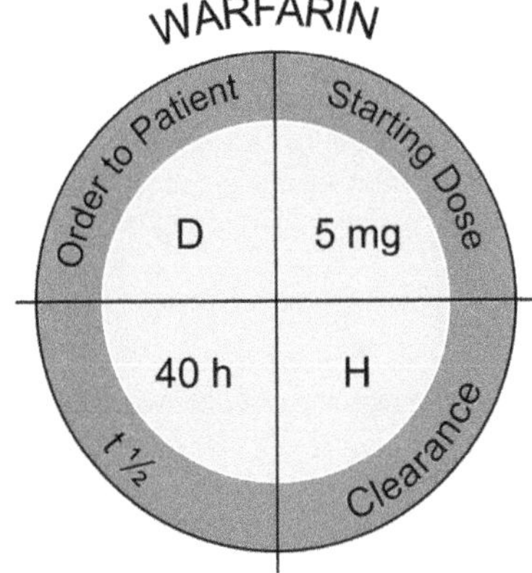

Pharmacologic Characteristics

- Vitamin K antagonist; inhibits clotting factors II, VII, IX, and X and protein C and S
- Nearly completely protein-bound (99%)
- Hepatic metabolism via CYP 2C9 pathway, with activity via 2C19, 1A2, and 3A4
- Half-life is ~40 hours, but variable based on age; discontinue drug 5 days prior to planned procedures

Dosing and Administration

- Starting dose 5 mg orally once daily but individualized dosing

- Reduce doses in patients with hepatic impairment, poor nutrition (decreased albumin results in higher free level), congestive heart failure, older age, and drug interactions
- Onset 24–72 hours after administration (factor II and X inhibition)
- Usually 5–7 days until fully therapeutic INR
- Warfarin is initiated with heparin bridging or alone. Any situation that could lead to recurrent hemorrhage quickly is a strong argument to increase the dose gradually and incrementally while closely monitoring the INR.
- Overlap parenteral therapy for 5 days when treating venous thromboembolism (irrespective of INR)

Monitoring

- No adjustment in patients with renal impairment
- INR monitoring is required when starting or stopping medications with possible interaction with warfarin
- Target INR of 2.5 for most indications
- Target INR of 3 for bi-leaflet, tilting-dish, or caged-ball valve
- Target INR of 3 for antiphospholipid antibody syndrome

Side Effects

- Skin necrosis
- "Purple toe" syndrome (from rapid depletion of coagulation factors)
- Possibility of hemorrhage anywhere (joints, gastrointestinal, hematuria, hemoptosis)

Factor Xa Inhibitors

Three factor Xa inhibitors are available in the United States: rivaroxaban, apixaban, and edoxaban. All three are approved for use in venous thromboembolic events (11) and to prevent strokes in non-valvular atrial fibrillation (NVAF). Edoxaban is the newest drug in this class. (Betrixaban- a fourth agent- is not yet readily available but approved for venous thromboembolic [VTE] prophylaxis.) All three medications have been compared with warfarin, but data are limited regarding the comparative efficacy and safety of the different factor Xa inhibitors. The 3-to-6-month mortality from bleeding can be up to 10% when used for deep venous thrombosis.

Anti-Xa chromogenic assays may test for the presence of Xa inhibitors, but there is often a delayed turnaround as the test is not generally available in hospital laboratories. INR and thromboelastography are not accurate. Andexanet alfa and aripazine may reverse factor Xa inhibitors and are currently undergoing phase III investigations.

Rivaroxaban PO

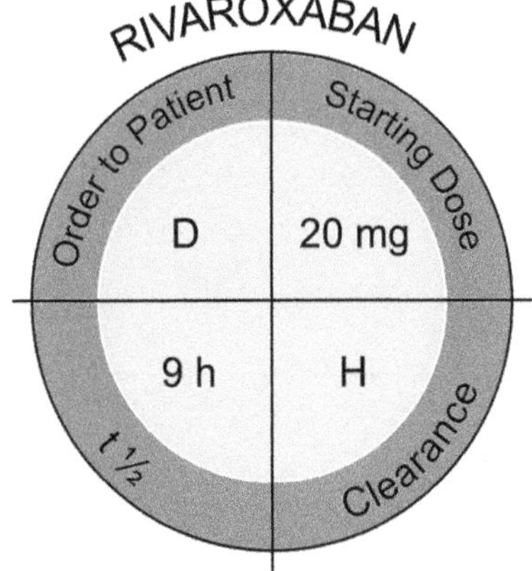

Pharmacologic Characteristics

- Factor Xa inhibitor
- Higher rate of gastrointestinal hemorrhage than warfarin
- Lower cerebral hemorrhage risk than warfarin
- Similar efficacy in stroke prevention when compared to warfarin
- Hold 3–5 days prior to planned procedures (dependent on renal function)

Dosing and Administration

- 20 mg/day for NVAF
- 15 mg bid × 21 days, then 20 mg/day for VTE treatment
- 10 mg/day for VTE prophylaxis following hip or knee replacement
- 15 mg orally once daily if CrCl < 50 ml/min

Monitoring

- Drug affects INR (false elevation), and not a useful metric
- Not dialyzable
- No adjustment in patients with minor liver disease without coagulopathy
- PT or anti-factor Xa assays may be used for a qualitative measure. No therapeutic range has been established for quantifiable dose response
- Undetectable Xa levels exclude clinically relevant drug concentrations
- Hold drug for 48 hours prior to planned procedures

Side Effects

- Possibility of hemorrhage anywhere (joints, gastrointestinal, hematuria, hemoptysis)
- Higher rate of gastrointestinal hemorrhage compared to warfarin

Apixaban PO

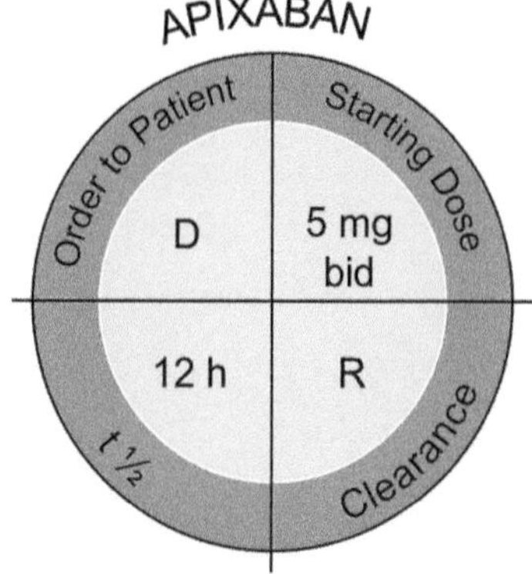

Pharmacologic Characteristics

- Factor Xa inhibitor
- Hold drug 2–4 days prior to planned procedures (dependent on renal function)

Dosing and Administration

- 5 mg bid for NVAF
- 2.5 mg bid for NVAF (age >80 creatinine >1.5 or weight <60 kg)
- 10 mg bid × 7 days, then 5 mg bid for VTE treatment
- 2.5 mg bid for VTE prophylaxis

Monitoring

- PT/INR and aPTT are all prolonged with apixaban
- Therapeutic ranges have not been established, but anti-Xa levels have been used to guide decisions
- Not dialyzable
- Not studied in patients with renal dysfunction
- No dose adjustments for patients with minor liver disease; avoid in those with severe impairment
- Avoid in patients with BMI > 40 or weight > 120 kg (not studied)

Side Effects

- Possibility of hemorrhage anywhere (joints, gastrointestinal, hematuria, hemoptosis)
- Lower rate of both gastrointestinal and cerebral hemorrhages when compared to warfarin

Edoxaban PO

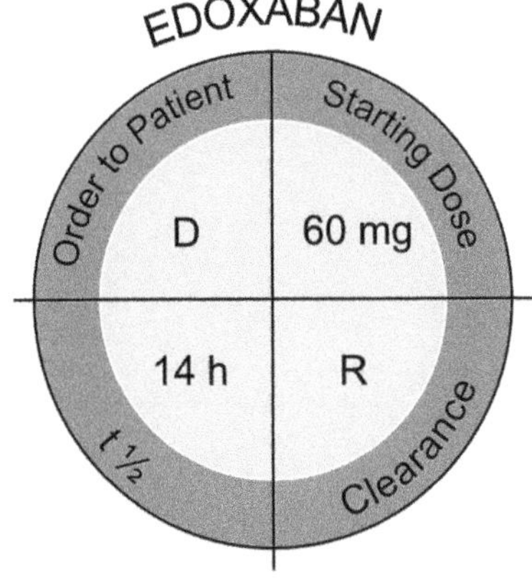

Pharmacologic Characteristics

- Factor Xa inhibitor
- Hold drug 2–4 days prior to planned procedures (depending on renal function)

Dosing and Administration

- 60 mg orally once daily
- For patients with renal dysfunction, decrease dose to 30 mg/day with CrCl 15–50 ml/min; not recommended with CrCl <15 ml/min
- Avoid use in patients with CrCl >95 ml/min

Monitoring

- No adjustments in patients with liver impairment but should avoid in those with severe liver failure
- Prolongs PT and aPTT
- No reference range available but anti-Xa gives a quantifiable dose response
- Not dialyzable

Side Effects

- Possibility of hemorrhage anywhere (joints, gastrointestinal, hematuria, hemoptosis)

Fondaparinux SC

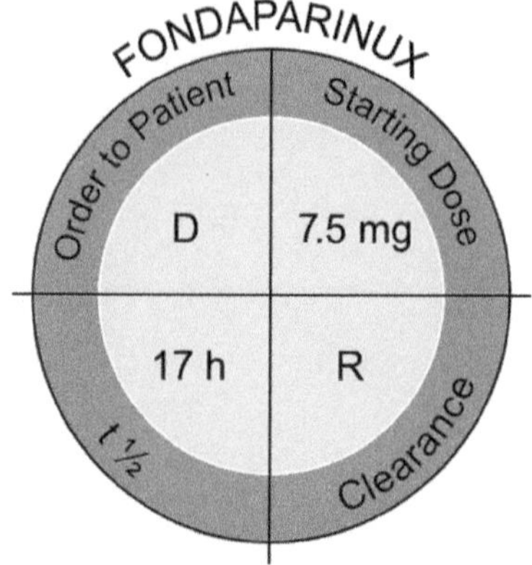

Pharmacologic Characteristics

- Synthetic pentasaccharide factor Xa inhibitor
- Antithrombin-mediated inhibition of factor Xa; inhibits thrombin formation and clot propagation
- For heparin-induced thrombocytopenia with need for deep venous thrombosis prophylaxis (Alternative options shown in Table 7.3)
- Probably as effective as LMWH in preventing venous thromboembolism

Dosing and Administration

- 7.5 mg subcutaneously once daily (5 mg/day if weight < 50 kg, and 10 mg/day if weight > 100 kg)
- Anti-Xa levels at 3 hours after dose: 0.4–0.5
- Avoid when CrCl <30 ml/min

Monitoring

- No dosage adjustments in patients with mild or moderate hepatic dysfunction. Use with caution in those with severe hepatic dysfunction.
- PT and aPTT do not measure degree of anticoagulation

Side Effects

- Thrombocytopenia (3% incidence < 50,000–100,000 platelets)
- Limited data for reversing fondaparinux in the event of major bleeding. PCC can provide some reversal of the drug. Andexanet alfa is being marketed for reversing anticoagulation effects of fondaparinux

Thrombin Inhibitors

Dabigatran has a rapid mode of action with a peak at 0.5 to 2 hours. It is used for elective total hip or knee arthroplasty to prevent deep venous thrombosis. It is also used for the treatment of nonvalvular atrial fibrillation. Most bleeding events are treated by withholding drugs. Idarucizumab is approved in the United States as a specific reversal agent for dabigatran (13). Both PT and INR have low sensitivity to anticoagulation with dabigatran. However, a normal aPTT may indicate a low serum level of dabigatran, and the same applies to thrombin time (TT). There are no specific monitoring tests available to assess the degree of anticoagulation with dabigatran.

Dabigatran PO

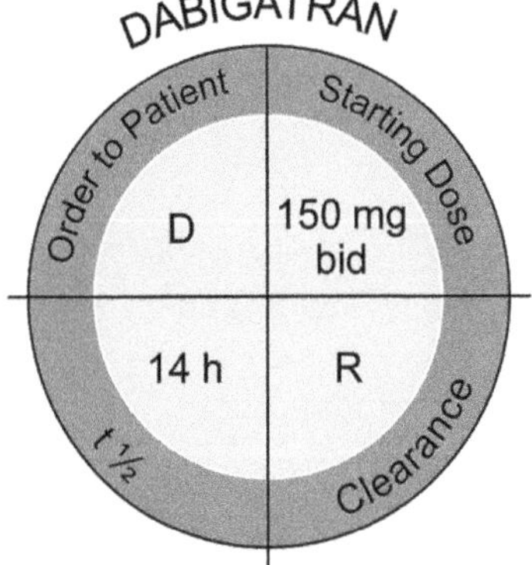

Pharmacologic Characteristics

- Direct thrombin inhibitor
- Greater risk of bleeding events in patients with poor renal function (even when dose is adjusted)

Dosing and Administration

- Dose 150 mg twice a day for NVAF and VTE
- Dose 75 mg twice a day if CrCl <50 ml/min in NVAF
- Prior to planned procedures, hold for 3–5 days

Monitoring

- INR may give some qualitative information on dose (INR < 1.3 indicates minimal drug effect)
- Bleeding risk
- Stroke or thromboembolism recurrence
- Can be dialyzed off in the event of emergent anticoagulation reversal

Side Effects

- Gastrointestinal hemorrhage (double the risk with warfarin)
- Intracranial hemorrhage (less than warfarin)
- Possibility of hemorrhage anywhere (joints, gastrointestinal, hematuria, hemoptosis)

Bivalirudin IV

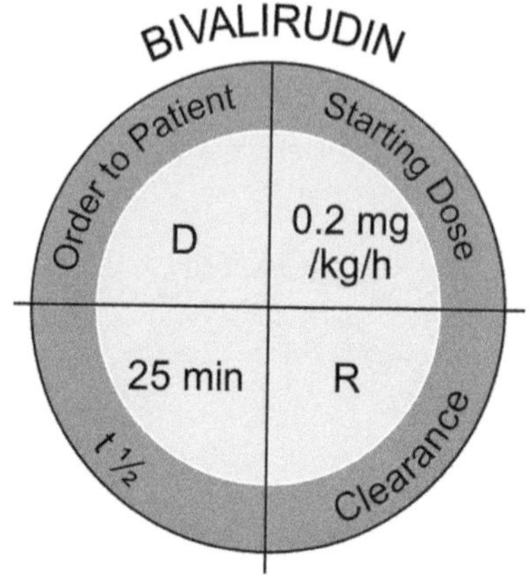

Pharmacologic Characteristics

- Synthetic thrombin inhibitor
- For heparin induced thrombocytopenia and need for therapeutic anticoagulation

Dosing and Administration

- Infusion: 0.2 mg/kg per hour IV for HIT
- Renal impairment: for CrCl < 30 ml/min, reduce infusion rate to 0.04 mg/kg per hour
- No adjustments in patients with hepatic dysfunction; titrate dose to aPTT goal

Monitoring

- aPTT (1.5–2.5 x baseline)
- Hemorrhage risk (e.g., bruising, epistaxis)

Side Effects

- Possibility of hemorrhage anywhere (joints, gastrointestinal, hematuria, hemoptosis)

Argatroban IV

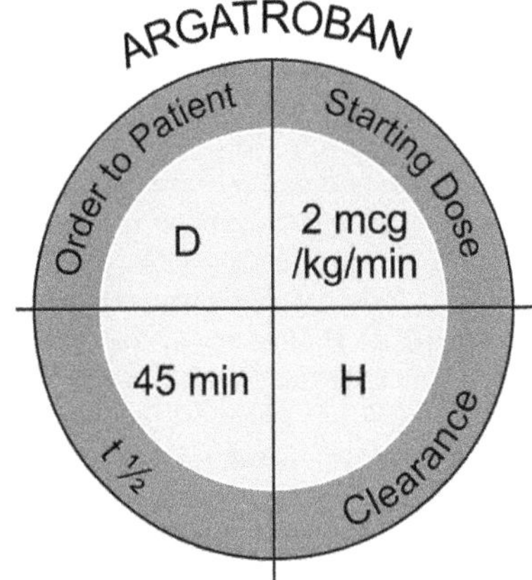

Pharmacologic Characteristics

- Selective thrombin inhibitor
- Action not dependent upon thrombin III level (in contrast to heparin)
- Immediate onset
- Hepatically cleared via CYP3A4/5

Dosing and Administration

- 2 mcg/kg per minute infusion for HIT
- Maximum rate: 10 mcg/kg per minute
- No dosage adjustments in patients with renal dysfunction
- Reduced dose in patients with hepatic dysfunction
- Hemodialysis has some effect on drug clearance

Monitoring

- Titrate to aPTT goals (1.5–3 times baseline)
- INR: false elevation—target INR of 4 prior to discontinuing infusion when transitioning to warfarin

Side Effects

- Major and minor bleeding episodes
- Chest pain
- Hypotension
- Dyspnea

Hemorrhage from Anticoagulants and Drug Reversal

INR correction is controversial if it is mildly elevated (INR values of 2–3) and if the patient is not noticeably bleeding. The benefits of reversal in actively bleeding patients are presumably improved outcomes and reduced mortality. In patients with a cerebral hemorrhage, spontaneous or traumatic, reduced hemorrhagic expansion after INR correction has not been consistently demonstrated. Most patients in the neurosciences ICU have serious cerebral hemorrhages or life-threatening traumatic injury (12). With each drug, it is important to understand the mode of action, clearance, half-life, concurrent medication use, and use in the presence of hepatic or renal impairment. Some drugs can be removed with hemodialysis or continuous renal replacement therapy, but this takes time to set up with likely too much delay. Information about reversal of antiplatelet agents and thrombolytics is found in Chapters 8 and 9.

Reversal of Vitamin K Antagonists in Life Threatening Bleeding

Vitamin K IV

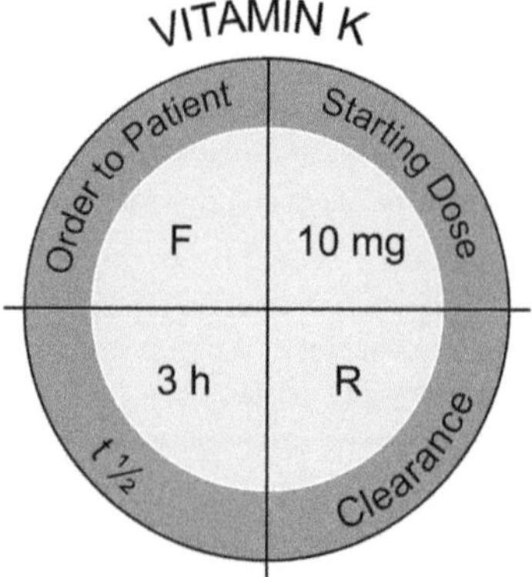

Pharmacologic Characteristics

- Provides re-synthesis of coagulation factors II, VII, IX, and X
- Protracted effect on INR reduction for 5-7 days
- No rapid effect with subcutaneous, intramuscular, or oral routes
- Combine with FFP, PCC, for warfarin reversal
- Not indicated with thrombin or factor Xa inhibitor reversal

Dosing and Administration

- 10 mg IV infusion for full reversal

Monitoring

- Any dose >5 mg will compromise the effect of restarting warfarin
- Allergic reaction
- INR
- Ongoing, active bleeding

Side Effects

- Anaphylactic reaction in 3 per 10,000 doses

Fresh-Frozen Plasma (FFP) IV

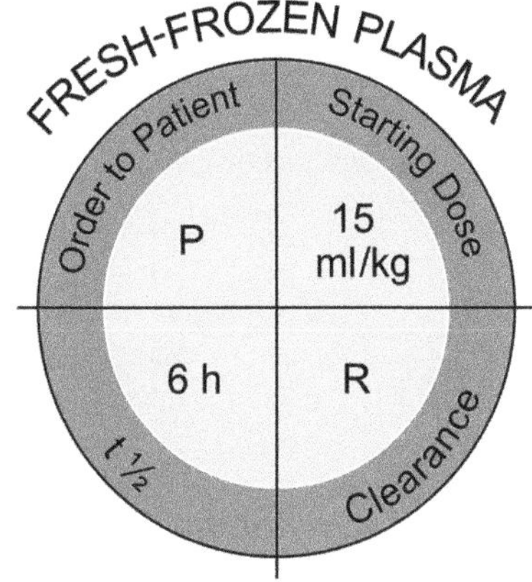

Pharmacologic Characteristics

- Contains all of the coagulation factors
- Protracted correction of INR up to 30 hours
- Duration: 6 hours
- ABO compatible, 10 minutes for ABO typing
- Delayed treatment due to thawing (~30 minutes)

Dosing and Administration

- 15 ml/kg
- Number of units administered relates to INR (Table 7.4)

Table 7.4 Reversal of INR with FFP

INR	FFP
1.5–1.9	1 unit
2–3	2 units
3–4	3 units
4–8	4 units

Adapted from Fakheri, R.J., *Formula for fresh frozen plasma dosing for warfarin reversal*. Mayo Clinic Proc, 2013. *88*: 440.

- INR correction below 1.5 not is possible (FFP has INR of 1.5)

Monitoring

- Goal INR ≤1.3 (often in combination with other reversal agents)
- Large volume (1–2 liters): use caution in patients with congestive heart failure
- After 3 units, patients are seriously at risk of fluid overload

Side Effects

- Increased transfusion-related reactions (acute lung injury [TRALI] and transfusion-associated circulatory overload [TACO])
- Anaphylaxis is relatively common, particularly in patients with IgA deficiency
- No viral inactivation (risk of infection)

Prothrombin Complex Concentrate (PCC) IV

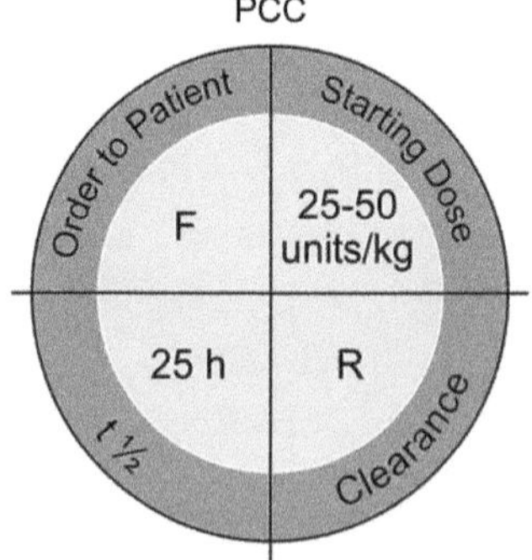

Pharmacologic Characteristics

- Three-factor PCC contains factor II, IX, and X (with a trace of heparin) and non-therapeutic levels of factor VII
- Four-factor PCC has additional factor VII, protein C, and protein S
- Rapid reversal in minutes (within 10–30 minutes, depending on which factor product is used—quicker with four-factor PCC)
- 5 minutes to reconstitute lyophilized product (when stored at room temperature)
- Duration of action: 12 or more hours

Table 7.5 Schedule for Dosing PCC by Initial INR		
INR	**Three-Factor PCC Dose**	
>4.0	50 IU/kg	
3.3–4.0	45 IU/kg	
2.6–3.2	40 IU/kg	
2.1–2.5	35 IU/kg	
1.7–2.0	30 IU/kg	
1.4–1.6	25 IU/kg	
INR	**Four-Factor PCC Dose**	**Max. Dose**
<2	Dosing unknown	Unknown
2 to <4	25 IU/kg	2,500 IU
4–6	35 IU/kg	3,500 IU
>6	50 IU/kg	5,000 IU

Dosing and Administration

- Typical weight-based dosing (may vary from 25 to 50 IU/kg; see Table 7.5)
- Rate of administration varies (~15 minutes for 1,000 IU): three-factor (e.g., Bebulin®)—100 units/min; four-factor (e.g., Kcentra®)—0.12 ml/kg per minute to maximum rate of 8.4 ml/min
- Fixed dose PCC (1000-2000 units) may be as effective, particularly with INR less than 2, but more data are needed before it can be universally accepted into practice (15)
- Give with Vitamin K to prevent rebound INR increase in warfarin-associated hemorrhage

Monitoring

- Goal INR ≤1.3
- Contraindicated in patients with disseminated intravascular coagulopathies, fibrinolysis, or other coagulopathies
- ABO typing not required
- Virus inactivated, but risk of infection still present

Side Effects

- Risk of venous thrombosis is 3%

Recombinant Factor VIIa IV

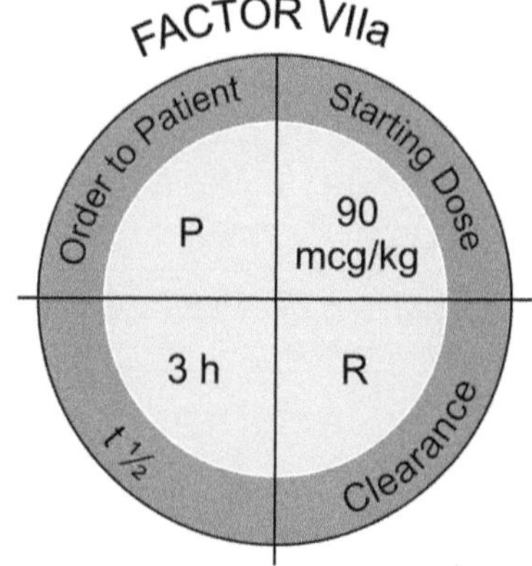

Pharmacologic Characteristics

- Rapid INR reversal
- Largely replaced by PCC
- Consider use for fondaparinux reversal
- Increases the activity of extrinsic tissue factor coagulation

Dosing and Administration

- Dose 90 mcg/kg, given IV push over 2–5 minutes

Monitoring

- INR every 4 hours
- Goal INR ≤1.3

Side Effects

- High venous thrombosis rate, up to 10%
- Risk of arterial thrombosis is 5%
- Thrombosis rate is dose-related

Other Reversal Strategies

Reversal of heparin and LMWH is common practice. The reversal of the direct oral anticoagulants is not fully established and a moving target with more antidotes awaiting. The reversal of IV tPA for symptomatic intracranial hematoma (2–6%) is discussed in Chapter 8.

Reversal of Heparin and Low-Molecular Weight Heparins

- Protamine sulfate in UFH: 1 mg for every 100 units of heparin, maximum 50 mg over 10 minutes (5 mg/min). Can increase to 1.5 mg for every 100 units of heparin if aPTT is elevated above goal. Complete reversal.
- Protamine 1 mg per 1 mg of enoxaparin, when administered within the previous 8 hours; maximal dose of protamine is 50 mg. Otherwise, 0.5 mg protamine for every 1 mg enoxaparin if >8 hours. Partial reversal.

Reversal of Factor Xa Inhibitors

- Activated charcoal, 50 g within 2 hours after administration of factor Xa inhibitors
- PCC or recombinant factor VIIa
- Four-factor PCC, 50 U/kg if intracerebral hemorrhage occurred within three to five half-lives of drug administration
- Four-factor PCC should be used over factor VIIa (lower risk of thrombotic events)
- Hemodialysis not effective

Reversal of Direct Thrombin Inhibitors

- Activated charcoal (within 2 hours of ingestion)
- Idarucizumab specific for dabigatran 2.5 g × 2 doses
- Should be given if dabigatran was given within three to five half-lives of the drug and no renal failure
- Three-factor or four-factor PCC if idarucizumab unavailable
- Hemodialysis can be considered
- No need for or measurable effect of factor VIIa or FFP (14)

Key Pointers

1. Heparin is currently best monitored with anti-factor Xa assays.
2. Heparin often causes mild thrombocytopenia, but may consider less common antibody-mediated heparin induced thrombocytopenia.
3. Factor Xa inhibitors (e.g., rivaroxaban, apixaban, edoxaban) have been used for both prevention and treatment of deep venous thrombosis.
4. Drug reversal of vitamin K antagonist-associated hemorrhage is best achieved with PCC and vitamin K 10 mg IV.
5. Activated charcoal can be considered for DOAC-induced hemorrhage if last dose was ingested within last 2 hours.

References

1. Wilson, D., et al., *Outcome of intracerebral hemorrhage associated with different oral anticoagulants*. Neurology, 2017. **88**: 1693–1700.
2. Costin, J., et al., *The new oral anticoagulants: clinical use and reversal agent development*. ISBT Science Series, 2015. **10**: 324–331.
3. Eikelboom, J.W., et al., *Idarucizumab: the antidote for reversal of dabigatran*. Circulation, 2015. **132**: 2412–2422.
4. Greinacher, A., Thiele, T. and Selleng, K. *Reversal of anticoagulants: an overview of current developments*. Thromb Haemost, 2015. **113**: 931–942.
5. Huisman, M.V. and Fanikos, J. *Idarucizumab and factor Xa reversal agents: role in hospital guidelines and protocols*. Am J Emerg Med, 2016. **34**: 46–51.
6. Nutescu, E.A., et al., *Management of bleeding and reversal strategies for oral anticoagulants: clinical practice considerations*. Am J Health Syst Pharm, 2013. **70**: 1914–1929.

7. Pollack, C.V., Jr., et al., *Idarucizumab for dabigatran reversal*. N Engl J Med, 2015. **373**: 511–520.
8. Siegal, D.M., et al., *Andexanet alfa for the reversal of factor Xa inhibitor activity*. N Engl J Med, 2015. **373**: 2413–2424.
9. Joy, M., et al., *Safety and efficacy of high-dose unfractionated heparin for prevention of venous thromboembolism in overweight and obese patients*. Pharmacotherapy, 2016. **36**: 740–748.
10. Babin, J.L., Traylor, K.L. and Witt, D.M. *Laboratory monitoring of low-molecular-weight heparin and fondaparinux*. Semin Thromb Hemost, 2017. **43**: 261–269.
11. Patel, M.R., et al., *Rivaroxaban versus warfarin in nonvalvular atrial fibrillation*. N Engl J Med, 2011. **365**: 883–891.
12. Won, S.Y., Dubinski, D., Bruder, M. et al., *Acute subdural hematoma in patients on oral anticoagulant therapy: management and outcome*. Neurosurg Focus, 2017. **43**: E12.
13. Grottke, O., et al., *Efficacy of prothrombin complex concentrates for the emergency reversal of dabigatran-induced anticoagulation*. Crit Care, 2016. **20**: 115.
14. Frontera, J.A., et al., *Guideline for reversal of antithrombotics in intracranial hemorrhage: a statement for healthcare professionals from the Neurocritical Care Society and Society of Critical Care Medicine*. Neurocrit Care, 2016. **24**: 6–46.
15. Zemrak, W.R., Smith, K.E., Rolfe, S.S. et al., *Low-dose prothrombin complex concentrate for warfarin-associated intracranial hemorrhage with INR less than 2.0*. Neurocrit Care, 2017. 27:334–340.

Chapter 8

Antifibrinolytics and Thrombolytics

Antifibrinolytics, usually tranexamic acid (TXA), are used to prevent rebleeding of recently ruptured intracranial aneurysms because fibrinolysis is considered the main mechanism of rebleeding. Many neurosurgical practices administer several doses of an antifibrinolytic agent while planning for immediate surgery or coiling of the aneurysm (1,2). Antifibrinolytics have now also been introduced to treat recurrent subdural hematoma.

In acute ischemic stroke with disability, intravenous alteplase (IV tPA) is the main fibrinolytic drug, and there is strong proof of its benefit in many types of strokes (3). A more recent study compared tenecteplase with alteplase and found similar benefit, although most ischemic strokes in this clinical trial were mild (NIH Stroke Scale [NIHSS] score < 7) (4). IV tPA remains the standard of care in acute ischemic strokes even if patients undergo endovascular retrieval of a clot (5–7). There is an ongoing debate whether its use is still justified in "known" large-vessel occlusion (8), now that access to endovascular procedures in the United States has markedly increased over the last decade (9). Depending on selection criteria and now CT perfusion mismatch rather than time—endovascular treatment is feasible in a sizable number of patients with large vessel occlusion (30,31). Unfortunately, there remains a failure to recognize stroke and failure to act quickly even when a stroke is diagnosed. Thrombolysis using telestroke services has become common practice and as a result its use has increased (11).

Basic Mechanisms and Targets

There is a finely orchestrated balance between activation of the coagulation cascade leading to thrombin and the fibrinolytic system dissolving clots. Fibrinolysis depends on plasminogen-activation inhibitors. Tranexamic acid (TXA) binds to plasminogen (at the lysine site), which prevents plasminogen activation on fibrin, thus blocking fibrinolysis (Fig. 8.1). On the other hand, recombinant tissue plasminogen activator (tPA) binds to plasminogen and activates fibrinolysis. The two drugs are closely related. (TXA is the drug of choice to counter IV tPA-associated hemorrhage.)

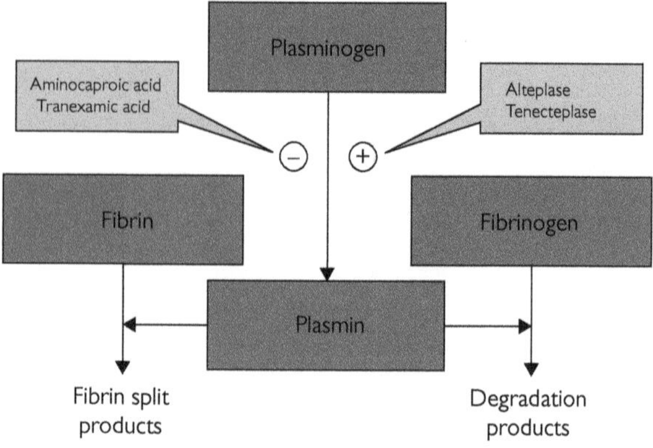

Figure 8.1 Mechanism of fibrinolysis and antifibrinolysis

Antifibrinolytics

TXA and epsilon-aminocaproic acid are used for several indications in the care of patients with complex conditions and has a role in treatment of immediate life-threatening bleeding (32). TXA is often used in patients with post-operative bleeding to substantially reduce blood transfusion requirements, but this claim has been refuted in those undergoing hip replacements (12).

The major indication for antifibrinolytics is to prevent rebleeding in aneurysmal hemorrhage. The risk of rebleeding in subarachnoid hemorrhage (SAH) is estimated at 15% within the next 12 to 24 hours. Evidence of improved outcome for SAH treated with antifibrinolytics is wanting (2,13,14), but the rebleeding rate was very low (1.5%) in a study using short-term epsilon-aminocaproic acid (15) and 2.7% in a study with a loading dose of 4 g of epsilon-aminocaproic acid and continuation with an infusion of 1 g/hr. Most U.S. practices use short-term TXA. An overview of its efficacy in SAH is shown in Box 8.1.

Box 8.1 Tranexamic Acid in Subarachnoid Hemorrhage

- 1 g IV, followed by 1 g IV every 6 hours (1)
- No increase in early deep venous thrombosis, pulmonary embolism, or myocardial infarction (14)
- May reduce rebleeding only if administered ultra-early
- May increase cerebral infarction when given more frequently than every 6 hours and for several days

Box 8.2 Tranexamic Acid in Subdural Hematoma

- 1 g IV loading and 1 g infused over 8 hours
- Effect on reduced need for surgery unknown
- Reduced mortality, especially when administered early
- No impact on contusion expansion or developing contusions (17)

TXA has been used both to resolve chronic subdural hematoma (without evacuation surgery) and to prevent reaccumulation after surgery. The use of TXA in chronic subdural hematomas is currently being studied in a clinical trial (TRACS) (16). The efficacy of TXA in subdural hematoma is shown in Box 8.2.

Tranexamic Acid (TXA) IV

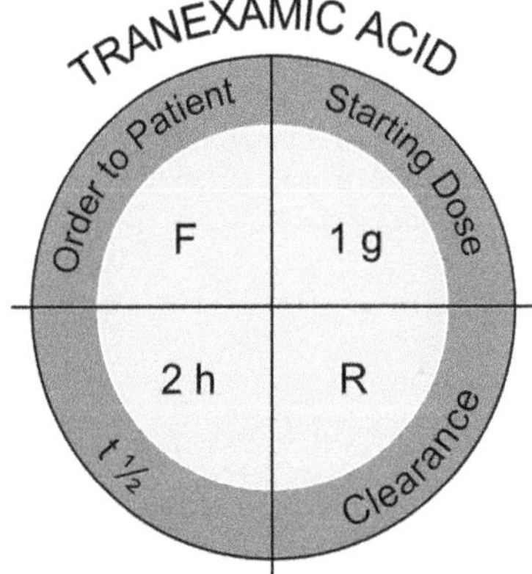

Pharmacologic Characteristics

- Synthetic derivative of the amino acid lysine
- Forms a reversible complex that displaces plasminogen from fibrin, resulting in the inhibition of fibrinolysis
- Competitive inhibitor of plasminogen activation; noncompetitively inhibits plasmin at high concentrations
- TXA is 6–10 times more potent than epsilon-aminocaproic acid
- Onset of action: 5–10 minutes
- Duration of fibrinolysis inhibition: up to 17 hours

Dosing and Administration

- In SAH: 1 g IV and 1 g IV 6 hours later up to 72 hours or until aneurysm has been secured (1 gr IV followed by infusion of 1 gr IV for 8 hours is current investigated in the ULTRA trial) (18)
- Total dose: 4–6 g IV daily

- In trauma, 1 g IV loading over 10 minutes and 1 g infused over 8 hours with maximum rate of infusion 100 mg/min; do not administer faster than 1 ml/min to avoid hypotension (19–21)
- In thrombolytic-induced hemorrhage: 10–15 mg/kg IV over 20 minutes
- Dosage adjustment in patients with renal failure but not in those with hepatic failure

Monitoring

- May prolong thrombin time
- Increases serum fibrin split products
- Reduced D-dimer value
- Drug interactions include any additional agents that may increase thrombotic risk profile

Side Effects

- Hypotension (from rapid IV push administration)
- Mild headache, gastrointestinal upset
- Thrombotic risk is increased with prior use of hormonal contraceptives and in patients with prior hypercoagulable profiles
- Seizures (rare), most often reported after major cardiovascular surgery and with high and repeated doses
- Isolated reports of severe hypersensitivity reactions

Epsilon-Aminocaproic Acid IV

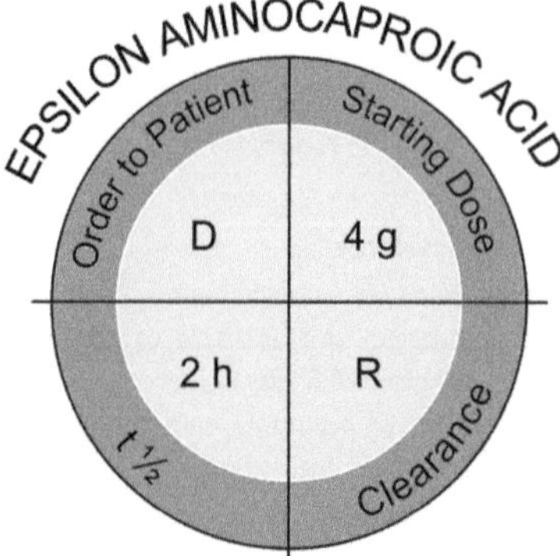

Pharmacologic Characteristics

- Much less potent than TXA
- Inhibits fibrin degradation by competitively binding to plasminogen, preventing its activation and fibrinolysis
- Less commonly used than TXA

Dosing and Administration

- 4–5 g IV bolus over 60 minutes followed by 1 g/hr infusion for 8 hours or until bleeding stops; continue infusion for <72 hours
- Discontinue infusion 4 hours prior to cerebral angiogram and 2 hours prior to endovascular treatment of aneurysm
- May accumulate in patients with renal dysfunction
- No dose adjustment in patients with liver disease

Monitoring

- Creatine phosphokinase levels (with prolonged use)
- Fibrinogen levels after infusion
- Renal indices

Side Effects

- Anaphylaxis
- Hypotension, bradycardia, arrhythmia if given IV push (discouraged)
- Thrombotic events including arterial events and pulmonary emboli
- Muscle necrosis, rhabdomyolysis
- Seizures
- Myoglobinuria

Fibrinolytics

Alteplase (tPA) is the only therapy approved by the U.S. Food and Drug Administration (FDA) for the treatment of acute ischemic, disabling stroke. Use has been shown to improve functional disability scores at 6 months. If an ischemic stroke in the posterior or anterior circulation seems clinically likely, an NIHSS score of 5 or more triggers the use of IV tPA. Posterior circulation stroke may present with serious symptoms not included in the NIHSS, and clinical judgment remains important (10). Decisions should not be made solely on the basis of the NIHSS score but on the basis of a complete neurologic assessment.

As previously noted, there are some questions about the efficacy of IV tPA in patients with large-vessel occlusions. Endovascular retrieval may be needed, and the additional cost of IV tPA could be substantial, although costs vary among U.S. institutions (22–24). Acute recanalization of carotid or middle cerebral artery occlusions with IV tPA is successful in only one in 10 patients and much less likely in patients with intracranial/extracranial (tandem) occlusions with a high clot burden (25). IV tPA could potentially delay the time interval from imaging to the start of the endovascular procedure by 30 minutes in one trial (26). Another unanswered question is whether to continue the IV tPA infusion if the artery has been recanalized and it is unknown if IV tPA further increases the risk of hemorrhagic conversion.

Once the decision has been made, working a fast "time to needle" remains a major challenge. Drug preparation of alteplase remains time-consuming, but better coordination will reduce the time to administration substantially. The current benchmark to administer thrombolytics is within 2 hours of stroke onset. Quicker (<30 minutes) access to IV thrombolytics remains a phenomenal challenge. Prehospital management through telemedicine with emergency medical services increases the frequency of thrombolytics administration. Delays have been identified mostly in the time between the computed tomography (CT) scan and thrombolytic administration, and this period between brain imaging and alteplase delivery requires close communication among emergency physicians, neurologists, nurses, pharmacists, and the patient's family. Failure to communicate on a timely basis with the pharmacist, failure to obtain definitive reading of the CT scan (when no neurologist or telestroke program is available), failure to obtain consent, or failure to communicate to the patient's nurse can all easily result in running out the clock.

Intravenous alteplase can be administered after certain inclusion criteria are met (e.g., major disability within 4.5 hours of onset). Patients who meet eligibility criteria in acute stroke receive alteplase with set goals (usually 60 minutes from the first evaluation and after interpretation of the CT scan). Disability criteria are shown in Box 8.3.

Contraindications have changed and remain relative (Box 8.4). This applies to age (no contraindication), prior hemorrhage (able to treat if it occurs), trauma (when considered minor), prior stroke (minor), and diabetes. However, strict blood pressure control and no evidence of ongoing coagulopathy (abnormal platelet levels, International Normalized Ratio [INR], or activated partial thromboplastin time [aPTT]) remain major preconditions.

There are several situations in which thrombolysis could jeopardize the patient's outcome. Not all are absolute contraindications, and decisions may have to be tailored for each individual. Several clinical situations may still be debated, but most physicians will hesitate and some will proceed with the use of thrombolytics (Box 8.5).

Box 8.3 Disability Criteria to Consider Administration of Alteplase

- Any NIHSS score >5
- Severe aphasia (NIHSS score of 3 in speech evaluation)
- Hemiparesis without ability to overcome gravity
- Severe ataxia
- Acute diplopia

Box 8.4 Contraindications to Alteplase for Acute Ischemic Stroke Within 3 Hours of Symptom Onset

Clinical Contraindications

- Major head trauma or stroke within the previous 3 months
- Sustained hypertension >185 mmHg systolic or >110 mmHg diastolic
- Active internal bleeding
- Blood glucose level <50 mg/dl and symptoms resolve with administration of dextrose
- History of intracranial hemorrhage
- Major surgery or serious trauma within the previous 14 days
- Acute bleeding diathesis
  - Platelet count <100 × 10^9/L
  - Heparin or heparin products received within 48 hours resulting in elevated aPTT or anti-Xa.
  - Anticoagulation resulting in INR >1.7
  - Current use of direct thrombin inhibitors or factor Xa inhibitors with elevated laboratory test results (e.g., aPTT, thrombin time [TT], ecarin clotting time [ECT], or anti-factor Xa activity assays)
- Pregnancy
- Gastrointestinal or urinary tract hemorrhage within the previous 21 days
- Acute myocardial infarction within the previous 3 months

Radiographic Contraindications

- Established sizable cerebral infarction (hypodensity of more than one-third of the middle cerebral artery territory)
- Intracranial hemorrhage

Box 8.5 Weighing Risks vs. Benefits of Alteplase Administration

- Improving substantially but still potentially disabling stroke
- Complete hemianopia (only)
- Administration early postpartum period (<14 days)
- Unknown platelet count (low probability of abnormal test)
- Low-dose, prophylactic low-molecular-weight heparin
- Gastrointestinal bleeding with treated source
- Large, unruptured intracranial aneurysm
- Dementia, but independent or assisted living
- Diabetic, hemorrhagic retinopathy

Thrombolytics

Alteplase IV

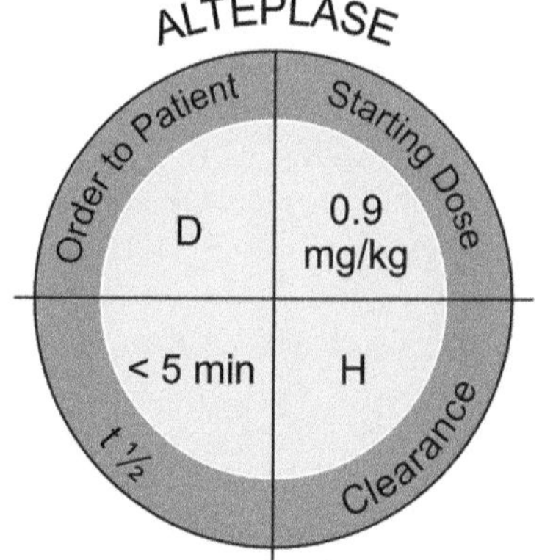

Pharmacologic Characteristics

- Engineered by DNA technology
- Enhances the conversion of plasminogen to plasmin
- Plasmin degrades fibrinogen and fibrin in the thrombus
- Duration of effect: 80% cleared from body within 10 minutes; fibrinolytic activity persists for up to 1 hour
- Half-life: 5 minutes

Dosing and Administration

- 0.9 mg/kg actual body weight
- Maximum dose of 90 mg
- 10% of total dose in bolus over 1 minute (maximum 9 mg)
- 90% of total dose in 1-hour infusion (maximum 81 mg)
- Important to flush the IV line with 50 ml 0.9% NaCl at the same rate of the infusion to ensure that the entire dose of alteplase has been infused
- Drug clearance is mediated by the liver, but no dose adjustments are needed in patients with hepatic dysfunction (very rapidly cleared from circulation)

Monitoring

- NIHSS check every 15 minutes for 2 hours, then every 30 minutes for 6 hours, then hourly (until 24 hours) after administration
- Keep blood pressure controlled: before tPA, systolic blood pressure <185 mmHg and diastolic blood pressure <110 mmHg; after tPA, systolic <180 mmHg and diastolic <105 mmHg
- Aspirin, 81 or 325 mg, 24 hours later with no evidence of major hemorrhage or hemorrhagic conversion

Side Effects

- Angioedema (1–8%)
  - Patients already taking angiotensin-converting enzyme (ACE) inhibitors are at high risk of developing angioedema
  - Angioedema is typically mild and transient. Several options for treatment are shown in Box 8.6

Box 8.6 Treatment of tPA-Associated Angioedema

- Stop infusion with new lip swelling
- Intubation if laryngeal involvement or stridor (may be nasal intubation)
- Immediate 0.3 mg intramuscular (IM) epinephrine, 10 mg IV dexamethasone, and 50 mg IV diphenhydramine
- Continue with prednisone 60 mg/day in 5-day taper

- Intracranial hemorrhage (ICH)
  - Incidence of symptomatic ICH 2–6%
  - ICH increased in patients with higher serum glutamic oxaloacetic transaminase (SGOT) level (>80), higher NIHSS score (>20), higher systolic blood pressure (>180 mmHg), higher blood glucose level (≥150 mg/dl), Asian ethnicity, (28)
  - A combination of drugs is needed to treat tPA-associated ICH (Box 8.7)

Box 8.7 Treatment of tPA-Associated Cerebral Hematoma

- Stop infusion with high suspicion before CT confirmation (29)
- 1 g TXA IV
- Reduce systolic blood pressure to 160 mmHg or lower
- Cryoprecipitate (10 units)—to increase fibrinogen and factor VIII levels
- 0.15 units/kg transfusion of platelets (6–8 units)
- Prothrombin complex concentrate (PCC) or factor VIIa (not proven, but an option)

Post-Alteplase Care

A major issue is to immediately manage blood pressure after IV alteplase administration. The American Heart Association/American Stroke Association guideline provides a target blood pressure of less than 180/105 mmHg in the first 24 hours after alteplase administration. This can be achieved with IV labetalol or a preferred proactive approach of an IV infusion of nicardipine.

There are a number of additional rules with alteplase administration:

- Strict bedrest 12–24 hours
- No bladder catheterization during infusion and 30 minutes after the infusion
- No central venous access, arterial puncture, or nasogastric tube for 24 hours
- No aspirin or other antiplatelet agents for 24 hours after alteplase administration (except in endovascular procedure leading to stent placement)
- No subcutaneous heparin or low-molecular-weight heparin until repeat CT shows no hemorrhage transformation

Key Pointers

1. TXA may have a role in reducing aneurysmal rerupture, but only when administered promptly.
2. TXA may prevent enlargement of a subdural hematoma or recurrence.
3. TXA has a defined role in counteracting the effect of IV tPA in the setting of thrombolysis-associated hemorrhage.
4. IV tPA remains the gold standard, even in patients who are candidates for immediate endovascular clot retrieval.
5. The most compelling indication for IV tPA remains any functionally significant disability from acute stroke.

References

1. Hillman, J., et al., *Immediate administration of tranexamic acid and reduced incidence of early rebleeding after aneurysmal subarachnoid hemorrhage: a prospective randomized study.* J Neurosurg, 2002. **97**: 771–778.
2. Roos, Y., *Antifibrinolytic treatment in subarachnoid hemorrhage: a randomized placebo-controlled trial. STAR Study Group.* Neurology, 2000. **54**: 77–82.
3. Sandercock, P.A.G. and Ricci, S. *Controversies in thrombolysis.* Curr Neurol Neurosci Rep, 2017. **17**: 60.
4. Logallo, N., et al., *Tenecteplase versus alteplase for management of acute ischemic stroke (NOR-TEST): a phase 3, randomized, open-label, blinded endpoint trial.* Lancet Neurol, 2017. **16**: 781–788.
5. Fiorella, D.J., et al., *Thrombectomy for acute ischemic stroke: an evidence-based treatment.* J Neurointerv Surg, 2015. **7**: 314–315.
6. Hirsch, J.A., et al., *Case volumes of intra-arterial and intravenous treatment of ischemic stroke in the USA.* J Neurointerv Surg, 2009. **1**: 27–31.
7. Saver, J.L., et al., *Stent-retriever thrombectomy after intravenous t-PA vs. t-PA alone in stroke.* N Engl J Med, 2015. **372**: 2285–2295.
8. Chandra, R.V., et al., *Does the use of IV tPA in the current era of rapid and predictable recanalization by mechanical embolectomy represent good value?* J Neurointerv Surg, 2016. **8**: 443–446.

9. Adeoye, O., et al., *Recombinant tissue-type plasminogen activator use for ischemic stroke in the United States: a doubling of treatment rates over the course of 5 years.* Stroke, 2011. **42**: 1952–1955.
10. Braksick, S.A. and Wijdicks, E.F. *An NIHSS of 0 and a very disabling stroke.* Neurocrit Care, 2016. **26**: 444–445.
11. Kepplinger, J., et al., *Safety and efficacy of thrombolysis in telestroke: a systematic review and meta-analysis.* Neurology, 2016. **87**: 1344–1351.
12. Goobie, S.M. and Frank, S.M. *Tranexamic acid: what is known and unknown, and where do we go from here?* Anesthesiology, 2017. **127**: 405–407.
13. Roos, Y.B., et al., *Antifibrinolytic therapy for aneurysmal subarachnoid haemorrhage.* Cochrane Database Syst Rev, 2003(2): CD001245.
14. Baharoglu, M.I., et al., *Antifibrinolytic therapy for aneurysmal subarachnoid haemorrhage.* Cochrane Database Syst Rev, 2013(8): CD001245.
15. Harrigan, M.R., et al., *Short-term antifibrinolytic therapy before early aneurysm treatment in subarachnoid hemorrhage: effects on rehemorrhage, cerebral ischemia, and hydrocephalus.* Neurosurgery, 2010. **67**: 935–940.
16. Iorio-Morin, C., et al., *Tranexamic Acid in Chronic Subdural Hematomas (TRACS): study protocol for a randomized controlled trial.* Trials, 2016. **17**: 235.
17. Shakur, H., et al., *Effect of tranexamic acid in traumatic brain injury: a nested randomised, placebo controlled trial (CRASH-2 Intracranial Bleeding Study).* BMJ, 2011. **343**: d3795.
18. Germans, M.R., et al., *Ultra-early Tranexamic Acid after Subarachnoid Hemorrhage (ULTRA): Study Protocol for a Randomized Controlled Trial.* Trials, 2013. **16**: 14:143.
19. Morrison, J.J., et al., *Military Application of Tranexamic Acid in Trauma Emergency Resuscitation (MATTERs) study.* Arch Surg, 2012. **147**: 113–119.
20. Roberts, I., et al., *The importance of early treatment with tranexamic acid in bleeding trauma patients: an exploratory analysis of the CRASH-2 randomized controlled trial.* Lancet, 2011. **377**: 1096–1101.
21. Shakur, H., et al., *Effects of tranexamic acid on death, vascular occlusive events, and blood transfusion in trauma patients with significant hemorrhage (CRASH-2): a randomized, placebo-controlled trial.* Lancet, 2010. **376**: 23–32.
22. Ganesalingam, J., et al., *Cost-utility analysis of mechanical thrombectomy using stent retrievers in acute ischemic stroke.* Stroke, 2015. **46**: 2591–2598.
23. Manchikanti, L. and Hirsch, J.A. *Patient Protection and Affordable Care Act of 2010: a primer for neurointerventionalists.* J Neurointerv Surg, 2012. **4**: 141–146.
24. Turk, A.S., et al., *Comparison of endovascular treatment approaches for acute ischemic stroke: cost effectiveness, technical success, and clinical outcomes.* J Neurointerv Surg, 2015. **7**: 666–670.
25. Tsivgoulis, G., et al., *Successful Reperfusion With Intravenous Thrombolysis Preceding Mechanical Thrombectomy in Large-Vessel Occlusions.* Stroke, 2018. **49**: 232–235.
26. Menon, B.K., et al., *Optimal workflow and process-based performance measures for endovascular therapy in acute ischemic stroke: analysis of the Solitaire FR thrombectomy for acute revascularization study.* Stroke, 2014. **45**: 2024–2029.
27. Demaerschalk, B.M., et al., *Scientific rationale for the inclusion and exclusion criteria for intravenous alteplase in acute ischemic stroke: A statement for healthcare professionals from the American Heart Association/American Stroke Association.* Stroke, 2016. **47**: 581–641.

28. Menon, B.K., et al., *Risk score for intracranial hemorrhage in patients with acute ischemic stroke treated with intravenous tissue-type plasminogen activator.* Stroke, 2012. **43**: 2293–2299.

29. Frontera, J.A., et al., *Guideline for reversal of antithrombotics in intracranial hemorrhage: A statement for healthcare professionals from the Neurocritical Care Society and Society of Critical Care Medicine.* Neurocrit Care, 2016. **24**: 6–46.

30. Mokin, M., Pendurthi, A., Ljubimov, V. et al., *ASPECTS Large Vessel Occlusion, and Time of Symptom Onset: Estimation of Eligibility for Endovascular Therapy.* Neurosurgery, 2017 Jul 6. doi:10.1093/neuros/nyx352. [Epub ahead of print]

31. Nogueira, R.G., Jadhav, A.P., Haussen, D.C. et al., *Thrombectomy 6 to 24 Hours after Stroke with a Mismatch between Deficit and Infarct.* N Engl J Med, 2018. **378**: 11–21.

32. Gayet-Ageron, A., Prieto-merino, D., Ker, K. et al., *Effect of treatment delay on the effectiveness and safety of antifibrinolytics in acute severe hemorrhage: a meta-analysis of individual patient-level data from 40 138 bleeding patients.* Lancet, 2017. pii: S0140-6736(17)32455-8.

Chapter 9

Antiplatelet Agents

In the neurosciences ICU and stroke units, there is little other use for antiplatelet agents than the pharmacologic management of patients with ischemic stroke (1–6). They are typically prescribed for patients who have had a transient ischemic attack (TIA), given that a TIA is a major risk factor for future stroke—up to a 4% annual risk, with the highest risk in the first 90 days following the event (7,8). The benefit of aspirin is strongest in the first 6 weeks after TIA or ischemic stroke; aspirin administration reduces the risk by more than 50%, justifying early initiation of therapy (9). However, there are acute indications for antiplatelet agents. Dual antiplatelet therapy is standard in patients with acute carotid artery recanalization and subsequent stenting for a residual stenosis. Furthermore, endovascular interventions associated with procedure-related thrombi are treated with intravenous antiplatelet agents, most frequently with abciximab.

Clinical Trials on Antiplatelet Agents in Stroke

Several landmark studies have evaluated the optimal duration and dose of antiplatelet therapy in stroke prevention (10–14). Dual antiplatelet therapy with aspirin and clopidogrel is recommended in certain mechanisms of stroke (e.g., intracranial artery atherosclerosis) but is not recommended for long-term stroke prevention.

The MATCH trial, with more than 7,500 patients, studied whether the addition of aspirin to clopidogrel could have a greater benefit than clopidogrel alone. The study found no greater benefit for stroke prevention but did find a substantial increase in the risk of bleeding with dual antiplatelet therapy when administered for more than 1 year (15).

The CHANCE trial evaluated more than 5,100 patients with TIA or minor stroke. Patients received clopidogrel 300 mg as a loading dose, followed by clopidogrel 75 mg daily for 90 days with or without aspirin concurrently for 21 days, or aspirin monotherapy 75 mg daily for 90 days. Stroke occurred in 8.2% of patients taking dual antiplatelet therapy and in 11.7% of those taking aspirin monotherapy, a small but statistically significant difference (16). The incidence of hemorrhagic stroke did not differ between the two groups. The CAPRIE trial showed no significant benefit of clopidogrel over aspirin in stroke patients, but improved outcomes in the combined risk of stroke, myocardial infarction, and vascular death, with similar adverse events (e.g., bleeding, neutropenia) (12). Clopidogrel is used as an alternative for anticoagulation in atrial fibrillation (with aspirin) when patients cannot receive anticoagulation (ACTIVE-A trial) (17). The combination of dipyridamole and aspirin is approved for stroke prevention but has not shown to be superior to clopidogrel alone (PRoFESS trial) (18).

The ARCH trial was a prospective, randomized, controlled open-label trial in patients with nondisabling ischemic stroke or TIA with at least 4 mm of atherosclerotic plaque in the thoracic aorta on echocardiography(10). Patients were randomly assigned to receive aspirin (75–150 mg/day) plus clopidogrel 75 mg/day or warfarin (International Normalized Ratio [INR] 2.0–3.0). After a median follow-up of 3.4 years, the rate of stroke and other vascular events was 7.6% in patients receiving aspirin plus clopidogrel and 11.3% in patients receiving warfarin. The incidence of major hemorrhage was not significantly different but trended higher in the warfarin group (2.3% in the aspirin-plus-clopidogrel group and 3.4% in the warfarin group).

The ongoing POINT trial (13) is a randomized study in "high risk" TIA (ABCD2 score >4) or minor stroke to determine the outcomes of major vascular effects using the combination of a 600-mg loading dose of clopidogrel, followed by a dosage of 75 mg/day and low-dose aspirin for 90 days.

Current Recommendations for Antiplatelet Agents

- Ischemic stroke (or TIA) outside thrombolysis window: aspirin 75–325 mg/day orally within 48 hours of hospitalization
- Ischemic stroke treated with intravenous (IV) or intra-arterial (IA) thrombolysis: no aspirin before thrombolysis and for 24 hours thereafter
- Lacunar syndrome: aspirin 325 mg/day, clopidogrel 75 mg/day, or aspirin/extended-release dipyridamole monotherapy 200/25 mg orally twice daily
- Intracranial artery atherosclerosis: aspirin 325 mg/day and clopidogrel 75 mg/day for 3 months; then monotherapy with aspirin, and high-intensity statin therapy (e.g., atorvastatin 80 mg/day or rosuvastatin 20 mg/day)
- Aortic atherosclerotic plaque including mobile plaque: aspirin 325 mg/day and clopidogrel 75 mg/day and high-intensity statin therapy
- Carotid endarterectomy: aspirin 75–325 mg/day or clopidogrel 75 mg/day
- Carotid artery stenting: loading clopidogrel (300 mg) and dual therapy (with clopidogrel plus aspirin) for 30 days, then aspirin monotherapy 325 mg/day with high-intensity statin therapy
- Carotid artery dissection: aspirin 325 mg/day (19)

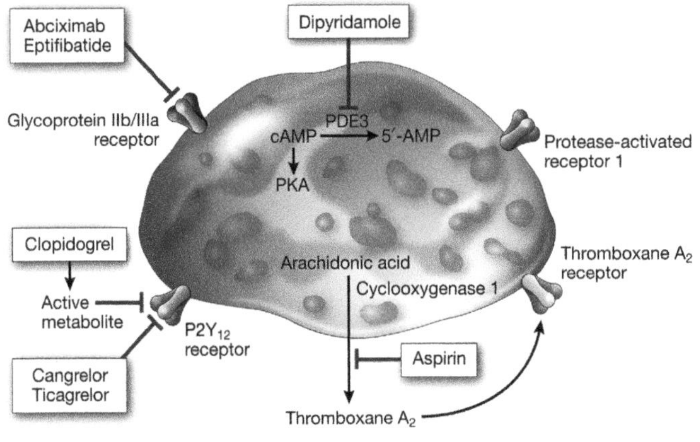

Figure 9.1 Mechanism of action of antiplatelet agents

Antiplatelet Agents

Aspirin is widely used. Several thienopyridines are on the market. Ticlopidine is no longer available in the United States. The drug most commonly used in secondary stroke prevention in patients already on aspirin is clopidogrel. Ticagrelor has not been extensively studied in stroke. Prasugrel is contraindicated in stroke (20). The major targets of antiplatelet drugs are summarized in Figure 9.1.

Aspirin PO

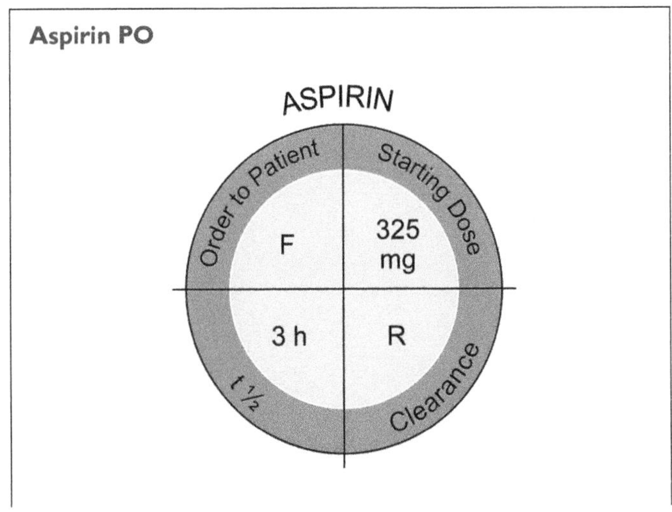

Pharmacologic Characteristics

- Irreversibly inhibits cyclooxygenase 1 (COX-1) and 2 enzymes, resulting in irreversible inhibition of thromboxane A_2
- Reduced thromboxane A_2 synthesis reduces platelet aggregation
- Irreversible inhibition of COX-1 will last 7–10 days after a single dose
- Peak plasma concentration within 30 minutes, platelet inhibition as early as 1 hour after administration (non–enteric-coated formulation). Chewing tablets will result in peak plasma concentration in 20 minutes (non–enteric-coated formulation)
- Half-life (dose-dependent): 3 hours with doses of 300–600 mg, and 10 hours with larger doses
- Avoid use in patients with severe hepatic dysfunction due to increased risk of bleeding

Dosing and Administration

- 75–325 mg/day orally
- 300 mg rectal suppository
- Chewable formulation when administered as monotherapy in low dose (e.g., 81 mg once daily)
- Administer with food to minimize gastrointestinal upset

Monitoring

- Bleeding
- Stroke recurrence
- Platelet reactivity to assess for resistance (incomplete inhibition of COX-1 enzyme)

Side Effects

- Gastrointestinal ulcer (may affect 1 in 3 patients and higher doses)
- Upper gastrointestinal tract bleeding
- Thrombocytopenia, pancytopenia
- Anaphylaxis with angioedema
- Hearing loss and tinnitus with very high doses (e.g., up to 4 g/day) and in patients with diminished renal function

Clopidogrel PO

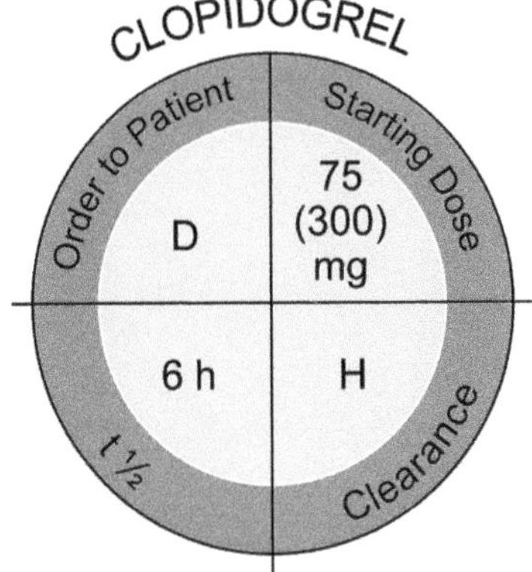

Pharmacologic Characteristics

- Irreversibly blocks $P2Y_{12}$ receptor, blocks adenosine diphosphatase activation, disrupts stability of platelet aggregation, and prevents activation of glycoprotein (GP) IIb/IIIa receptor complex
- Onset within 2 hours (for 300-600 mg loading dose)
- Duration of action: 5–10 days

Dosing and Administration

- 75 mg once daily for most indications
- 300 mg loading dose in TIA and minor stroke within 24 hours of symptom onset
- 300–600 mg loading dose in carotid stenting
- No dosage adjustment in patients with renal dysfunction, but higher platelet activity in patients with end-stage renal disease
- No dosage adjustment in patients with hepatic dysfunction

Monitoring

- Signs of bleeding
- Complete blood cell count
- Drug–drug interactions with CYP2C19 inhibitors (e.g., omeprazole, cimetidine, fluoxetine, ketoconazole, fluconazole)—may lead to treatment failure from incomplete clopidogrel activation

Side Effects

- Abnormal bruising or bleeding
- Hemorrhage after injury
- Pruritus

Ticagrelor PO

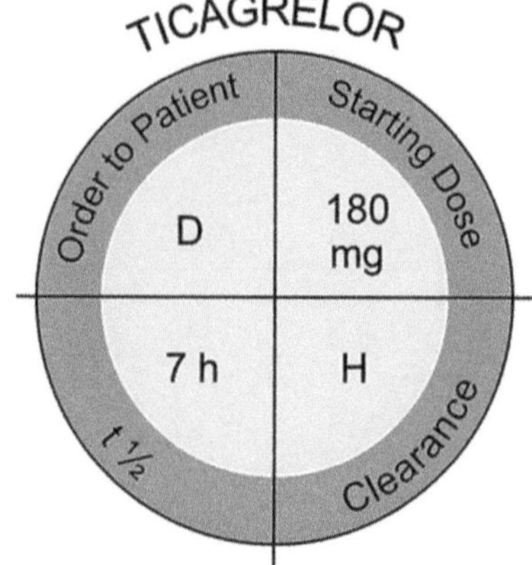

Pharmacologic Characteristics

- Reversibly blocks $P2Y_{12}$ receptor, blocks adenosine diphosphatase activation, disrupts stability of platelet aggregation, and prevents activation of glycoprotein (GP) IIb/IIIa receptor complex
- Due to reversible platelet binding, platelet function depends on serum ticagrelor levels
- Crushing tablet increases peak effect time, with slightly higher drug concentration
- Peak effect 88% at 2 hours

Dosing and Administration

- 180 mg load, followed by 90 mg twice daily
- Maximal aspirin dose of 100 mg with ticagrelor (reduced effectiveness of ticagrelor with larger aspirin doses)
- No dosage adjustments in patients with renal dysfunction
- No dosage adjustments in patients with hepatic dysfunction, but avoid in severe liver failure

Monitoring

- Respiratory signs
- Bleeding, bruising
- Renal function

Side Effects

- Bleeding, major and minor hemorrhage
- Dyspnea
- Bradycardia
- Increase in serum creatinine

Dipyridamole/Aspirin PO

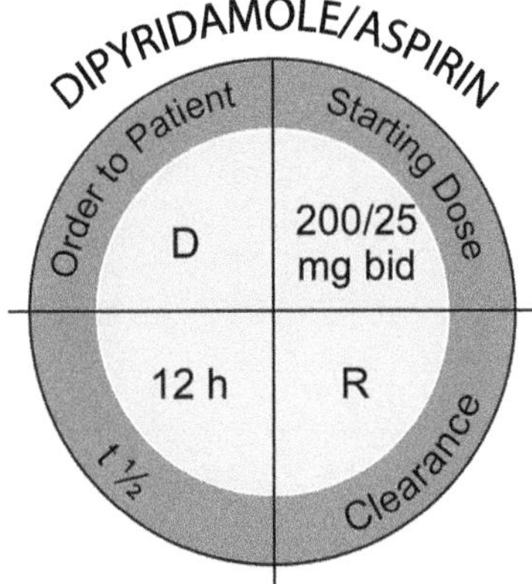

Pharmacologic Characteristics

- Phosphodiesterase inhibitor; increases levels of cyclic adenosine monophosphate (cAMP), which potentiates antiplatelet effect of prostacyclin
- Product not interchangeable with two individual components

Dosing and Administration

- 200/25 mg proprietary capsule orally twice daily
- Must be swallowed whole (extended-release capsule)
- No dosage adjustment is needed in patients with renal dysfunction, but avoid with creatinine clearance (CrCl) <10 ml/min
- No dosage adjustment is needed in patients with liver dysfunction, but avoid use with severe liver failure

Monitoring

- Bleeding, major and minor hemorrhage
- Dysphagia (need to swallow capsules whole)

Side Effects

- Headache (in nearly half of patients)
- Gastrointestinal upset (in nearly a third of patients)
- Bleeding risk

Cilostazol PO

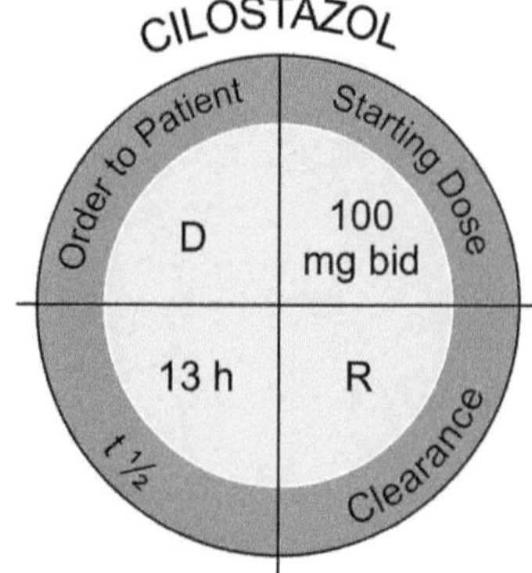

Pharmacologic Characteristics

- Phosphodiesterase-3 inhibitor
- Reversibly inhibits platelet aggregation
- Effective for stroke prevention, mainly in Asian populations
- Recommended third-line agent after clopidogrel or dipyridamole/aspirin for stroke prevention
- Mainly used for intermittent claudication prevention
- Anti-atherogenic properties
- Contraindicated in patients with heart failure

Dosing and Administration

- 100 mg by mouth twice daily
- Reduce dose to 50 mg by mouth twice daily if given with CYP2C19 inhibitors (e.g., fluconazole, omeprazole, voriconazole) or CYP3A4 inhibitors (e.g., diltiazem, erythromycin, ketoconazole, clarithromycin, ritonavir)
- No dose adjustment is needed in patients with renal dysfunction; but not studied in end-stage renal disease
- No dose adjustment is needed in patients with liver dysfunction, but use with caution in severe liver failure

Monitoring

- Platelets
- New cardiac murmurs
- Electrocardiograph (EKG)

Side Effects

- Headache
- Diarrhea
- Cardiac dysrhythmias
- Thrombocytopenia, leukopenia
- Risk of infection

Glycoprotein IIb/IIIa Inhibitors

These drugs prevent platelet aggregation by inhibiting fibrinogen and von Willebrand factor. They also prevent early adhesion of platelets to vessel walls and inhibit the final pathway of platelet aggregation. They are reserved for use in patients with embolic complications during diagnostic cerebral angiography or as a result of endovascular procedures.

Abciximab IV

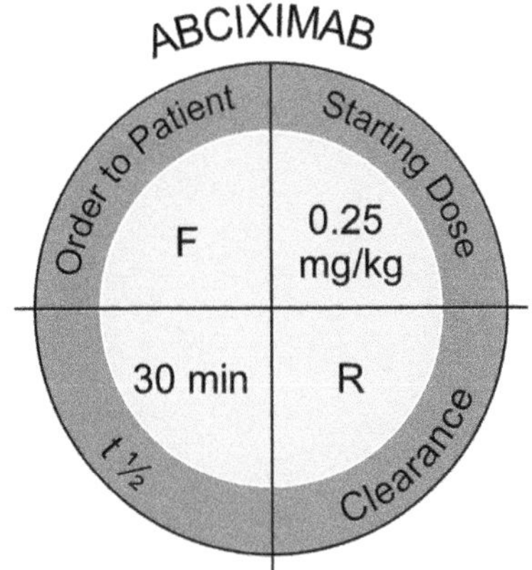

Pharmacologic Characteristics

- Humanized monoclonal antibody against GPIIb/IIIa receptor (21)
- Immediate onset
- Platelet aggregation decreased to <20% at 10 minutes
- Platelet function, completely blocked for 24 hours, improves over 48 hours after administration but may remain abnormal for up to 7 days
- Remains in circulation for up to 10 days in a platelet-bound state

Dosing and Administration

- 0.25 mg/kg bolus over 10 minutes, followed by 0.125 mcg/kg per minute (maximum 10 mcg/min) for 12 hours
- No dosage adjustments needed in patients with renal or hepatic dysfunction

Monitoring

- Prothrombin time, activated partial thromboplastin time
- Complete blood count
- Platelet count at baseline, 2–4 hours after bolus dose, and at 24 hours
- Bleeding, abnormal bruising

Side Effects

- Hypotension
- Nausea
- Hemorrhage
- Antibody development
- Thrombocytopenia (affects <5% of patients but can be serious; greater risk with recurrent administration of any GPIIb/IIIa antagonist)

Eptifibatide IV

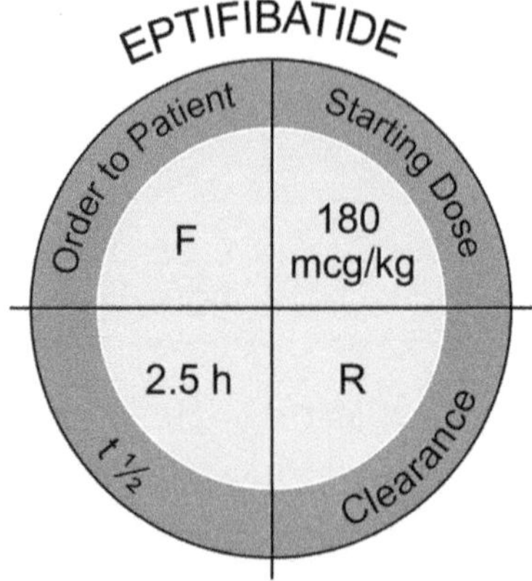

Pharmacologic Characteristics

- Cyclic heptapeptide inhibitor of platelet GPIIb/IIIa receptor; reversibly blocks platelet aggregation as a result of blocking binding of fibrinogen and von Willebrand factor to the receptor
- Immediate onset (80% platelet inhibition at 5 minutes), maximum effect in 1 hour
- Platelet function normalizes after 4–8 hours of drug discontinuation

Dosing and Administration

- 180 mcg/kg bolus (maximum 22.6 mg), followed by 2 mcg/kg per minute infusion (maximum 15 mg/hr)
- Maximum infusion rate 1 mcg/kg per minute (7.5 mg/hr) if CrCl < 50 ml/min (same bolus dose)
- No dosage adjustments in patients with hepatic dysfunction
- Contraindicated in patients with end-stage renal disease

Monitoring

- Prothrombin time, activated partial thromboplastin time
- Complete blood count
- Platelet count at baseline, 2–4 hours after bolus, and at 24 hours
- Bleeding

Side Effects

- Hemorrhage, major and minor
- Thrombocytopenia (rare)
- Hypotension

Tirofiban IV

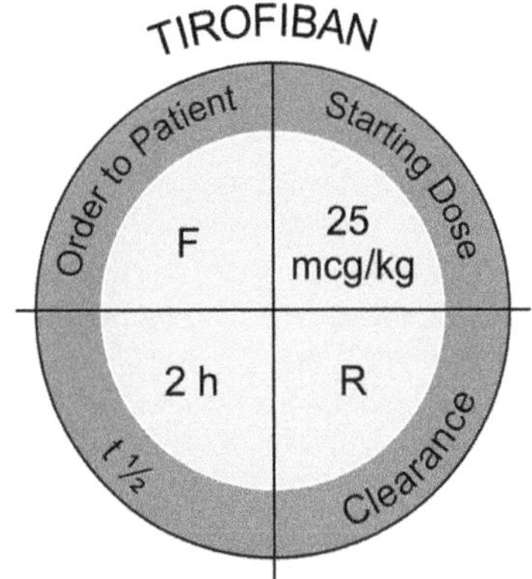

Pharmacologic Characteristics

- Reversible GPIIb/IIIa receptor antagonist, resulting in dose-dependent inhibition of platelet aggregation
- Onset rapid (70–90% platelet inhibition at 5 minutes)

Dosing and Administration

- 25 mcg/kg over 3–5 minutes, followed by 0.15 mcg/kg per minute up to 18 hours
- Reduce maintenance infusion to 0.075 mcg/kg per minute when CrCl $\leq$ 60 ml/min

Monitoring

- Prothrombin time, activated partial thromboplastin time
- Complete blood count
- Clinical signs of hemorrhage
- Renal function
- Platelet count at baseline and 6 hours after initiation

Side Effects

- Bleeding
- Thrombocytopenia (rare)

Testing Platelet Function

Measurement of bleeding time assesses platelet function, but it has been considered inaccurate and poorly reproducible. Light-transmission measurement of agonist-induced platelet aggregation (optical aggregometry) is currently considered the standard of care, with good reproducibility. Other options are whole blood aggregometry or point-of-care rapid platelet function (VerifyNow®) or TEG platelet mapping. Platelet function testing is used fairly commonly in clinical practice and requires less technical expertise to perform. It is used to test platelet function in patients taking aspirin who are also taking P2Y12 inhibitors or GPIIb/IIIa inhibitors.

Antiplatelet Agent Resistance

Poor patient compliance may be more common than antiplatelet resistance. Patients with antiplatelet resistance are at higher risk of recurrent cardiovascular or cerebrovascular events. The prevalence of aspirin resistance is nearly 25% but can be as high as 60% (22). Possible causes of aspirin resistance are related to COX-1 pathway thromboxane A_2 production, poor absorption, inadequate dosing, and drug interactions. Ibuprofen and other nonsteroidal anti-inflammatory drugs (NSAIDs) can reduce the effect of antiplatelet agents. Clopidogrel resistance is associated with the CYP2C19*2 genotype and is particularly high in Asian populations. In Caucasians, the prevalence is 5% to 30% (23) (Box 9.1).

Routine platelet function testing for antiplatelet resistance is not recommended. Blood aggregometry may identify resistance (PFA-100); the VerifyNow® Aspirin assay measures agglutination of fibrinogen-coated beads with the patient's platelets. Thromboelastography is an alternative method to assess platelet function over time.

Box 9.1 Factors Associated with Antiplatelet Agent Resistance
Female sex
Increasing age
Diabetes
High plasma triglyceride levels
Low hemoglobin levels
NSAIDs
Elevated norepinephrine levels
Cigarette smoking
Hypercholesterolemia
Polymorphisms affecting COX-1 (e.g., 50T), COX-2 (-765C), TXA_2 synthase

Discontinuation of Antiplatelet Agents Before Procedures

The risks of postoperative bleeding in patients taking antiplatelet agents vary: They are high in neurosurgical procedures but low in diagnostic procedures. Any surgical intervention involving biopsy or tissue removal warrants discontinuation of aspirin 5 to 7 days prior to the procedure. The duration of holding thienopyridines prior to a high-risk procedure is 5 days (clopidogrel), 3 to 5 days (ticagrelor), or 7 days (prasugrel).

Clinical Urgency While on Antiplatelet Agents

Urgent reversal is needed if hemorrhage occurs or if an urgent procedure such as ventriculostomy is required in a patient taking an antiplatelet agent. Intracranial hemorrhage—particularly when lobar or subdural—may require neurosurgical evacuation. With systemic hemorrhage, such as gastrointestinal hemorrhage, endoscopy or other specific diagnostic surgical interventions may be needed to find the bleeding source. It is important to establish the time of the last dose given to the patient and to calculate five half-lives, which would estimate residual drug effect. Complete blood count should be repeated to determine possible large blood loss (24).

There are no specific reversal agents for patients taking antiplatelet drugs. Platelet infusions are an option, but their effects remain to be seen. One apheresis unit ("six pack") increases platelets by 30,000 to 60,000. Most neurosurgeons will administer one or two "six packs" before surgery or ventriculostomy placement, but its benefits and risks are not known. In the PATCH trial, platelet transfusion in patients with cerebral hemorrhage found no benefit and more adverse effects (25). Another option is desmopressin (0.3–0.4 mcg/kg in a single IV dose) (26), which increases von Willebrand factor, factor VIII, and pro-coagulant platelets.

In patients treated for abciximab-associated hemorrhage, platelet transfusion should be strongly considered also because thrombocytopenia may occur (up to 5% of patients).

Key Pointers

1. Aspirin alone remains the mainstay therapy for secondary stroke prevention.
2. Dual antiplatelet therapy is needed after carotid artery stenting.
3. Platelet transfusion may be needed if thrombocytopenia is caused by GPIIb/IIIa inhibitors.

4. The benefits of platelet transfusion to reverse the actions of antiplatelet drugs are unknown in many clinical situations and may actually lead to more side effects.
5. Desmopressin may reverse the effect of antiplatelet drugs in the presence of cerebral hemorrhage.

References

1. Taylor, G., et al., *Is platelet transfusion efficient to restore platelet reactivity in patients who are responders to aspirin and/or clopidogrel before emergency surgery?* J Trauma Acute Care Surg, 2013. **74**: 1367–1369.
2. Oprea, A.D. and Popescu, W.M. *Perioperative management of antiplatelet therapy*. Br J Anaesth, 2013. **111** Suppl 1: i3–17.
3. Antithrombotic Trialists, C., et al., *Aspirin in the primary and secondary prevention of vascular disease: collaborative meta-analysis of individual participant data from randomised trials*. Lancet, 2009. **373**: 1849–1860.
4. Topol, E.J., Byzova, T.V. and Plow, E.F. *Platelet GPIIb-IIIa blockers*. Lancet, 1999. **353**: 227–231.
5. Eisert, W.G., *Dipyridamole in antithrombotic treatment*. Adv Cardiol, 2012. **47**: 78–86.
6. Gresele, P., Momi, S. and Falcinelli, E. *Anti-platelet therapy: phosphodiesterase inhibitors*. Br J Clin Pharmacol, 2011. **72**: 634–646.
7. Cheng-Ching, E., et al., *Update on pharmacology of antiplatelets, anticoagulants, and thrombolytics*. Neurology, 2012. **79**(13 Suppl 1): S68–76.
8. Kapil, N., et al., *Antiplatelet and anticoagulant therapies for prevention of ischemic stroke*. Clin Appl Thromb Hemost, 2017. **23**: 301–318.
9. Rothwell, P.M., et al., *Effects of aspirin on risk and severity of early recurrent stroke after transient ischaemic attack and ischaemic stroke: time-course analysis of randomised trials*. Lancet, 2016. **388**: 365–75.
10. Amarenco, P., et al., *Clopidogrel plus aspirin versus warfarin in patients with stroke and aortic arch plaques*. Stroke, 2014. **45**: 1248–1257.
11. Bhatt, D.L., et al., *Clopidogrel and aspirin versus aspirin alone for the prevention of atherothrombotic events*. N Engl J Med, 2006. **354**: 1706–1717.
12. Gent, M., et al., *A randomised, blinded, trial of clopidogrel versus aspirin in patients at risk of ischaemic events (CAPRIE). CAPRIE Steering Committee*. Lancet, 1996. **348**: 1329–1339.
13. Johnston, S.C., et al., *Platelet-oriented inhibition in new TIA and minor ischemic stroke (POINT) trial: rationale and design*. Int J Stroke, 2013. **8**: 479–483.
14. Wang, Y., et al., *Clopidogrel with aspirin in acute minor stroke or transient ischemic attack*. N Engl J Med, 2013. **369**: 11–19.
15. Diener, H.C., et al., *Aspirin and clopidogrel compared with clopidogrel alone after recent ischemic stroke or transient ischemic attack in high-risk patients (MATCH): randomized, double-blind, placebo-controlled trial*. Lancet, 2004. **364**: 331–337.
16. Pan, Y., et al., *Risks and benefits of clopidogrel-aspirin in minor stroke or TIA: Time course analysis of CHANCE*. Neurology, 2017. **88**: 1906–1911.
17. Connolly, S.J., et al., *Effect of clopidogrel added to aspirin in patients with atrial fibrillation*. N Engl J Med, 2009. **360**: 2066–2078.

18. Diener, H.C., et al., *Effects of aspirin plus extended-release dipyridamole versus clopidogrel and telmisartan on disability and cognitive function after recurrent stroke in patients with ischaemic stroke in the Prevention Regimen for Effectively Avoiding Second Strokes (PRoFESS) trial: a double-blind, active and placebo-controlled study.* Lancet Neurol, 2008. **7**: 875–884.

19. Kennedy, F., et al., *Antiplatelets vs anticoagulation for dissection: CADISS nonrandomized arm and meta-analysis.* Neurology, 2012. **79**: 686–689.

20. Udell, J.A., et al., *Prasugrel versus clopidogrel in patients with ST-segment elevation myocardial infarction according to timing of percutaneous coronary intervention: a TRITON-TIMI 38 subgroup analysis (Trial to Assess Improvement in Therapeutic Outcomes by Optimizing Platelet Inhibition with Prasugrel-Thrombolysis In Myocardial Infarction 38).* JACC Cardiovasc Interv, 2014. **7**: 604–612.

21. Tcheng, J.E., *Clinical challenges of platelet glycoprotein IIb/IIIa receptor inhibitor therapy: bleeding, reversal, thrombocytopenia, and retreatment.* Am Heart J, 2000. **139**(2 Pt 2): S38–45.

22. Hovens, M.M., et al., *Prevalence of persistent platelet reactivity despite use of aspirin: a systematic review.* Am Heart J, 2007. **153**: 175–181.

23. Mijajlovic, M.D., et al., *Clinical consequences of aspirin and clopidogrel resistance: an overview.* Acta Neurol Scand, 2013. **128**: 213–219.

24. Makris, M., et al., *Guideline on the management of bleeding in patients on antithrombotic agents.* Br J Haematol, 2013. **160**: 35–46.

25. Baharoglu, M.I., et al., *Platelet transfusion versus standard care after acute stroke due to spontaneous cerebral haemorrhage associated with antiplatelet therapy (PATCH): a randomised, open-label, phase 3 trial.* Lancet, 2016. **387**: 2605–2013.

26. Desborough, M.J., et al., *Desmopressin for treatment of platelet dysfunction and reversal of antiplatelet agents: a systematic review and meta-analysis of randomized controlled trials.* J Thromb Haemost, 2017. **15**: 263–272.

Chapter 10

Immunosuppression and Immunotherapy

Immune modulation in the neurosciences intensive care unit mostly involves high-dose corticosteroids, plasma exchange, and intravenous immunoglobulin (IVIG). A common indication for use of corticosteroids is a recent diagnosis of a glioma or a metastasis, particularly if there is mass effect. Corticosteroids are also the treatment of choice in patients with acute metastatic epidural spinal cord compression.

In acute neuromuscular disorders, plasma exchange and IVIG are commonly used in Guillain-Barré syndrome, acute worsening in chronic inflammatory demyelinating polyneuropathy and myasthenia gravis but with a variable immediate response.

More recently, immune modulation has been considered essential in autoimmune encephalitis despite lack of controlled clinical trials. In these disorders, which are now better characterized, a combination of corticosteroids, IVIG, plasma exchange, rituximab, or cyclophosphamide is suggested (1).

Neurologic complications can also emerge from immunotherapy for cancer, which mostly relates to checkpoint inhibitor immunotherapy. There is a defining clinical picture of major—sometimes fatal—neurologic side effects.

Corticosteroids

The common indications for use of corticosteroids in general critical care are shown in Box 10.1. A recent study found that although hydrocortisone did not reduce the risk of septic shock, the incidence of delirium was significantly reduced (3).

Common indications for use in neurocritical illness are severe brain edema surrounding malignant (glioma) or benign (meningioma) brain

Box 10.1 Critical Care Indications for Corticosteroids

- Adrenal insufficiency
- Acute respiratory distress syndrome
- Chronic obstructive pulmonary disorder exacerbation
- Transplantation
- Thyroid storm
- Myxedema coma

Box 10.2 Neurocritical Care Indications for Corticosteroids

- Newly diagnosed glioma
- Central nervous system metastases
- Central nervous system vasculitis
- Autoimmune encephalitis
- Fulminant bacterial meningitis
- Pituitary apoplexy
- Rapidly progressing demyelinating conditions
- Myasthenia crisis

tumors, acute cerebral vasculitis, autoimmune encephalitis, acute bacterial meningitis, transverse myelitis, and acute neuromuscular disorders particularly myasthenia gravis (Box 10.2). Corticosteroids are frequently used in patients with neurologic complications of cancer. Neurosurgeons typically use corticosteroids after performing a craniotomy to reduce cerebral edema. A rare but urgent indication for the use of corticosteroids is pituitary apoplexy (hemorrhage into a pituitary adenoma). The recommendations for dexamethasone use in patients with primary brain tumors are shown in Table 10.1.

A frequently asked question is whether corticosteroids are beneficial in patients with severe traumatic brain injury. Since a landmark study in the 1980s (5), additional studies found no benefit or increased mortality (6). Corticosteroids are used in some practices to reduce cerebral edema surrounding a cerebral hematoma or hemorrhagic infarct and in particular edema that has become symptomatic. There are no data for short-term use and no recent data for long-term use. Corticosteroids are used commonly in patients with central nervous system inflammatory disorders. In bacterial meningitis, to be effective, corticosteroids must be administered prior to the first dose of antibiotics. Corticosteroids reduce mortality—but not

Table 10.1 Recommendations for Dosing and Tapering of Dexamethasone in Patients with Brain Tumors

Clinical Scenario	Recommended Dose of Dexamethasone	Recommended Taper
Worsening focal signs	4–8 mg/day (given as single dose or twice daily)	Goal is to taper to lowest dose at which the patient remains asymptomatic
Radiographic or clinical evidence of critical mass effect	Initial one-time dose of 10 mg IV, followed by 4 mg every 6 hours (orally or IV)	Should be postponed until surgery
Postoperatively	16 mg/day, given two to four times daily (orally or IV)	In asymptomatic postoperative patients, reduce dose over 5–7 days by 50% every 1–2 days

Based on data from reference 4.

disabling neurologic deficits—from tuberculosis meningitis or *Streptococcus pneumoniae* meningitis but not *Haemophilus influenzae* or *Neisseria meningitidis* (7). There was an additional benefit of corticosteroids reducing the incidence of hearing loss in children and adults in "high-income" countries (7). Corticosteroids have no proven effect (or proven adverse effect) in patients with viral encephalitis.

Corticosteroids are established as the initial treatment modality of choice for patients with acute metastatic epidural spinal cord compression. Corticosteroids decrease spinal cord edema and may have a tumoricidal effect with certain neoplasms (e.g., lymphoma). A single randomized controlled trial showed improved ambulation (by 20%) using 96 mg of intravenous dexamethasone followed by 96 mg/day orally for 3 days and then a 10-day taper along with radiotherapy (8). Comparative studies have suggested that lower doses (10 mg dexamethasone load, followed by 16 mg/day and a taper) may be equivalent and associated with fewer side effects (9).

As a rule, comparative corticosteroid equivalents are prednisone 5 mg = dexamethasone 0.75 mg = methylprednisolone 4 mg. Dexamethasone is generally preferred for CNS indications amongst neurointensivists, neurosurgeons and neurooncologists.

Dexamethasone IV

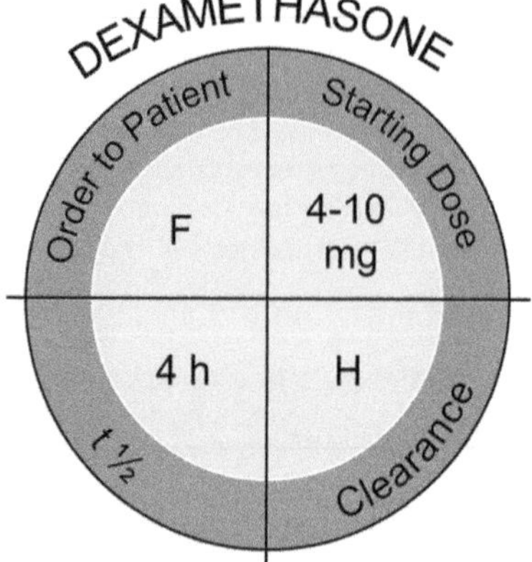

Pharmacologic Characteristics

- Dampens the inflammatory cascade (i.e., prostaglandins, leukotrienes) and proliferation of inflammatory cells
- Reduces vascular endothelial growth and tumor neovascularization
- Decreases cerebral edema
- Metabolized through the liver via CYP450 enzymes. Enzyme inducers of CYP3A4 (particularly barbiturates, carbamazepine, phenytoin) change availability
- Oral bioavailability varies from 60% to 100%

- Half-life: 1–5 hours (IV), 3–5 hours (orally)
- Time to peak: 5–10 minutes (IV), 1–2 hours (orally) (10–12)

Dosing and Administration

- 10 mg IV (over 5–10 minutes) followed by 4 mg IV or orally every 6 hours

Monitoring

- Blood glucose level (augmentation of hepatic gluconeogenesis, inhibition of glucose uptake into adipose tissues)
- Serum transaminases
- Skin breakdown

Side Effects

- Non-ketotic hyperosmolar state for predisposed patients
- Emotional lability to acute psychosis, insomnia
- Increased appetite (weight gain with chronic use)
- Skin rash, perineal irritation with rapid IV push
- Abdominal distention
- Gastrointestinal hemorrhage from ulceration
- Anaphylaxis with angioedema, fluid retention, and hypertension
- Increased infection risk
- Leukocytosis without infection (neutrophilia)
- Myopathy
- Osteopenia with long term use
- Impaired wound healing

Prednisone PO

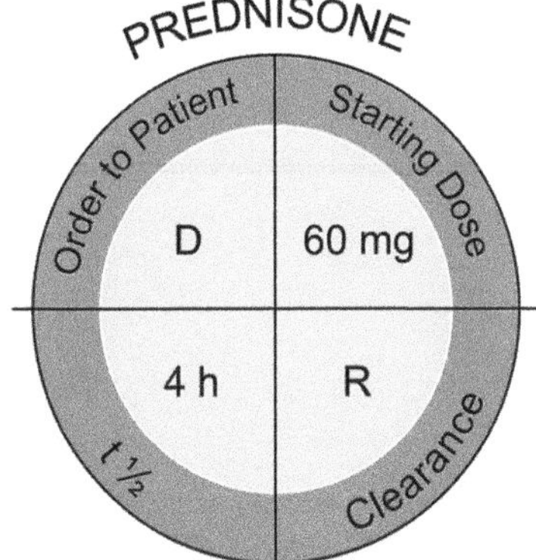

Pharmacologic Characteristics

- Most commonly used corticosteroid, but no significant mineralocorticoid action

- Time to peak: 2 hours
- Hepatically metabolized to active form, prednisolone

Dosing and Administration

- 60 mg once daily for inflammatory/immunologic response, up to 1 mg/kg per day in acute neurology diseases (e.g., myasthenia gravis or central nervous system vasculitis)
- When used for <7–10 days, tapering is not required
- Administer with food to avoid gastrointestinal upset

Monitoring

- Blood glucose level (augmentation of hepatic gluconeogenesis, inhibition of glucose uptake into adipose tissues)
- Serum transaminases

Side Effects

- Psychiatric manifestations (improved sense of well-being, euphoria, hypomania, insomnia), usually with prednisone doses >20 mg/day
- Increased appetite (weight gain with chronic use)
- Gastrointestinal intolerance
- Increased infection risk
- Leukocytosis without infection (neutrophilia)
- Hypokalemia
- Hypernatremia (from fluid retention)
- Impaired wound healing
- Cataracts and glaucoma (long-term use)
- Myopathy and osteoporosis (long-term use)
- Iatrogenic Cushing's disease (long-term use)

Methylprednisolone IV

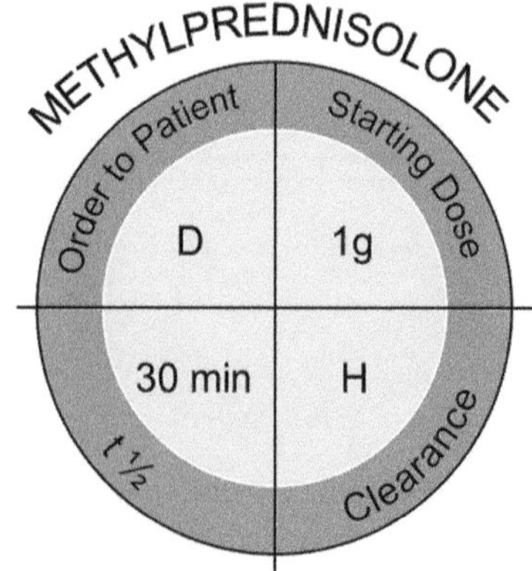

Pharmacologic Characteristics

- Used for acute neurologic exacerbations such as multiple sclerosis, autoimmune encephalitis, myasthenia gravis
- High doses of methylprednisolone have been used to treat acute spinal cord injury, but the data no longer recommend this strategy
- Onset: within 1 hour
- Duration (single dose): up to 2 weeks
- Half-life: 30 minutes (IV), 2.5 hours (orally)

Dosing and Administration

- 1,000 mg IV infusion once daily for 5 days
- Medrol® Dosepak™: 4 mg methylprednisolone tablets (5-day taper from 24 mg/day to 4 mg/day)

Monitoring

- Hyperglycemia
- Serum transaminase levels
- Hypoalbuminemia

Side Effects

- Blood glucose levels (augmentation of hepatic gluconeogenesis, inhibition of glucose uptake into adipose tissues)
- Emerging hypertension
- Psychiatric manifestations
- Hypokalemia
- Hypernatremia (from fluid retention)
- Acute nausea with oral formulations

Cyclophosphamide PO

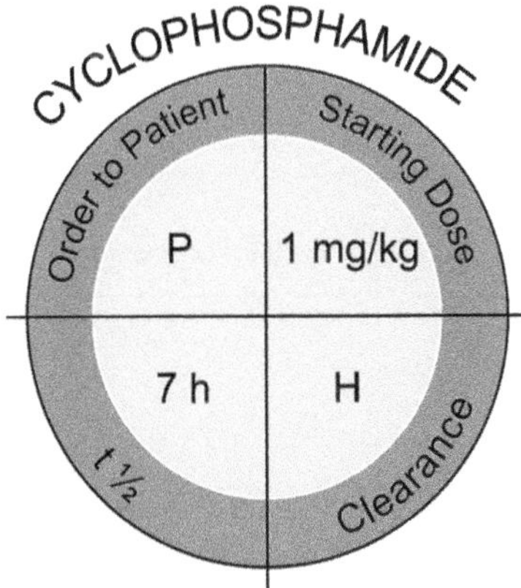

Pharmacologic Characteristics

- Alkylating agent; prevents cell division
- Requires consent due to high likelihood of sterility
- Indications: progressive multiple sclerosis, B-cell lymphoma, myasthenia gravis, cerebral vasculitis, NMDA-R–positive encephalitis
- Given alone or combined with other immunotherapies (e.g., cortico steroids, IVIG, plasma exchange)
- Metabolized in liver to active drug and via CYP2B6, CYP2C9, and CYP3A4 enzymes

Dosing and Administration

- 1–2 mg/kg per day orally in two divided doses
- Alternatively, 500–1,000 mg/m^2 per month IV (0.6–1 g/m^2)
- No dosage adjustments in patients with renal or hepatic dysfunction but greater risk of toxicity (reduced metabolism to active metabolite in hepatic dysfunction and hence decreased efficacy)
- Pre- and post-hydration with intravenous normal saline recommended with high dose IV therapy

Monitoring

- Hydration
- Renal function indices
- Complete blood count and transaminase levels
- Transaminase levels three times upper limit: use 75% of dose

Side Effects

- Vomiting (very common and premedication with antiemetics recommended)
- Bone marrow depression
  - Febrile neutropenia
  - Leukopenia
  - Thrombocytopenia
- Stomatitis
- Hemorrhagic cystitis (prevented with mesna, hydration or bladder irrigation)
- Bladder cell cancer
- Alopecia
- Azoospermia, abnormal oogenesis (counseling for infertility needed)

Rituximab IV

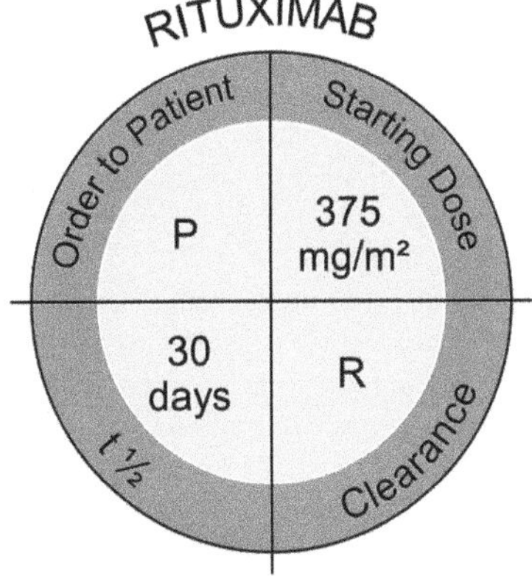

Pharmacologic Characteristics

- Monoclonal antibody directed against CD20 antigen of B-lymphocyte and leading to cell apoptosis
- Indications: Autoimmune encephalitis, refractory myasthenia gravis, neuromyelitis optica spectrum disorders

Dosing and Administration

- 1 g IV with repeat in 2 weeks
- Repeat every 6 months
- Alternatively, 375 mg/m^2 every 4 weeks, then every 1–3 months
- Titrate infusion every 30 minutes to a maximum of 400 mg/hr, starting at 50 mg/hr
- No adjustments needed in renal or hepatic dysfunction (not fully studied)
- Hepatitis B antigen prior to therapy due to fatal hepatitis B reactivations

Monitoring

- Monitor complete blood count with differential
- Monitor liver function test results
- Serious or fatal transfusion reactions may occur

Side Effects

- Lymphocytopenia, anemia, neutropenia
- Headache
- Skin rash and pruritus
- Nausea and diarrhea
- Increased transaminase levels
- Hypersensitivity with angioedema
- Higher infection risk (increased risk for tuberculosis and pneumocystis)

- Infusion reactions (hypotension, fever, chills, bronchospasm; premedicate with corticosteroids, acetaminophen, and diphenhydramine)
- Hepatitis B reactivation
- Progressive multifocal leukoencephalopathy (rare)

Plasma Exchange

Neurologic indications for plasma exchange are shown in Table 10.2. Therapeutic apheresis is generally accepted as a supportive therapy in Guillain-Barré syndrome and myasthenia crisis, but other indications for use in neurologic disorders have been categorized by the American Society of Apheresis (13):

Category I: apheresis is standard but not mandatory in all cases
Category II: apheresis generally accepted but supportive therapy
Category III: insufficient evidence of benefit

Plasma exchange is performed through a venous access and using a large apheresis catheter (Quinton-Mahurkar), generally at 1.25 volume exchange per procedure. The estimated plasma volume is

$$0.07 \times \text{weight}\,(\text{in kg}) \times (1 - \text{hematocrit}).$$

Plasma is replaced with 5% albumin, an albumin–saline combination, saline, or fresh-frozen plasma. Scheduled apheresis has been determined on the basis

Table 10.2 ASFA Category I and II Indications for Apheresis (13)

Indication for Apheresis	**ASFA Category**
Acute inflammatory demyelinating polyneuropathy (Guillain-Barré syndrome)	I
Chronic inflammatory demyelinating polyradiculoneuropathy	I
Lambert-Eaton myasthenic syndrome	II
Multiple sclerosis	
Acute central nervous system inflammatory demyelinating disease	II
Neuromyelitis optica	II
Myasthenia gravis	I
Paraproteinemic polyneuropathies	
Demyelinating polyneuropathy with IgG/IgA	I
Polyneuropathy with IgM	II
Rasmussen's encephalitis	II

of estimated changes in IgM and IgG levels. Within 2 days, the plasma IgG level returns to 40% to 50% of the pre-apheresis level. In most instances, a full course of five standard exchanges is recommended.

Complications and urgent interventions include the following:

- Citrate-induced hypocalcemia and metabolic alkalosis
  - Treatment: 10-ml ampule of 10% calcium chloride IV over 30 minutes
- Anaphylactic reaction
  - Epinephrine 0.2–0.5 mg given intramuscularly (IM)
  - Diphenhydramine 50 mg IV
  - Ranitidine 50 mg IV
- Transfusion-related acute lung injury (TRALI)
- Infectious risk of viral transmission
- Thromboembolism (central line placement)
- Pneumothorax (central line placement)
- Hypotension (may need vasopressors temporarily)
- Electrolyte abnormalities (fluid volume shifts)

Intravenous Immunoglobulin

Since both plasmapheresis and IVIG can be used to manage specific neurocritical illnesses, there is little in the literature to support one therapy over the other as the initial option.

Several IVIG preparations are available in the United States, and formulations differ based on IgA content, osmolality, and sodium and sugar content (Box 10.3). No sucrose is found in Gammaplex, Bivigam, Octagam, Gamunex C, Gammagard Liquid, Gammagard S/D, Gammaked, Flebogamma, Privigen, and Hizentra.

Box 10.3 IVIG Preparations Available in the United States*

Carimune NF™ (CSL Behring AG, Bern, Switzerland)

- pH 6.4–6.8
- Traces of IgA and IgM lyophilized powder in 6- and 12-g sizes
- Osmolality: in sterile water for injection, 192–768 mOsmol/kg; in 0.9% NaCl, 498–1,074 mOsmol/kg; in D5W, 444–1020 mOsmol/kg
- 1.67 g sucrose and <20 mg NaCl per gram protein

Flebogamma DIF™ (Grifols USA, Inc., Los Angeles, CA)

- pH 5–6
- Trace amounts of IgA (<100 mcg/ml)
- 5%, 10% liquid preparation containing IgG 100 mg/ml; 5-g, 10-g, 20-g vials
- Trace amounts of sodium (<3.2 mmol/L) and IgM

Box 10.3 (Continued)

- Contains 5 g D-sorbitol in 100 ml (10%) of product
- Osmolality: 240–370 mOsm/kg

Gammagard Liquid™ (Baxalta Inc., Westlake, CA)

- pH 4.6–5
- Average IgA content <3.2 mcg/ml in 10% solution
- 10% liquid in 1-g, 2.5-g, 5-g, 10-g, 20-g, and 30-g bottles
- Osmolality: 240–300 mOsmol/kg
  - No sugar, no sodium added

Gammagard S/D™ (Baxter/Hyland, Deerfield, IL)

- pH 6.8 ± 0.4 in 5% solution
- IgA content <2.2 mcg/ml in 5% solution
- Lyophilized powder in 5% and 10% concentrations; 5-g and 10-g bottles
- Sodium content in mEq/ml of 0.85%
- Contains IgM in trace amounts
- Additives in 5% solution include 0.3% albumin, 2.25% glycine, and 2% glucose

Gammar-P IV™ (Armour, Blue Bell, PA)

- pH 6.8 ± 0.4
- IgA content <25 mcg/ml
- Lyophilized powder in 5% concentration
- Sodium content in mEq/ml of 0.5%

Gamimune-N™ (Miles, Elkhart, IN; Bayer, Cologne, Germany)

- pH 4–4.5
- IgA content 270 mcg/ml
- Sterile solution in 5% and 10% concentrations
- Sodium content in mEq/ml considered trace amount (incompatible in saline)
- Not sugar-glycine based
- Advanced viral removal and inactivation technologies used in manufacturing; solvent detergent treated
- Contraindicated with history of prior systemic allergic reaction to IVIG products or a history of IgA deficiency
- Additives in 5% solution include 9–11% maltose; in 10% solution, 0.16–0.24 M glycine

Gammaked™ (Grifols Therapeutics Inc., Research Triangle Park, NC)

- pH 4.0–4.5
- IgA content ~46 mcg/ml

Box 10.3 (Continued)

- 10% liquid in 1-g (10 ml), 2.5-g, 5-g, 10-g, and 20-g bottles
- Trace amounts of sodium
- Osmolality: 258 mOsm/kg

Gamunex-C™ (Grifols Therapeutics Inc., Research Triangle Park, NC)

- pH 4–4.5
- Contains trace amounts of IgM and IgA (average 46 mcg/ml)
- 10% sterile solution supplied in 1-g (10 ml), 2.5-g, 5-g, 10-g, 20-g, 40-g bottles
- 9–11% protein in 0.16–0.24 M glycine
- Preservative-free
- No sugar
- Osmolality: 285–295 mOsmol/kg

Iveegam EN™ (Baxter Healthcare Corporation, Westlake Village, CA)

- pH 7.0
- IgA content <10 μg/ml; trace amounts of IgM
- Lyophilized power in 5% concentration
- Sodium content in mEq/ml of 0.3%
- Prepared using modified Cohn-fractionation process combined with hydrolase treatment and polyethylene glycol precipitation
- Additives in 5% solution include 5% glucose and 0.3% NaCl

Octagam S/D™ (Octaphama USA Inc., Hoboken, NJ)

- pH 4.5–5.0
- Contains trace amounts of IgA (106 mcg/ml) and even lower amounts of IgM
- 10% liquid solution (100 mg protein/10 ml solution); 2-g, 5-g, 10-g, and 20-g vials
- IV filter size: 0.2–200 microns
- Osmolality: 310–380 mOsmol/kg
- Contains maltose 90 mg/ml
- Contains no preservatives or sucrose
- No more than 30 mmol/L sodium

Polygam S/D™ (Baxter/Hyland for American Red Cross, Washington, DC)

- pH 6.8
- IgA content <1.2 mcg/ml
- Lyophilized powder in 5% and 10% concentrations

Box 10.3 (Continued)

- Sodium content in mEq/ml of 0.85%
- Manufactured by the Cohn-Oncley cold ethanol fractionation process followed by ultrafiltration and ion exchange chromatography; solvent detergent treated; sterile, freeze-dried preparation of highly purified IgG derived from large pools of human plasma
- Additives in 5% concentration include 0.3% albumin, 2.25% glycine, and 2% glucose

Privigen™ (CSL Behring AG, Bern, Switzerland)

- pH 4.8 (range 4.6–5.0)
- IgA content <25 mcg/ml
- 10% IgG solution in 5-g, 10-g, 20-g, and 40-g vials
- Osmolality: 320 mOsmol/kg (range 240–440)
- 250 mmol/L L-proline (non-essential amino acid)
- No sucrose or maltose
- No preservatives
- Trace amounts of sodium

Sandoglobulin™ (Sandoz, Vienna, Austria)

- pH 6.6
- IgA content 720 mcg/ml
- Lyophilized powder in 6 g or 12 g protein; reconstituted to 3% or 6% solution
- Sterile, highly purified polyvalent antibody product that contains, in concentrated form, all IgG antibodies regularly occurring in donor population
- Produced by cold alcohol fractionation from plasma of volunteer U.S. donors; fractionation includes several filtration steps performed in presence of filter aids; filtration used for separation of cold ethanol precipitate
- Additives per gram of IgG include 1.67 g sucrose and <20 mg NaCl
- Trace amounts of IgM

Venoglobulin-I™ or Venoglobulin-S™ (Alpha Therapeutic, Los Angeles, CA)

- pH 5.2–5.8
- IgA content 15–50 mcg/ml
- Sterile solution in 5% and 10% concentrations
- Sodium content <1 mEq/ml
- Prepared using cold alcohol fraction, polyethylene glycol bentonite fraction, and ion exchange chromatography; solvent detergent treated
- Additives in 5% solution include 5% sorbitol and 0.13% albumin; in 10% solution, 5% sorbitol and 0.26% albumin

*Manufacturer-provided information

With IVIG, premedication with diphenhydramine, 25 mg orally, should be considered in patients at risk for anaphylactic transfusion reactions, and certainly in patients who experienced a reaction with previous exposure. Avoid shaking or freezing the prepared product and mixing products from different manufacturers.

Immunoglobulin IV

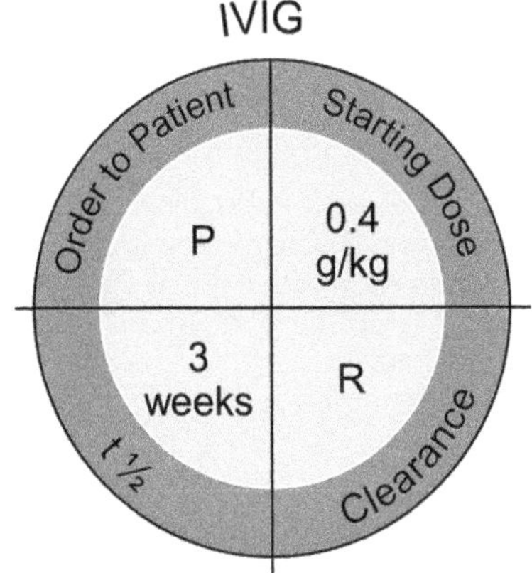

Pharmacologic Characteristics

- Suppression of neutralization of cytokines by specific antibodies in IVIG
- Neutralizing IgG antibodies against bacterial, viral, parasitic agents
- Blockade of leukocyte-adhesion molecules
- Passive immunity by increased antibody titer and antigen–antibody reaction potential
- Anti-idiotypic antibodies directed against idiotypes on circulating auto-antibodies
- Clearance of immunocomplex deposits
- Alterations in regulatory T-cells
- Peak immune response of IVIG occurs in 3–4 weeks
- Expensive

Dosing and Administration

- In myasthenia gravis and Guillain-Barré syndrome, 2 g/kg per course, dosed over 2–5 days (i.e., 1 g/kg daily × 2 days, but much preferred 0.4 g/kg daily × 5 days)
- Dosage of IVIG is typically adjusted to ideal body weight in obese patients but is based on actual weight in underweight patients
- Each product has its own titration recommendations. The purpose of titrating the infusion rate is to minimize potential anaphylactic

reactions (given human blood product). Titration must be repeated with each subsequent dose, as every dose is different
- Requires a dedicated IV line for administration

Monitoring
- Urticaria
- Nausea and vomiting
- Muscle spasm
- Chills, cold sweats, shaking (transfusion-related reactions)
- New headaches

Side Effects
- Adverse reactions in 20% to 50% of patients treated with IVIG
- Stevens-Johnson syndrome
- Aseptic meningitis
- Anaphylaxis in IgA-deficient patients (this is rare and mostly treated with epinephrine and high-dose corticosteroids)
- Transfusion volume overload and related lung injury (TACO and TRALI)
- Thromboembolic events (both arterial and venous), preventable with adequate hydration
- Renal complications in patients with preexisting renal failure and prior diabetes
    - Spontaneous resolution of renal complications within 10 days after discontinuation of IVIG
    - Dialysis may be needed in some instances
    - More likely in products containing sucrose
- Pseudo-hyponatremia
- Hemolysis and neutropenia
- Infection risk (pooled human donors, blood product)

Checkpoint Inhibitor Immunotherapy

Immunotherapy has great promise in treating patients with melanoma, renal cell carcinoma, non-small cell lung cancer, head and neck cancer, urethral carcinoma, and Hodgkin's lymphoma. The drugs are divided into those involving programmed cell death and PD1-linked receptors (e.g., pembrolizumab, nivolumab) or cytotoxic T-lymphocyte–associated antigen for antibody (e.g., ipilimumab). These drugs have been associated with a unique set of neurologic sequelae (e.g., Guillain-Barré syndrome, myasthenia gravis, posterior reversible encephalopathy syndrome, aseptic meningitis, transverse myelitis, enteral neuropathy autoimmune encephalitis) (14,15,16). These neurologic adverse effects occur in about 1% to 3% of patients being treated with checkpoint immunotherapy. Treatment consists of discontinuing causative immunotherapy and high-dose corticosteroids or IVIG, but treatment paradigms are not well defined.

Other Therapeutic Targets in Autoimmune Neurology

Several of these drugs are used in patients with myasthenia gravis and in patients with myasthenia who were temporarily worsening and monitored in the neurosciences unit or in 'crisis' on a ventilator. Pyridostigmine is the key drug in myasthenia gravis, but its use is often briefly stopped in endotracheally intubated patients and restarted during ventilator weaning.

Pyridostigmine PO

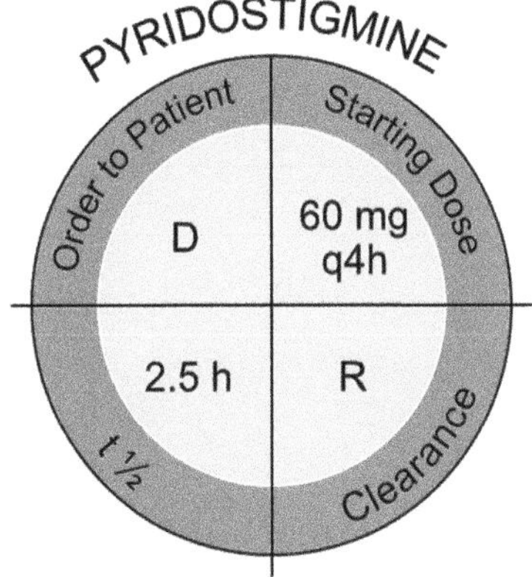

Pharmacologic Characteristics

- Acetylcholinesterase inhibitor; prevents breakdown of acetylcholine in the neuromuscular junction
- Onset: 30 minutes (oral), 2–5 minutes (IV)
- Duration: 3–4 hours (oral)

Dosing and Administration

- Dosing very individualized
- Not for use in mechanically ventilated patients
- Use half the dose in patients on bilevel positive airway pressure (BiPAP)
- 60–600 mg/day, divided five or six times/day
- Sustained-release tablets
  - Administer one or two times/day
  - Provide overnight dosing
  - Use in conjunction with immediate-release formulation
  - Do not crush

- Injection route
  - Dosed at 1/30th total daily dose of oral option
  - IM only route
  - Risk of cardiac arrest with IV route
  - Continuous infusion: 1–2 mg/hr; maximum 4 mg/hr (rarely used and concerning option)
- No adjustments in patients with renal or liver dysfunction

Monitoring

- Blood pressure and heart rate
- Cholinergic effects

Side Effects

- SLUDGE: salivation, lacrimation, urination, defecation, gastrointestinal cramping, emesis
- Bradycardia with excessive dosing

Azathioprine PO

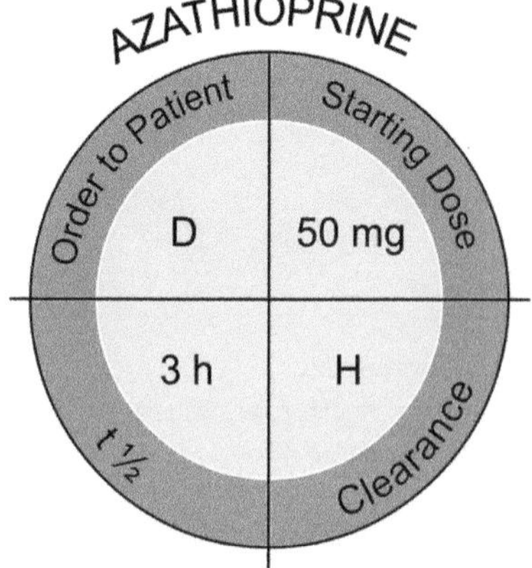

Pharmacologic Characteristics

- Antimetabolite prodrug (metabolized to 6-mercaptopurine)
- Suppresses T-cells more than B-cells
- Potent anti-inflammatory action
- Off-label use for myasthenia gravis and multiple sclerosis

Dosing and Administration

- 50 mg/day once orally, titrated to 2.5 mg/kg per day
- Obtain thiopyridine methyltransferase (TPMT) genotyping and phenotyping prior to starting therapy (assess potential toxicity from ability to metabolize); patients who are deficient in enzyme are at higher risk for toxicity

* No dosage reductions for patients with renal or hepatic dysfunction, with the exception of oliguric renal transplant recipients (then reduce the dose)

Monitoring

* Complete blood count with differential
* Transaminase levels: toxicity usually occurs within the first 6 months of therapy
* Greater risk of myelosuppression when administered with xanthine oxidase inhibitors (e.g., allopurinol)
* Renal function

Side Effects

* Infection risk
* Malignancy from chronic immunosuppression
* Gastrointestinal intolerance (administer with meal to minimize)
* Progressive multifocal leukoencephalopathy has been reported

Mycophenolate Mofetil PO

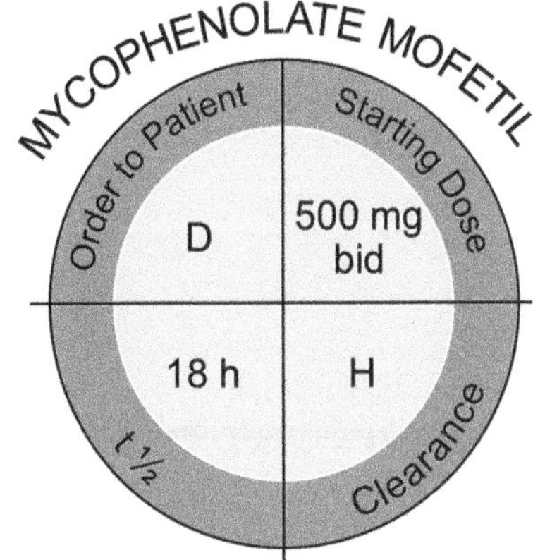

Pharmacologic Characteristics

* T- and B-lymphocyte inhibitor
* Off-label use for myasthenia gravis
* Not dialyzable

Dosing and Administration

* 500 mg orally twice daily on empty stomach (food decreases rate but not extent of absorption), up to 1,500 mg orally twice daily
* Ensure safe handling of medication prior to administration (teratogenic risk for healthcare providers)
* Use with azathioprine not recommended

- No dosage adjustments needed in patients with renal or hepatic dysfunction
- Hepatically cleared, active metabolites

Monitoring

- Risk Evaluation Mitigation Strategy (REMS) program with risk of fetal loss during first trimester; obtain pregnancy test prior to initiating therapy; provide appropriate counseling for pregnancy prevention
- Complete blood count with differential
- Transaminase levels
- Electrolyte levels (hyper/hypokalemia, hypocalcemia, hypomagnesemia reported in post-transplant patients)
- Renal function: higher levels of active metabolite noted in patients with diminished renal function

Side Effects

- Leukopenia, infection
- Progressive multifocal leukoencephalopathy
- Hyperglycemia
- Elevated lactate dehydrogenase levels
- Hypertension
- Peripheral edema
- Gastrointestinal intolerance (diarrhea, ulceration, hemorrhage, perforation)

Key Pointers

1. Corticosteroids have no use in patients with cerebral hematoma or traumatic brain or spinal cord injury.
2. Corticosteroids reduce mortality from *Streptococcus pneumoniae* meningitis.
3. Corticosteroids are the treatment of choice in patients with epidural spinal cord compression.
4. Plasma exchange and IVIG have equally efficacy in Guillain-Barré syndrome and myasthenia gravis.
5. Checkpoint immunotherapy is associated with neurologic syndromes.

References

1. Graus, F., et al., *A clinical approach to diagnosis of autoimmune encephalitis.* Lancet Neurol, 2016. **15**: 391–404.
2. Abdel-Moez, W., et al., *Corticosteroids in the ICU.* Int Anesthesiol Clin, 2009. **47**: 67–82.

3. Keh, D., et al., *Effect of hydrocortisone on development of shock among patients with severe sepsis: the HYPRESS randomized clinical trial.* JAMA, 2016. **316**: 1775–1785.
4. Ly, K.I. and Wen, P.Y. *Clinical relevance of steroid use in neuro-oncology.* Curr Neurol Neurosci Rep, 2017. **17**: 5.
5. Braakman, R., et al., *Megadose steroids in severe head injury. Results of a prospective double-blind clinical trial.* J Neurosurg, 1983. **58**: 326–330.
6. Hoshide, R., et al., *Do corticosteroids play a role in the management of traumatic brain injury?* Surg Neurol Int, 2016. **7**: 84.
7. Brouwer, M.C., et al., *Corticosteroids for acute bacterial meningitis.* Cochrane Database Syst Rev, 2015: CD004405.
8. Sorensen, S., et al., *Effect of high-dose dexamethasone in carcinomatous metastatic spinal cord compression treated with radiotherapy: a randomised trial.* Eur J Cancer, 1994. **30A**: 22–27.
9. Cole, J.S. and Patchell, R.A. *Metastatic epidural spinal cord compression.* Lancet Neurol, 2008. **7**: 459–466.
10. Carmeliet, P. and Jain, R.K. *Molecular mechanisms and clinical applications of angiogenesis.* Nature, 2011. **473**: 298–307.
11. Forster, C., et al., *Glucocorticoid effects on mouse microvascular endothelial barrier permeability are brain specific.* J Physiol, 2006. **573**(Pt 2): 413–425.
12. Roth, P., Happold, C. and Weller, M. *Corticosteroid use in neuro-oncology: an update.* Neurooncol Pract, 2015. **2**: 6–12.
13. Shelat, S.G., *Practical considerations for planning a therapeutic apheresis procedure.* Am J Med, 2010. **123**: 777–784.
14. Haddox, C.L., et al., *Pembrolizumab induced bulbar myopathy and respiratory failure with necrotizing myositis of the diaphragm.* Ann Oncol, 2017. **28**: 673–675.
15. Jaeger, B., et al., *Respiratory failure as presenting symptom of necrotizing autoimmune myopathy with anti-melanoma differentiation-associated gene 5 antibodies.* Neuromuscul Disord, 2015. **25**: 457–460.
16. Gu Y, Menzies AM, Long GV, et al. *Immune mediated neuropathy following checkpoint immunotherapy.* J Clin Neurosci, 2017. **45**: 14–17.

Chapter 11

Antimicrobial Therapy for Central Nervous System Infections

Broad-spectrum antibiotics—those that are bactericidal and able to penetrate the blood–brain barrier—must be administered in any patient with a suspected central nervous system (CNS) infection, before the results of diagnostic tests to pinpoint the cause are known. Even when the inflammation starts to subside, high-dose antimicrobials need to be continued to ensure adequate eradication. In acute bacterial meningitis, early management (i.e., within 1 hour after admission) with antibiotics and corticosteroids is key (1).

Treatment for viral encephalitis is often for herpes simplex virus (HSV) infection, and intravenous (IV) acyclovir should be continued while awaiting definitive polymerase chain reaction (PCR) results on cerebrospinal fluid (2). There are many other infectious encephalitides, such as viral or mosquito- or tick-borne. Supportive management is often the only option in these cases.

Treatment for fungal CNS infections is well defined but is indicated only in extreme situations and in complex immunocompromised patients. Treatment is needed for months and causes significant toxicity and adverse effects. The costs are enormous; therefore, these drugs should generally not be preemptively used.

Proven CNS infections are infrequently seen in the neurosciences intensive care unit (ICU), and antibiotic use for suspected CNS infection is far more common. Antibiotics with good CNS penetration are listed in Table 11.1. Treatment often requires one or a few antimicrobials but we have added alternatives for reference.

Bacterial Meningitis

The clinical diagnosis of bacterial meningitis remains difficult, with many cases missed early. Pneumococcal meningitis remains overwhelmingly the most common type and follows some prior infection (e.g., otitis or pneumonia). Pneumococcal meningitis is also more common in patients with malnutrition, alcoholism, asplenia, diabetes, chronic renal disease, or multiple myeloma, and in patients younger than 2 years or older than 65 years. The CSF profile of bacterial meningitis remains the best indicator of infection and shows marked pleocytosis with reduced glucose and increased

Table 11.1 Antibiotics with Good CNS Penetration and Doses for CNS Infections

Amikacin 5 mg/kg q8h IV	**Ampicillin** 2 g q4h IV*	**Aztreonam** 2 g q6–8h IV
Cefepime 2 g q8h IV	**Cefotaxime** 2 g q4–6h IV*	**Ceftazidime** 2 g q8h IV
Ceftriaxone 2 g q12h IV*	**Chloramphenicol** 1–1.5 g q6h IV	**Ciprofloxacin** 400 mg q8–12h IV
Daptomycin 6–10 mg/kg q24h IV	**Gentamicin** 1.7 mg/kg q8h IV	**Linezolid** 600 mg q12h IV
Meropenem 2 g q8h IV	**Moxifloxacin** 400 mg q24h IV	**Nafcillin** 2 g q4h IV
Oxacillin 2 g q4h IV	**Penicillin G** 4 million units q4h IV	**Rifampin** 600 mg q24h IV
Sulfamethoxazole/ trimethoprim 5–10 mg/kg/day (TMP component), q6h IV	**Tobramycin** 1.7 mg/kg q8h IV	**Vancomycin** 15–20 mg/kg q8–12h IV*

* Recommended as initial treatment choices

protein. Table 11.2 (1,3) shows the CSF findings in bacterial meningitis compared with those in viral, fungal, and tuberculous meningitis.

Empiric Antibiotic Use

Any patient suspected of having bacterial meningitis should receive vancomycin plus a third-generation cephalosporin. Corticosteroids are mandatory. Ampicillin is added in elderly patients, immunocompromised patients, or patients receiving immunomodulating therapy. Any patient with suspected bacterial meningitis should have two sets of blood cultures drawn prior to antibiotic and corticosteroid administration, followed by a computed tomography (CT) scan and, eventually, a CSF examination. A CT scan showing early brain edema warrants the administration of osmotic agents, such as mannitol or hypertonic saline (Chapter 5). Blood cultures must be obtained prior to antibiotic administration, as the likelihood of a positive blood culture declines after antibiotics, especially for meningococcus species. CSF Gram staining can detect bacteria with a yield of up to 90% in pneumococcal and meningococcal meningitis (4). Sensitivities will determine the antibiotic choice and dosage adjustment (Table 11.3).

Table 11.2 CSF Findings in Meningitis

	White Blood Cells	% Polynucleated Cells	Glucose (mg/dl)	Protein (mg/dl)
Bacterial	>1,000–5000	90–100	<40	>150
Viral	100–1,000	<50	40–60	50–100
Fungal	100–200	<50	30–40	100–500
TBC	100–200	<50	30–40	100–500

Table 11.3 Initial Therapy in Acute Bacterial Meningitis

Ceftriaxone	2 g IV	q12h	Dependent on culture
Vancomycin	20 mg/kg IV	q8–12h	Dependent on culture
Ampicillin	2 g IV	q4h	Dependent on culture
Dexamethasone	10 mg IV	q6h	Dependent on antibiotic timing
Mannitol	1 g/kg IV	q6h	Dependent on CT scan

PCRs have been increasingly used for the diagnosis of bacterial meningitis, with a reported sensitivity of 79% to 100% for *Streptococcus pneumoniae* meningitis and 91% to 100% for *Neisseria meningitidis*. Gram-negative organisms are uncommon in patients with community-acquired meningitis. Penetrating trauma can be associated with *Staphylococcus aureus, Staphylococcus epidermis*, or aerobic Gram-negative bacilli and is treated with vancomycin plus an anti-pseudomonal beta-lactam.

Antibiotics by Organisms

- *Streptococcus pneumoniae* (Gram-positive coccus)
  - Treatment (empiric): vancomycin + ceftriaxone or cefotaxime
  - Penicillin G if isolate susceptible
  - Alternative agents: chloramphenicol (beta-lactam allergy), fluoroquinolone (i.e., moxifloxacin or ciprofloxacin)
  - Duration: 10–14 days
- *Neisseria meningitides* (Gram-negative coccus)
  - Treatment (empiric): ceftriaxone or cefotaxime
  - Penicillin G if isolate susceptible
  - Alternative agents: chloramphenicol, fluoroquinolone (i.e., moxifloxacin or ciprofloxacin), aztreonam
  - Eradication of nasal organisms with rifampin or ciprofloxacin
  - Duration: 7 days
- *Listeria monocytogenes* (Gram-positive bacillus)
  - Treatment (empiric): ampicillin or penicillin G with or without aminoglycoside (added for synergy)
  - Alternative agent: sulfamethoxazole/trimethoprim
  - Duration: 21 days
  - Gentamicin can be discontinued if patient is clinically improved after 1 week
- *Haemophilus influenzae type B* (Gram-negative coccobacillus)
  - Treatment (empiric): cefotaxime or ceftriaxone
  - Alternative agents: chloramphenicol, cefepime, meropenem, fluoroquinolone (i.e., ciprofloxacin or moxifloxacin)
  - Duration: at least 7 days
- *Staphylococcus aureus* (Gram-positive coccus)
  - Treatment (empiric): vancomycin
  - Nafcillin or oxacillin if isolate susceptible (methicillin-sensitive *S. aureus* [MSSA])
  - Alternatives to vancomycin: linezolid, daptomycin (with rifampin), sulfamethoxazole/trimethoprim
  - Duration: 14 days

- Miscellaneous Gram-negative organisms (e.g., *Klebsiella pneumoniae, Enterobacteriaceae, Escherichia coli, Pseudomonas aeruginosa*)
  - Treatment (empiric): ceftriaxone or cefotaxime
  - Treat with meropenem, ceftazidime, or cefepime if *Pseudomonas* is suspected or if identified
  - More difficult to cure than Gram-positive organisms; a repeat CSF sample is recommended 2–3 days into therapy
  - Duration: 21 days

Adjunctive Therapy with Dexamethasone

- In adults with *Streptococcus pneumoniae* meningitis
- Increases favorable outcomes
- Does not reverse damage from cerebral edema or direct neuronal injury
- 10 mg IV every 6 hours for 4 days
- Administer 10–20 minutes prior to antibiotics
- Do not administer if antibiotics have already been initiated, as it is unlikely to improve outcomes
- Continue only if Gram stain shows diplococci, or if blood cultures are positive for *Streptococcus pneumoniae*

Viral, Fungal, and Parasitic Infections

A viral infection is the most common cause of acute encephalitis in adults. Epidemic outbreaks are produced by the seasonal spread of arboviruses (i.e., viruses transmitted by arthropod vectors, such as mosquitoes). These encephalitides are constrained to specific geographic locations. The West Nile virus has been identified as a cause of summer outbreaks of encephalitis in many countries.

HSV-1 is a cause of sporadic viral encephalitis in immunocompetent patients. It is suspected when febrile patients develop confusion associated with (focal) seizures or focal deficits. The diagnosis is established by confirming the presence of the virus in the CSF. PCR can detect HSV-1 DNA in the CSF with great sensitivity and specificity. If PCR results are negative but the clinical/radiologic presentation is suspicious for HSV-1 infection, the test should be repeated on a new CSF sample after 3 to 5 days.

Varicella zoster virus (VZV) occurs in approximately 2 out of 100,000 cases, usually presenting as ataxia merging into a more diffuse form. Cytomegalovirus (CMV) encephalitis is more common in developing countries and in immunodeficient patients, but the prevalence has declined due to treatment with antiretroviral therapy. All of these herpes viruses can be detected by PCR. An important additional virus to consider is human herpes virus 6 (HHV-6), which may have a clinical presentation almost identical to that of autoimmune encephalitis but is predominantly seen in transplant recipients. HHV-6 is the most common cause of post-transplant acute limbic encephalitis, mostly among recipients of allogeneic stem cell transplantation.

Arboviruses are seasonal because they are transmitted by arthropods, mosquitoes, ticks, and flies. Best known as West Nile virus, tick-borne encephalitis and Japanese encephalitis manifest during summer outbreaks. There are a number of other viral encephalitides associated with exposure to

Table 11.4 Antivirals in Acute Viral Encephalitis		
HSV encephalitis	Acyclovir	10 mg/kg q8h for 3 weeks
CMV encephalitis	Ganciclovir	5 mg/kg q12h for 4 weeks
VZV encephalitis	Acyclovir	10 mg/kg q8h for 3 weeks

animals, predominantly rodents. Hanta virus encephalitis is usually preceded by a respiratory-renal syndrome and thrombocythemia. Treatment options are very limited (Table 11.4).

Fungal and parasitic infections are threats in any patient with prolonged immunosuppression or hematologic-oncologic disorders. Transplant recipients have an unusual spectrum of opportunistic infections (Table 11.5) (5–7).

In the 2- to 6-month period after transplantation, patients are at highest risk for known immunocompromise-related CNS infections. These infections are typically *Aspergillus* species, *Nocardia*, or *Toxoplasma gondii* and, in occasional patients, are due to CMV, HSV, HHV-6, and VZV. Later infections, defined as those appearing after 6 months, are meningitis associated with *Cryptococcus neoformans, Histoplasma capsulatum*, or *Coccidioides immitis*; each of these infections is region-specific.

Cryptococcal meningitis should be considered early in patients with prior organ transplants and in those with human immunodeficiency virus (HIV) infection or acquired immune deficiency syndrome (AIDS). CSF examination should confirm the results of the serum latex agglutination test and positive cryptococcal antigens.

CNS infections with viruses, fungi, or parasites in immunocompetent individuals are rare. They are referred to as aseptic meningitis because of the lack of bacterial involvement. The course is usually self-limited and does not require any specific treatment. There are many causes of aseptic meningitis, including viral, fungal, parasitic, or drug-induced. Enteroviruses are the most common cause of viral meningitis; cryptococcus and coccidioides are the most common causes of fungal meningitis.

Treatment with antifungals is medically complicated and should not be started until the diagnosis is confirmed. The major infections in transplant recipients are summarized in Table 11.6.

Table 11.5 Clinical Presentation, Diagnosis, and Treatment of Opportunistic Infections

Infection	Special CSF Tests (Sensitivity/Specificity)	Treatment
Cryptococcal meningitis	Elevated opening pressure; cryptococcal antigen	Amphotericin B and flucytosine
Toxoplasma encephalitis	*T. gondii* PCR (50–80%/100%)	Pyrimethamine, folinic acid, and sulfadiazine *or* trimethoprim/sulfamethoxazole
Tuberculous meningitis	Culture and acid-fast bacilli stain (>80%)	Rifampin, isoniazid, pyrazinamide, ethambutol
Acute syphilitic meningitis	CSF VDRL (CSF FTA-ABS more sensitive but less specific)	Penicillin G, 3–4 million units q4h for 10–14 days

Table 11.6 CNS Infections in Transplant Recipients

Organism	Time from Transplant (months)	Presentation	CT or MRI	CSF
Listeria monocytogenes	1–6	Headache, stupor (prior abdominal cramps and diarrhea)	Meningeal enhancement only; commonly brainstem involvement	May be normal
Nocardia asteroïdes	1–6	Localizing findings: headache, stupor	Abscesses (may be solitary)	Pleocytosis
Aspergillus	1–6	Rapidly developing coma, seizures (prior lung infection)	Ring lesion, scattered hemorrhages	Pleocytosis
Cryptococcus neoformans	>6	Unexplained headache, fever, cognitive changes, rarely focal signs	Thalamus, basal ganglia; widespread miliary; no edema	Pleocytosis; may be normal
Toxoplasma gondii	>6	Seizures, stupor, rarely focal signs	Multiple lesions, subcortical meninges spared	Pleocytosis; may be normal

MRI: magnetic resonance imaging; CT: computed tomography; CSF; Cerebrospinal fluid.

The Pharmacology of Antibiotics

Ampicillin IV

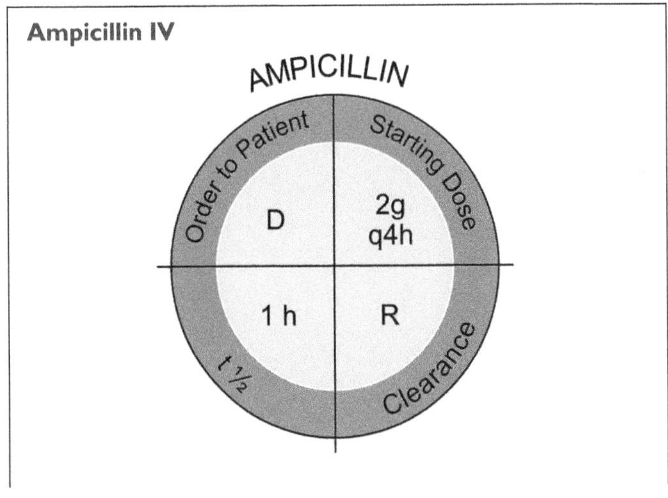

Pharmacologic Characteristics

- Semisynthetic penicillin
- Interrupts cell wall synthesis and cell wall integrity
- Bactericidal or bacteriostatic action depending on drug concentrations
- CSF penetration only occurs with inflamed meninges
- Drug of choice for *Listeria*, group B streptococcus, and enterococcus meningitis

Dosing and Administration

- 2 g IV every 4 hours; lengthen dosing interval depending on degree of renal dysfunction
- With vancomycin and third-generation cephalosporin for empiric coverage in patients 50-plus years of age
- Infuse over 15 minutes (rapid bolus increases likelihood of seizure)
- No dosage adjustments in patients with hepatic dysfunction

Monitoring

- Renal function
- Periodic complete blood counts
- Cultures

Side Effects

- Dermatologic: dermatitis, rash, urticaria
- Seizure (with rapid bolus administration and high serum levels)
- Increased liver function test results
- Interstitial nephritis (rare)
- Hematologic: agranulocytosis, eosinophilia, leukopenia, thrombocytopenia (rare)

Cefepime IV

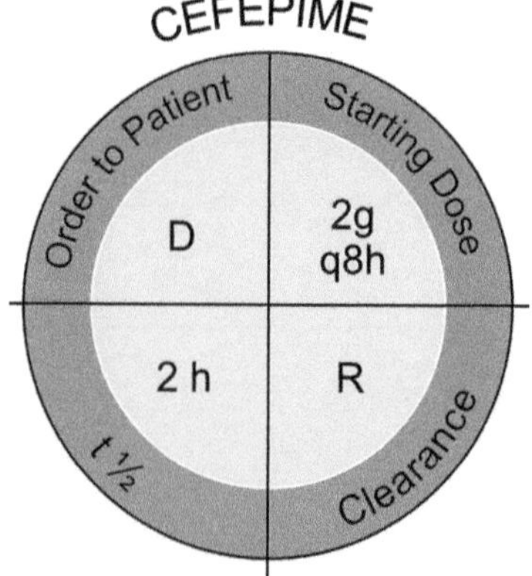

Pharmacologic Characteristics

- Fourth-generation cephalosporin
- Inhibits cell wall synthesis
- Metabolism: minimal

Dosing and Administration

- 2 g IV every 8 hours; decrease dose or lengthen interval in patients with renal dysfunction
- Give IV push over 5 minutes or infusion over 30 minutes
- Doses >4 g/day effective in *Pseudomonas* infections
- No dosage adjustments in patients with hepatic disease

Monitoring

- Cultures and sensitivities
- Renal function indices
- Allergic reactions

Side Effects

- Positive direct Coombs test without hemolysis
- Rash
- Neurotoxicity (reversible encephalopathy with myoclonus)
- Hypophosphatemia (rare)
- Mild thrombocytopenia and coagulopathy (rare)

Cefotaxime IV

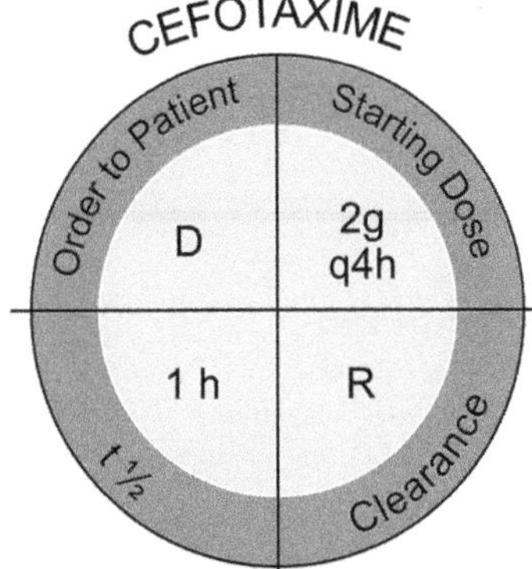

Pharmacologic Characteristics

- Third-generation cephalosporin
- Inhibits bacterial cell wall synthesis, has some activity in the presence of beta-lactamases
- Provides adequate CSF levels in meningitis

Dosing and Administration

- 2 g every IV 4–6 hours
- Decrease the dose in patients with renal dysfunction (lower dose or lengthen interval)
- Infusion over 15 minutes
- No dosage adjustments in patients with hepatic disease, though drug half-life may be slightly prolonged in those with hepatic impairment

Monitoring

- Complete blood count
- Renal function

Side Effects

- Hypersensitivity reaction
- Mild thrombocytopenia and coagulopathy (rare)
- Rash (rare)

Ceftriaxone IV

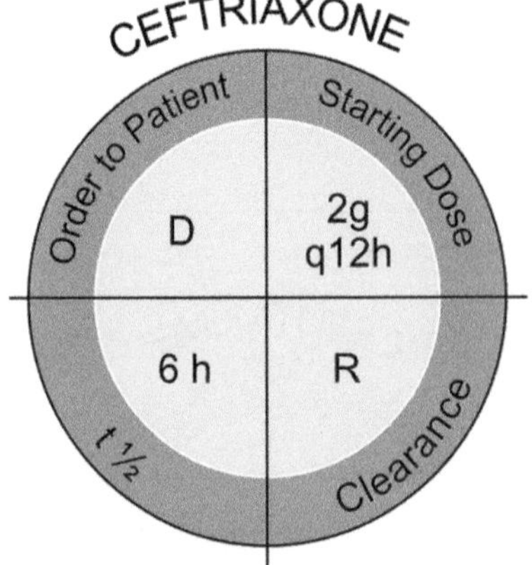

Pharmacologic Characteristics

- Third-generation cephalosporin
- Inhibits bacterial cell wall biosynthesis
- Distributed into the CNS, better penetration when meninges are inflamed

Dosing and Administration

- 2 g IV every 12 hours
- Maximal dosing in patients with hepatic and renal dysfunction: 2 g/day
- Infusion over 30 minutes, IV push over 1–4 minutes

Monitoring

- Liver function
- Signs of allergic reaction

Side Effects

- Eosinophilia, thrombocytopenia, leukopenia
- Gallbladder pseudolithiasis
- Diarrhea
- Increased liver function test results
- Pancreatitis secondary to biliary sludge
- Up to 3% incidence of allergic reaction (mild) with rare anaphylaxis
- Phlebitis

Daptomycin IV

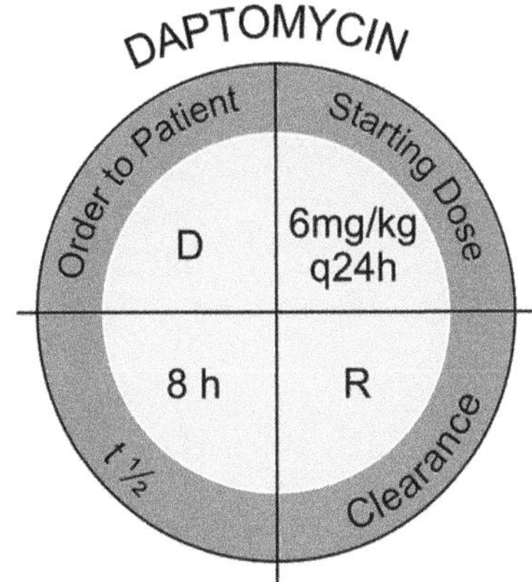

Pharmacologic Characteristics

- For patients who are allergic to penicillin and cannot receive vancomycin (due to resistance or allergy)
- Cyclic lipopeptide antibiotic, depolarizes cell membrane potential leading to RNA, DNA, and protein synthesis disruption
- Bactericidal properties, with concentration-dependent killing

Dosing and Administration

- 6–10 mg/kg IV once daily
- IV infusion over 30 minutes, or IV push over 2 minutes in adults
- Reduce interval to every-other-day administration if creatinine clearance (CrCl) is <30 ml/min
- No dosage reductions in patients with mild to moderate hepatic dysfunction; not studied in severe hepatic disease
- Incompatible with dextrose solutions

Monitoring

- Creatinine kinase levels weekly, or more often if receiving an HMG-CoA reductase inhibitor (e.g., atorvastatin, simvastatin)
- Renal function
- Blood pressure

Side Effects

- Elevated creatinine kinase levels leading to potentially severe rhabdomyolysis (increased risk when administered with HMG-CoA reductase inhibitors)
- Hypertension
- Pruritus
- Eosinophylic pneumonia (rare)
- Renal failure (rare)
- Insomnia

Gentamicin IV

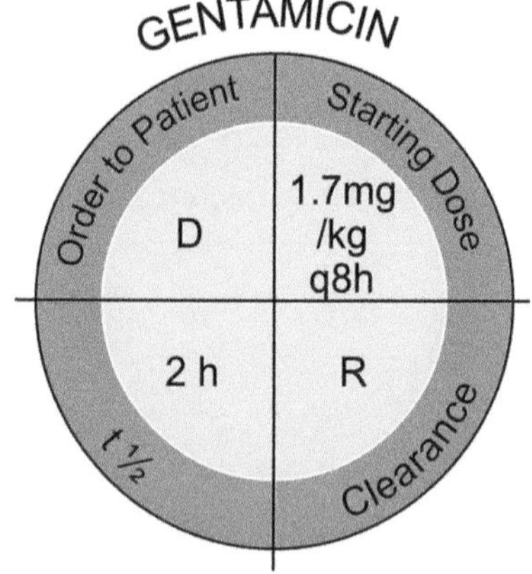

Pharmacologic Characteristics

- Aminoglycoside antimicrobial
- Inhibits protein synthesis, resulting in defective cell membranes
- Broad-spectrum activity against Gram-negative organisms
- Synergy against gram positive organisms with antimicrobials that inhibit cell wall synthesis
- Use caution in patients with myasthenia gravis or those receiving neuromuscular blocking agents
- Poor diffusion across blood–brain barrier; CSF levels depend on dose, rate of administration, and degree of meningeal inflammation
- CSF concentrations are small (10% of serum levels without meningeal inflammation and 25% with inflamed meninges)

Dosing and Administration

- 1.7 mg/kg IV every 8 hours
- Lengthen interval (every 12 or 24 hours) in patients with decreased renal function
- Intraventricular dose: 4–8 mg/day
- Infuse over 30 minutes

- Can be administered with pulse/extended-interval dosing (lower risk of nephrotoxicity)
- No dosage adjustments in patients with hepatic dysfunction

Monitoring

- Renal function
- Electrolytes (e.g., potassium, magnesium, calcium)
- Serum drug levels
  - Peak: 7–10 mcg/ml
  - Trough: 0.6–1.2 mcg/ml
  - Avoid peak levels > 12 mcg/ml and trough levels > 2 mcg/ml

Side Effects

- Nephrotoxicity
- Ototoxicity (dizziness and tinnitus first)
- Hematologic: granulocytopenia, thrombocytopenia
- Seizures/neurotoxicity

Meropenem IV

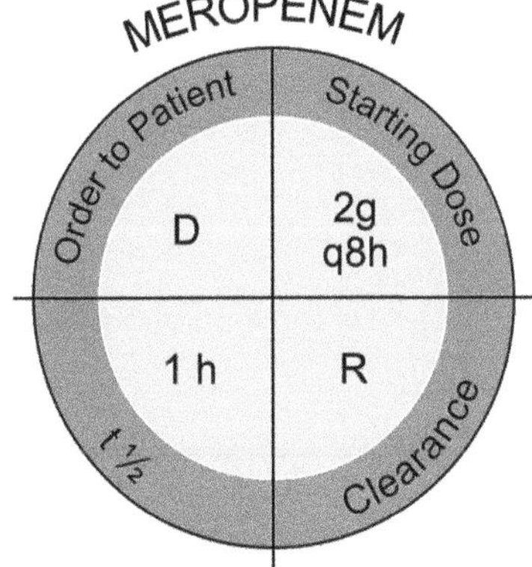

Pharmacologic Characteristics

- Inhibits cell wall synthesis
- Limited effectiveness against *Listeria monocytogenes*
- Achieves greater CSF concentrations with inflamed meninges

Dosing and Administration

- 2 g IV every 8 hours
- Lengthen interval or decrease dose in patients with renal dysfunction
- No dosage adjustments in patients with hepatic dysfunction
- Infuse over 15–30 minutes; give extended infusions over 3 hours (stability concerns if at room temperature); IV push over 3-5 minutes

Monitoring

- Complete blood count
- Renal function
- Liver function (with prolonged therapy)

Side Effects

- Headache
- Seizures (low risk)
- Nausea, diarrhea

Penicillin G IV

Pharmacologic Characteristics

- Interferes with cell wall synthesis
- Bactericidal activity against susceptible organisms
- Poor blood–brain barrier penetration even with inflamed meninges
- CSF concentration 2–6% of serum levels

Dosing and Administration

- 4 million units IV every 4 hours
- Can be given as continuous 24-hour infusion
- Give intermittent doses over 15–30 minutes
- Decrease total daily dose pending on degree of renal dysfunction
- No dosage adjustments in patients with hepatic dysfunction

Monitoring

- Renal function
- Cultures and sensitivities
- Complete blood count
- Electrolytes (potassium or sodium salt formulations)

Side Effects

- Localized phlebitis
- Seizures (with high doses)
- Hematologic: neutropenia
- Hypersensitivity reactions
- Interstitial nephritis

Rifampin IV

Pharmacologic Characteristics

- Broad-spectrum antibiotic with Gram-positive, Gram-negative, and anaerobic activity, as well as antifungal properties
- Bactericidal activity, inhibition of RNA-polymerase, prevents transcription of DNA to RNA
- CSF levels adequate in the presence of inflammation, ~20% of serum levels; highly lipophilic

Dosing and Administration

- 600 mg IV daily in combination with third-generation cephalosporin
- IV infusion over 30 minutes
- No dosage adjustments in patients with renal or hepatic disease

Monitoring

- Liver function
- Complete blood count
- Drug–drug interactions (i.e., strong inducer of CYP1A2, 2A6, 2C19, 2C8, 2C9, 3A4, and P-glycoprotein)

Side Effects

- Drug fever, eosinophilia, skin rashes (uncommon)
- Flu-like syndrome
- Hepatotoxicity
- Exudative conjunctivitis

Sulfamethoxazole/Trimethoprim (SMZ/TMP) IV

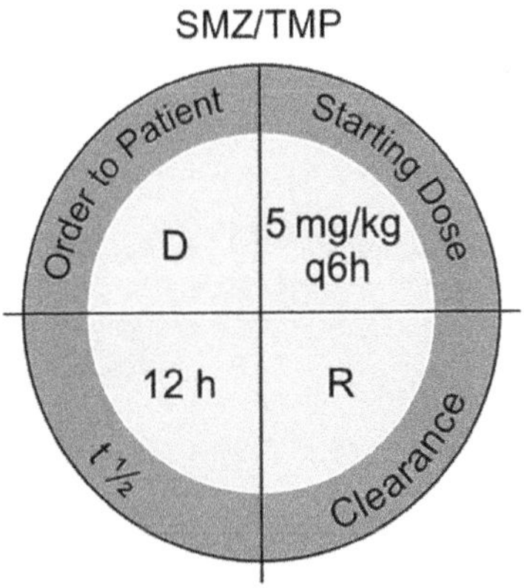

SMZ/TMP

Order to Patient	Starting Dose
D	5 mg/kg q6h
t ½	**Clearance**
12 h	R

Pharmacologic Characteristics

- Interferes with bacterial folic acid synthesis (SMZ), inhibits enzymes in the folic acid pathway (TMP)
- Often bactericidal, displays synergy when combined
- Good CSF penetration

Dosing and Administration

- 10–20 mg/kg/day TMP component, divided every 6 hours IV
- Reduce dose or lengthen administration interval in patients with renal dysfunction
- Administer over 60 minutes
- Large total volume administered daily (>1 L/day from drug alone)
- No dosage adjustments in patients with hepatic dysfunction
- SMZ undergoes extensive hepatic metabolism

Monitoring

- Drug rash
- Electrolytes (e.g., potassium)
- Renal function
- Fluid status (SMZ can inhibit carbonic anhydrase)
- Organism resistance (increasing to many organisms)
- Sulfonamide allergic reactions
- Drug interactions: can significantly increase INR in patients on vitamin K antagonists

Side Effects

- Hyperkalemia (TMP is structurally related to potassium-sparing diuretics): high doses
- Hyponatremia (rare)
- Photosensitivity
- Folic acid deficiency
- Hematologic: hemolytic anemia, agranulocytosis, leukopenia, thrombocytopenia
- Hepatotoxicity (rare)
- Hypoglycemia (rare)

Vancomycin IV

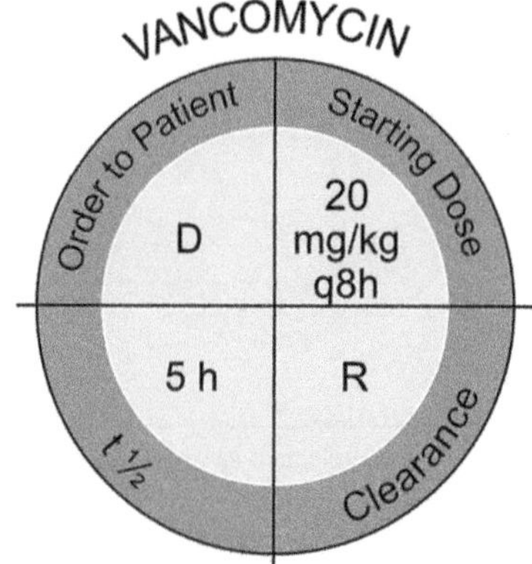

Pharmaceutical Characteristics

- Inhibits bacterial cell wall synthesis; glycopeptide antimicrobial
- Affects permeability of cell membranes and inhibits RNA synthesis
- Bactericidal for most Gram-positive organisms
- Erratic CNS penetration; penetration of blood–brain barrier improved with impaired meninges
- Synergistic activity when combined with other antimicrobials

- Mean inhibitory concentration (MIC) > 2 mcg/ml; otherwise, organism may be resistant, higher risk for treatment failure
- Concentrated up to 10 mg/ml in fluid-restricted patients
- CSF concentrations 15–19% of serum drug levels

Dosing and Administration

- 15–20 mg/kg IV
- Use adjusted body weight for dose calculation if body mass index (BMI) is >40 or weight is >120 kg
- Loading doses (i.e., 25–30 mg/kg) reserved for severe infections in critically ill patients
- Give 1 g over 1 hour, then increase infusion by 30 minutes for every 500 mg administered
- Intrathecal: 10–20 mg (1 mg/0.1 ml normal saline concentration)
- Dosing interval depends on patient's renal function and severity of infection (Table 11.7)

Table 11.7 Vancomycin Dosing Interval

Creatinine Clearance (ml/min)	Dosing Interval (hours)
>90	8
70–90	12*
35–69	24†
21–34	48
<20	72

* Consider q8h interval in severe infections.
† Consider q12h interval in severe infections and titrate to serum levels.

Monitoring

- No dosing adjustments in patients with liver dysfunction
- Trough levels at 15–20 mcg/ml
- Peak levels specifically in morbidly obese (peak goal 20–40 mcg/ml)
- Renal function
- Use of other concurrent nephrotoxic agents

Side Effects

- Ototoxicity (serum level >80 mcg/ml), increased risk with other ototoxic agents, may be permanent
- Nephrotoxicity (mostly when dosage adjustments are not done): doses >4 g/day, obesity, combination with other nephrotoxic agents
- Interstitial nephritis
- "Red man" syndrome: sudden, profound hypotension with flushing of face, neck, torso, and pruritus; premedicate with antihistamine (e.g., diphenhydramine) and decrease rate of infusion for subsequent doses
- Hypotension with flushing (with rapid administration)

- Hematologic: eosinophilia, neutropenia
- Rash
- Phlebitis
- Drug fever

Antivirals

Acyclovir IV

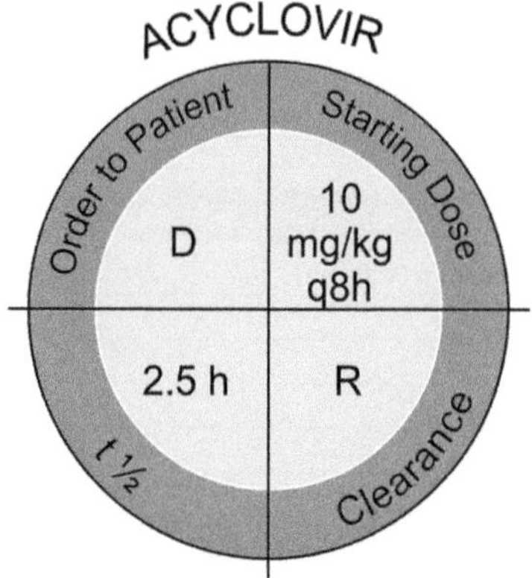

Pharmacologic Characteristics

- Synthetic purine nucleoside analog
- Inhibits DNA synthesis and viral replication
- Indicated for HSV-2 meningitis, VZV (immunocompromised), herpes zoster virus (immunocompromised)
- No effect in arboviral infections or CMV
- CSF concentrations ~50% of plasma levels

Dosing and Administration

- 10 mg/kg IV every 8 hours for 21 days (dosing based on ideal weight if obese, actual weight if underweight)
- Infuse over 1 hour; rapid administration increases nephrotoxicity
- Adequate hydration before and after infusions (200 ml 0.9% NaCl)
- Lengthen dosing interval in patients with renal impairment
- No dosage adjustments in patients with hepatic dysfunction

Monitoring

- Renal function
- Liver function
- Complete blood count

Side Effects

- Gastrointestinal: nausea and vomiting
- Nephrotoxicity
- Increase in liver function test results
- Neurotoxicity (e.g., tremors/myoclonus, confusion, drowsiness)
- Injection site inflammation

Ganciclovir IV

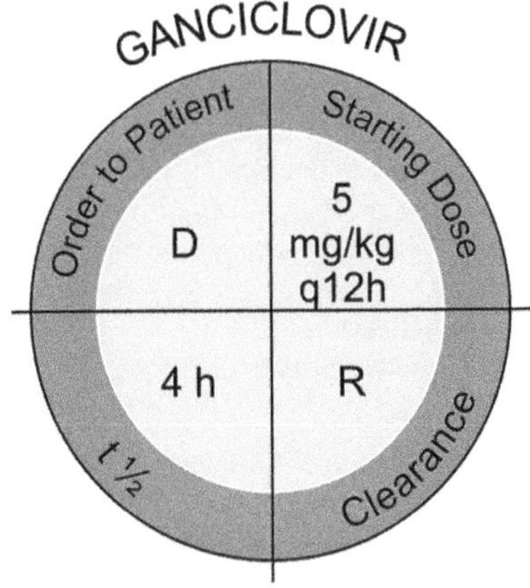

Pharmacologic Characteristics

- Acyclic nucleoside analog of deoxyguanosine inhibiting the replication of CMV and HSV; inhibits viral DNA synthesis
- Indicated for CMV encephalitis or viremia
- More toxicities than acyclovir

Dosing and Administration

- 5 mg/kg IV every 12 hours for 21–28 days
- Reduce dose and increase interval in patients with renal dysfunction
- No adjustments provided by the manufacturer in patients with hepatic dysfunction
- Infuse over 1 hour; rapid infusion increases toxicities and plasma levels

Monitoring

- Complete blood count with differential and platelets
- Renal function tests

Side Effects

- Fevers (occur in half of patients)
- Anemia
- Thrombocytopenia (common), leukopenia (common), neutropenia (uncommon)

- Diaphoresis
- Pruritus
- Diarrhea, vomiting, anorexia
- Increased serum creatinine levels

Antifungals

Amphotericin B IV

Pharmacologic Characteristics

- Fungistatic or fungicidal depending on drug concentration and organism
- Binds to fungus cell membrane, causing a change in permeability
- May require premedication with antihistamine, corticosteroid, acetaminophen, nonsteroidal anti-inflammatory drugs (NSAIDs), or meperidine to prevent transfusion-related reaction (e.g., rigors)
- CSF concentration <2.5% of serum levels; poor penetration regardless of inflammation
- Do not confuse with liposomal or lipid complex formulations

Dosing and Administration

- 0.5–1.5 mg/kg IV per day; 1–1.5 mg/kg IV over 4–6 hours every other day once therapy is established
  - Aspergillosis, rhinocerebral mucormycosis: 1–1.5 mg/kg IV per day; do not exceed 1.5 mg/kg IV per day
  - Histoplasmosis: 0.25–1 mg/kg IV per day
  - Cryptococcus: 0.7–1 mg/kg IV per day
- Test dose: 1 mg IV over 20–30 minutes
- Intrathecal: initially, 0.01–0.05 mg IV as single daily dose; may increase daily in increments of 0.025–0.1 mg IV as tolerated (maximum: 1.5 mg/day; with CSF improvement noted, decrease frequency on a weekly basis); intrathecal use generally discouraged
- Product infused over 2–6 hours
- Reduce dose by 50% or change to every-other-day dosing if drug-induced renal dysfunction occurs
- Poorly dialyzed
- No adjustments needed with hepatic dysfunction

Monitoring

- Renal function
- Liver function
- Complete blood count
- Electrolytes (especially magnesium and potassium)
- Transfusion reactions

Side Effects

- Nephrotoxicity

- Hypotension
- Hypokalemia, hypomagnesemia
- Nausea, vomiting, diarrhea
- Arthralgia, myalgia

Flucytosine PO

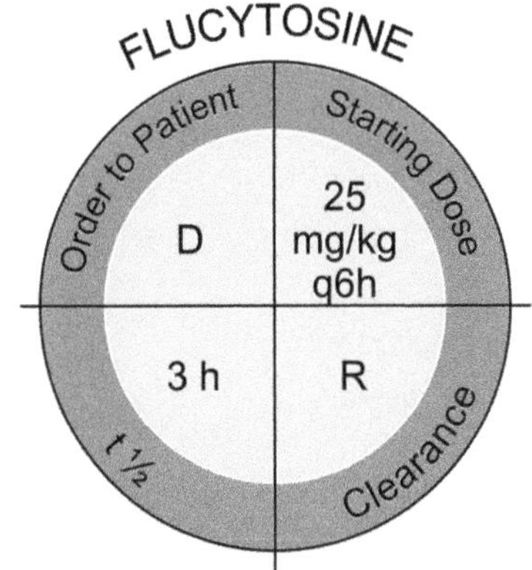

Pharmacologic Characteristics

- Penetrates fungal wall, converted to fluorouracil; competes with fungal RNA and protein synthesis
- Best to administer every 6 hours (vs. four times daily) to ensure consistent peak and trough levels
- Avoid monotherapy (high resistance)

Dosing and Administration

- CNS candidiasis: 25 mg/kg orally every 6 hours, with amphotericin B (liposomal), until stepdown therapy appropriate (use adjusted body weight for dose calculation in obese patients)
- Cryptococcal meningitis: 25 mg/kg per dose orally every 6 hours, with amphotericin B, for 4 weeks; if improving, step down to fluconazole maintenance
- Reduce dose or interval, depending on renal function; use with caution in patients with renal disease
- Markedly prolonged half-life in patients with renal dysfunction
- No dosage adjustments in patients with hepatic disease
- Very expensive oral formulation

Monitoring

- Trough level: 25–50 mcg/ml (not routinely obtained), peak level 50–100 mcg/mL; avoid levels >100 mcg/ml (bone marrow toxicity)
- Renal function

- Nausea and vomiting (administer capsules over 15 minutes)
- Hepatic function, toxicity (dose-related)
- Bone marrow toxicity (dose-related)
- Electrolytes

Side Effects

- Hematologic (e.g., agranulocytosis, anemia, bone marrow aplasia, leukopenia, pancytopenia, thrombocytopenia)
- Gastrointestinal: abdominal pain, nausea, vomiting, diarrhea
- Hallucinations (rare)
- Renal failure
- Cardiotoxicity, chest pain
- Hypokalemia
- Hepatotoxicity, abnormal liver function test results

Fluconazole IV or PO

Pharmacologic Characteristics

- Azole antifungal agent
- Interferes with fungal CYP450 activity; inhibits cell membrane formation; decreases ergosterol synthesis (component of fungal cell wall)
- Broad-spectrum activity against *Blastomycosis, Candida albicans, Coccidioidomycosis, Cryptococcus*
- CSF concentration ~50% of serum with normal meninges, increases to 80% during inflammation

Dosing and Administration

- Total daily dose the same for oral and IV administration
- *Candida* infection: 800 mg (12 mg/kg) on day 1, then 400 mg/day (6 mg/kg per day) for 14 days
- CNS blastomycosis: 800 mg once daily for 1 year or more (step-down therapy after response to amphotericin and flucytosine)
- Cryptococcal meningitis: 400-mg load, followed by 200 to 400 mg once daily for 10–12 weeks following negative culture
- CNS candidiasis: 400–800 mg/day (6–12 mg/kg per day) as step-down therapy after response to initial therapy (usually amphotericin with flucytosine); continue fluconazole until signs/symptoms and CSF/radiologic abnormalities have resolved
- Decrease load/maintenance dose and/or interval in patients with renal dysfunction
- No dosage adjustments are needed in patients with hepatic dysfunction, but use with caution
- Infuse over 1–2 hours, maximum rate: 200 mg/hr
- Use lean body weight for dosage calculations in morbidity obese patients

Monitoring

- Hepatic function
- Renal function

- Drug–drug interactions (strong inhibitor of CYP2C19)
- Electrocardiogram (EKG)

Side Effects

- Headache
- Hypokalemia
- Abdominal pain, diarrhea, nausea, vomiting
- Agranulocytosis, leukopenia, thrombocytopenia
- Hepatitis
- QT prolongation (high doses or in combination with other medications that can prolong QT leading to torsades de pointes)

Voriconazole IV

Pharmacologic Characteristics

- Azole antifungal, inhibition of CYP450 ergosterol synthesis resulting in fungal cell wall dysfunction/disruption
- Effective against *Aspergillosis*, most *Candida* species, *Coccidioidomycosis*
- CSF concentrations: 42–67% of serum levels

Dosing and Administration

- Empiric: 6 mg/kg IV every 12 hours × 2 doses, then maintenance 4 mg/kg every 12 hours
- Coccidioidal meningitis: 6 mg/kg IV every 12 hours × 2 doses, then 4 mg/kg every 12 hours maintenance; alternative: 200–300 mg orally every 12 hours (3–4 mg/kg); may reduce maintenance therapy to 3 mg/kg every 12 hours if unable to tolerate
- If patient shows no improvement on IV therapy, consider adding amphotericin B (liposomal)
- Infuse over 1–2 hours
- Administer oral product 1 hour before or after meals

Monitoring

- Therapeutic range for serious infections: 2–5 mcg/ml
- Drug–drug interactions
- EKG
- Renal function: avoid IV product in renal impairment (CrCl < 50 ml/min) due to decreased clearance of solubilizing vehicle in IV product
- Liver function
- Electrolytes

Side Effects

- Electrolyte abnormalities
- Hepatic failure (may be associated with jaundice)
- Pancreatitis
- Hallucinations
- Visual disturbances, photophobia
- Increase in serum creatinine level

- Nausea, vomiting, diarrhea
- Fever
- Prolonged QT (rare)
- Rash (rare)

Key Pointers

1. Blood cultures can be used to find the source of bacterial meningitis in over 60% of patients. They must be obtained prior to starting antimicrobial therapy or corticosteroids.
2. Vancomycin, ceftriaxone, and ampicillin are necessary for adequate antibiotic coverage in patients with a suspected bacterial meningitis who are over 50 years old.
3. Dexamethasone adjunctive therapy is warranted in deteriorating patients with bacterial meningitis associated with *Streptococcus pneumoniae*.
4. Acyclovir is indicated in any patient with suspected viral encephalitis awaiting CSF PCR results, but substantial adjustment and hydration in patients with renal dysfunction is warranted.
5. Antifungal therapy is medically complicated and should only be administered when there are severe clinical symptoms. Doses vary with different viral infections.

References

1. Tunkel, A.R., et al., *2017 Infectious Diseases Society of America's clinical practice guidelines for healthcare-associated ventriculitis and meningitis*. Clin Infect Dis, 2017 [E-pub before print].
2. Whitley, R.J., *Herpes simplex virus infections of the central nervous system*. Continuum (Minneap Minn), 2015. **21**(6 Neuroinfectious Disease): 1704–1713.
3. Segreti, J. and Harris, A.A. *Acute bacterial meningitis*. Infect Dis Clin North Am, 1996. **10**: 797–809.
4. Brouwer, M.C. and D. van de Beek, *Management of bacterial central nervous system infections*. Handb Clin Neurol, 2017. **140**: 349–364.
5. Albarillo, F. and P. O'Keefe, *Opportunistic neurologic infections in patients with acquired immunodeficiency syndrome (AIDS)*. Curr Neurol Neurosci Rep, 2016. **16**: 10.
6. Bowen, L.N., et al., *HIV-associated opportunistic CNS infections: pathophysiology, diagnosis and treatment*. Nat Rev Neurol, 2016. **12**: 662–674.
7. Dorsett, M. and Liang, S.Y. *Diagnosis and treatment of central nervous system infections in the emergency department*. Emerg Med Clin North Am, 2016. **34**: 917–942.

Chapter 12

Vasopressors and Inotropes

In the neurosciences ICU the right target of blood pressure remains a quandary. In hypotension, vasopressors and inotropes will maintain a mean arterial pressure (MAP) but are truly effective only in a volume-resuscitated patient (1). Vasopressors are also needed to improve cerebral perfusion in patients with severe cerebral vasospasm in subarachnoid hemorrhage, in patients with critical carotid or cerebral artery stenosis producing marginal compromised cerebral blood flow, or in patients who are maintained in drug-induced comas (e.g., in status epilepticus). The most common indication for the use of vasopressors in acutely ill neurologic patients—in a single bolus or short-term infusion—is to correct hypotension as a result of anesthetics, intravenous (IV) infusions of antiepileptic medications (i.e., propofol, fosphenytoin), or endotracheal intubation with a set of inducers.

In acute neurologic conditions, hypotension can be caused by septicemia, profound blood loss in traumatic brain injury with long bone fractures, abdominal trauma, or cardiac dysfunction from neurogenic stress cardiomyopathy (1–3). Acute new hypotension in a previously relatively stable neurologically injured patient commonly points to new bacteremia and sepsis, loss of vascular tone due to progression to brain death, and, in polytrauma patients, a bleeding source somewhere. The optimal systolic blood pressure or MAP remains debated and essentially unknown. Standard definitions of a MAP of approximately 65 mmHg may be insufficient in patients with a recent stroke and large-vessel occlusion and prior chronic kidney failure. Approximations of blood pressure goals are all that neurointensivists can achieve, and a reasonable goal is to maintain a MAP of at least 85 mmHg.

Mechanisms of Action

Vasopressors cause vasoconstriction while inotropes augment cardiac contractility. Both the alpha-1 receptor and the alpha-2 receptor cause vascular smooth-muscle contraction.

Beta-adrenergic receptors are divided into two groups: beta-1 adrenergic receptors stimulate sympathetic effect on heart rate and contractility while beta-2 adrenergic receptors mediate smooth-muscle relaxation and cause vasodilation. The alpha-1 adrenergic receptors are also located in the heart and increase contractility. Therefore, vasopressors, when compared to inotropes, have similarities in receptor physiology. Most

Table 12.1 Targets of Inotropes and Vasopressors

Receptor	Target	Response
Alpha-1	Vascular smooth muscle, ventricles	Vasoconstriction, increased contractility
Alpha-2	Vascular smooth muscle	Vasoconstriction
Beta-1	Sinoatrial (SA) and atrioventricular (AV) node Myocardium	Increased contractility and heart rate
Beta-2	Arterioles of heart, skin, lungs, skeletal muscle	Vasodilation

vasopressors stimulate the alpha-1 receptor on vascular smooth muscle, with the exception of vasopressin. This results in increased resistance and pressure in arteries and restores adequate perfusion. Vasopressors also improve cardiac function by improving coronary artery perfusion. This is particularly important in clinical situations such as pulmonary embolism or systolic cardiac failure. Moreover, the workings of inotropes are dose-dependent. Dopamine stimulates beta-1 adrenergic receptors and dopamine receptors at low doses but stimulates alpha-1 adrenergic receptors at high doses, with greater beta-1 receptor response. The mechanism of action is summarized in Table 12.1.

Another important concern is whether vasopressors can affect the brain vasculature. The intracerebral vessels, however, have minimal alpha-receptor densities. Moreover, there is no direct action of phenylephrine or epinephrine on intracerebral vessels because these vasoactive drugs do not cross the blood–brain barrier (4–8).

Vasopressors

Vasopressor use requires a central venous catheter. Peripheral administration of vasopressors may cause tissue necrosis. Thus, if vasopressors must be administered peripherally (i.e., if there is no other choice in a critical situation), they should be given at the lowest concentration available and only for a short period until central access can be obtained. Vasopressors carry the risk of tissue extravasation. Phentolamine can be used in the event of vasopressor-induced extravasation in many cases.

Four agents are commonly used in daily practice, and they are discussed here.

Norepinephrine IV

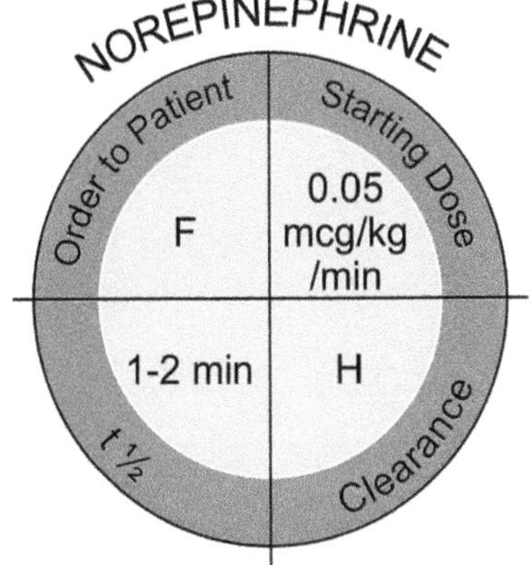

Pharmacologic Characteristics

- First-line agent in patients with septic shock (9,10)
- Potential benefit over dopamine in septic shock
- Potent beta-1 agonist (less than epinephrine)
- Potent alpha-1 agonist (more than epinephrine)
- Marked arterial and venous vasoconstriction
- Main effect is increased vascular resistance
- Increase in heart rate and contractility but not cardiac output

Dosing and Administration

- Starting infusion: 0.05 mcg/kg per minute
- Maximal infusion: 3 mcg/kg per minute
- Initial response: immediate, raises MAP in 1 minute

Monitoring

- Blood pressure
- Heart rate and rhythm

Side Effects

- Reflex bradycardia
- Tachydysrhythmias (with doses up to 30 mcg/min and beyond)
- Hypoperfusion (digital ischemia, gut)
- Tissue necrosis with long-term use or higher doses
- Headache

Phenylephrine IV

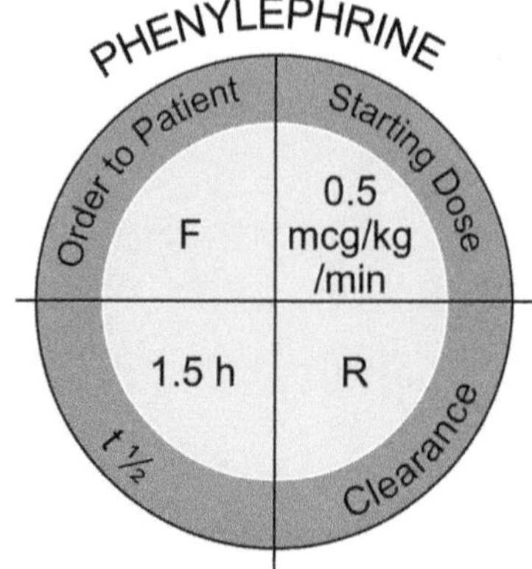

Pharmacologic Characteristics

- Pure alpha-adrenergic agonist activity
- Marked arterial vasoconstriction and increased systemic vascular resistance improve blood pressure
- Low arrhythmogenic potential

Dosing and Administration

- Bolus: 100–500 mcg every 10–15 minutes
- Infusion: 20–40 mcg/min or 0.5–1.4 mcg/kg per minute
- Higher doses used for shock (up to 6 mcg/kg per minute)
- Initial response: immediate, raises MAP in 1 minute

Monitoring

- Add to norepinephrine if serious arrhythmias occur, when there is good cardiac output or as salvage therapy.

Side Effects

- Reflex bradycardia
- Peripheral ischemia
- Decrease in cardiac output
- Risk of tissue necrosis with extravasation
- Digital necrosis, or dry gangrene from peripheral vasoconstriction

Epinephrine IV

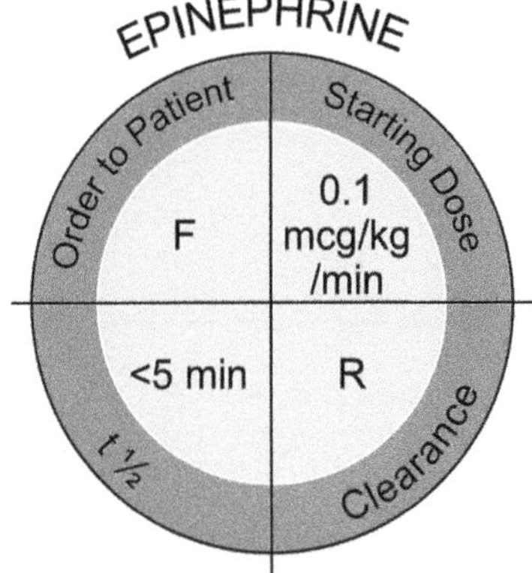

Pharmacologic Characteristics

- Often used for anaphylactic shock
- Second-line choice—after norepinephrine—for septic shock
- Potent beta-1 agonist (more than norepinephrine)
- Moderate alpha-1 agonist at low doses but potent alpha-1 agonist at high doses
- Marked increase in cardiac output and contractility
- Does not cross blood–brain barrier

Dosing and Administration

- Dose: 0.1–1 mcg/kg per minute

Monitoring

- Increased myocardial oxygen demand
- MAP

Side Effects

- Cardiac dysrhythmia (common)
- Myocardial ischemia
- Risk of tissue necrosis with extravasation

Vasopressin IV

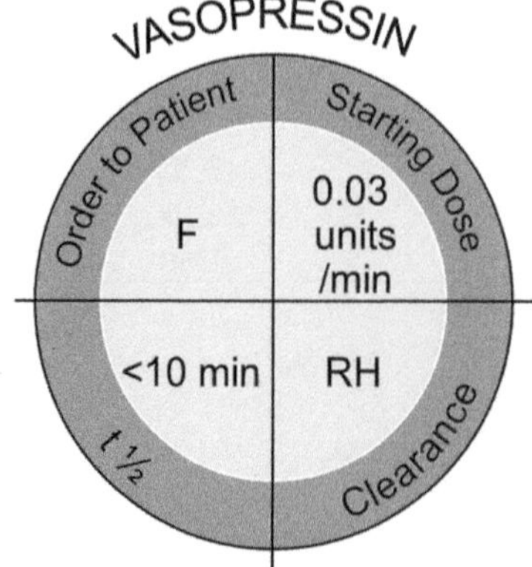

Pharmacologic Characteristics

- V1 receptors are responsible for vasoconstriction and are located on vascular smooth muscle and organs
- V2 receptors are responsible for water resorption and are located on the collecting duct of the renal tubule; decrease urine volume and increase osmolality
- No cerebral vasoconstriction
- No impact on cardiac output and heart rate
- No reflexive increase in vagal tone
- Less risk of cardiac arrhythmias than with other vasopressors
- Improves coronary flow
- Onset rapid, with peak within 15 minutes

Dosing and Administration

- Dose: 0.03–0.07 units/min

Monitoring

- Dose of vasopressin >0.03 units/min may cause coronary or mesenteric ischemia and should be reserved as salvage therapy.
- Dose needs tapering to avoid hypotension; decrease by 0.005 units/min every hour after blood pressure has been maintained for 8 hours.
- Consider use when there has been an inadequate response to one or two other catecholamines (i.e., norepinephrine-sparing effects).

Side Effects

- Hypoperfusion (gut ischemia)
- Cardiac dysrhythmias

Inotropes

Inotropes are used when there is evidence of myocardial dysfunction that has resulted in reduced cardiac output (11,12). Inotropes improve cardiac contractility and compensate for increased myocardial oxygen demand. Myocardial depression may be associated with significant vasodilatation (e.g., sepsis), which often results in combined use of vasopressors and inotropes (13,14).

Dopamine IV

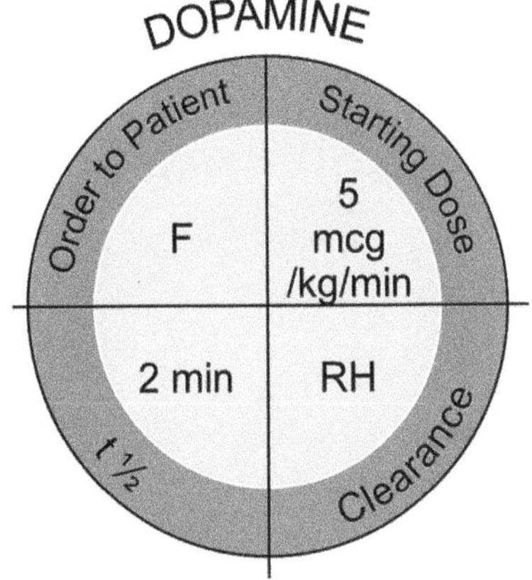

Pharmacologic Characteristics

- Commonly used inotropic agent, alone or in combination with vasopressors
- Augments renal blood flow (at low to moderate doses)
- Does not cross the blood–brain barrier
- Onset: 5 minutes
- Duration: 10 minutes

Dosing and Administration

- At doses of 1–2 mcg/kg per minute, it produces selective vasodilation in renal, mesenteric, cerebral, and coronary beds
- At doses of 5–10 mcg/kg per minute, it stimulates beta-1 and beta-2 adrenergic receptors and increases cardiac output
- At doses of 10–20 mcg/kg per minute, it loses its dopamine effects but has potent alpha-1 and beta-1 agonist activity and moderate beta-2 agonist activity

Monitoring

- Similar activity to norepinephrine at doses >15 mcg/kg per minute

- Doses >20 mcg/kg per minute may not have beneficial effects on blood pressure but may increase the frequency of arrhythmias
- If higher doses are needed, may need to consider using a more direct vasopressor (e.g., norepinephrine or epinephrine)

Side Effects

- In sepsis, increased short-term mortality when compared with norepinephrine
- More arrhythmic events than norepinephrine (15)
- Tachycardia, arrhythmias
- Risk of tissue necrosis with extravasation

Dobutamine IV

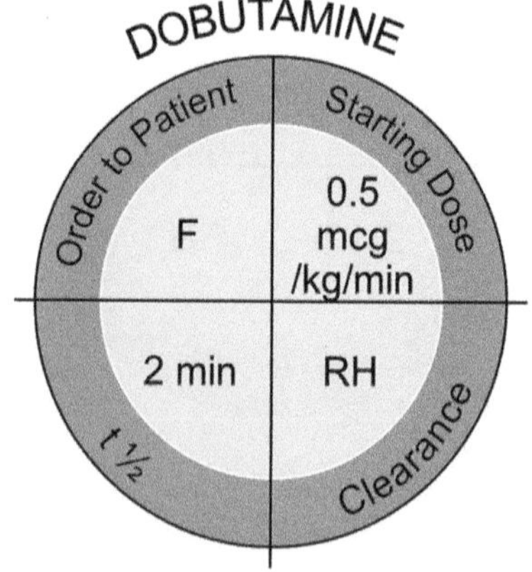

Pharmacologic Characteristics

- Used in cardiogenic shock or if there are ongoing signs of hypoperfusion
- Primarily beta-1 agonist activity
- Lower doses (up to 20 mcg/kg per minute) in patients with cardiac failure
- Onset: 1–10 minutes
- Peak effect: 10–20 minutes

Dosing and Administration

- Start at 0.5–1 mcg/kg per minute
- Maintenance: 2–15 mcg/kg per minute
- Maximum recommended dose is 20 mcg/kg per minute, but dosage can be as high as 40 mcg/kg per minute

Monitoring

- Cardiac output
- Blood pressure

Side Effects

- Tachyarrhythmias
- Myocardial ischemia
- Risk of tissue necrosis with extravasation

Milrinone IV

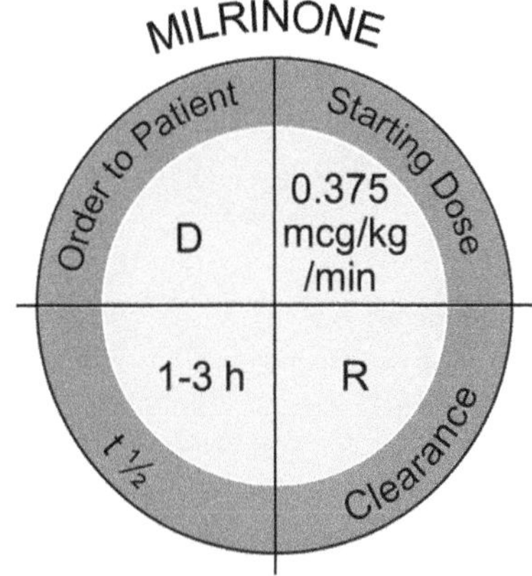

Pharmacologic Characteristics

- Phosphodiesterase inhibitor resulting in relaxation of cardiac and smooth vascular muscle by decreasing calcium stores available for muscle contraction
- Improves cardiac output without increasing oxygen consumption
- Relaxes vascular and tracheal smooth muscle
- Reduces left ventricular end-diastolic pressure
- In high doses may reduce cerebral vasospasm
- Onset: 5–15 minutes
- Duration: 1–3 hours

Dosing and Administration

- Dose: 0.375–0.75 mcg/kg per minute

Monitoring

- Heart rate
- Blood pressure
- Renal function

Side Effects

- Thrombocytopenia (reversible)
- Hepatotoxicity
- Supraventricular tachycardia
- Ventricular arrhythmias

Isoproterenol IV

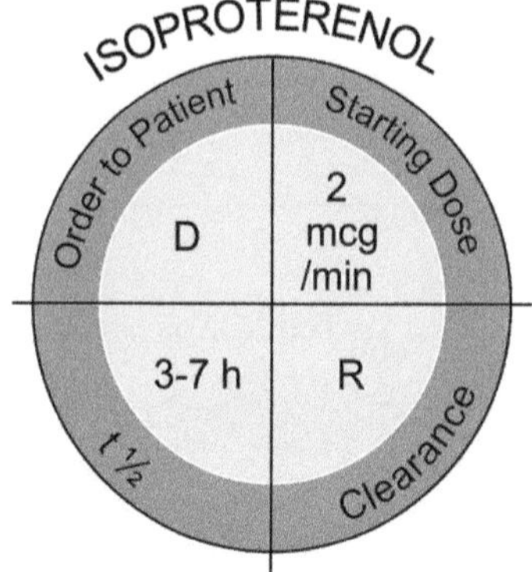

Pharmacologic Characteristics

- Potent beta-1 and beta-2 agonist
- Moderate decrease in MAP
- Relaxation of bronchial, gastrointestinal, and uterine smooth muscle
- Onset: immediate
- Duration: 10–15 minutes

Dosing and Administration

- Dose: 2–10 mcg/min or 0.05–0.2 mcg/kg per minute
- Used as an adjunct in vasoconstrictive and cardiogenic shock, low ejection fraction, bradyarrhythmias, refractory torsades de pointes

Monitoring

- Heart rate
- Blood pressure
- Electrocardiogram (EKG)

Side Effects

- Ventricular fibrillation
- Tachyarrhythmias
- Angina (marked increased in myocardial oxygen demand)
- Hypotension and syncope

Vasopressors and inotropes have different effects on blood pressure, cardiac contractility, and heart rate (Table 12.2).

Use in Clinical Practice

Generally, when the clinician is confronted with a patient with acute hypotension, a simplified thought process can go as follows:

1. Is hypotension due to decreased systemic vascular resistance (i.e., sepsis, acute withdrawal of corticosteroids, or recently administered anesthetics)?
2. Is hypotension due to decreased cardiac output (i.e., hypovolemia, left or right ventricular dysfunction)?

Hypotension (i.e., systolic blood pressure <70 mmHg and MAP <65 mmHg) presents with a decreased level of consciousness, oliguria, delayed capillary refill, and cooling of the skin. In addition, as a result of sudden tissue ischemia, serum lactate levels increase. Generally, hemodynamic instability is more likely to be a result of reduced afterload than poor cardiac contractility.

Pharmacotherapy of Shock

The approach includes fluid resuscitation, administration of packed red cells if the hemoglobin level is less than 7 g/dl or the hematocrit is less than 30%, correction of any hypothermia, and use of vasopressors. Some practices prefer to use norepinephrine; others prefer to use dopamine or dobutamine, alone or in combination with vasopressin. Most physicians will use 200-mcg phenylephrine boluses in the intensive care unit to correct brief declines in blood pressure. This is immediately followed by a continuous infusion of phenylephrine at a dosage of 0.5 to 9 mcg/kg per minute while proceeding with a central line placement for norepinephrine use if no central access has yet been established. If a bedside cardiac ultrasound shows evidence of poor contractility, dopamine infusion can then replace one vasopressor.

Vasopressin is added quickly if there is no adequate response to norepinephrine and phenylephrine. It provides a vasopressor-sparing effect. Vasopressin infusions are often started at a lower rate of 0.01 units/min and titrated to the desired MAP or blood pressure goal.

There are several disease-specific recommendations depending on the type of shock. Cardiogenic shock is best first treated with dobutamine and dopamine in combination to improve inotropy (often at a dosage of 7.5 mcg/kg per minute each). Norepinephrine is needed if this does not result in blood pressure stabilization or if the patient's systolic blood pressure remains below 70 mmHg. In vasodilatory shock, epinephrine or norepinephrine is used and is frequently combined with vasopressin.

Patients with vasodilatory or hypovolemic shock should receive aggressive fluid resuscitation (quick administration of 1–2 L of crystalloids and transfusion of red blood cells). A serum lactic acid level can be used as guidance; a level of more than 4 mmol/L indicates tissue hypoperfusion and requires aggressive hemodynamic support. If the blood pressure target is not achieved, norepinephrine is supplemented with low-dose vasopressin. Phenylephrine is not a good choice in septic shock because it can reduce cardiac output, and septic patients may already have myocardial dysfunction. Patients with septic shock who do not quickly respond to these

Table 12.2 Effects of Vasopressors and Inotropes

Agent	Alpha-1	Alpha-2	Beta-1	Beta-2	Dopamine	Hemodynamic Effects				
						MAP	Heart Rate	Cardiac output	SVR	PCWP
Dopamine										
1–3 mcg/kg per minute	–	–	+	–	++++	↔	↔	↔	↔	↔
3–10 mcg/kg per minute	–	–	++++	++	++++	↔			↔ or –	↔
>10 mcg/kg per minute	+++	–	++++	+	–					
Norepinephrine										
0.02–3 mcg/kg per minute	++++	++	++	–	–		↔	↔		
Phenylephrine										
0.5–9 mcg/kg per minute	++++	+	–	–	–		↔	↔ or –		
Epinephrine										
0.01–0.05 mcg/kg per minute	+	++	++++	++	–			↔	↔ or –	↔
>0.05 mcg/kg per minute	+++	++++	+++	+	–					
Vasopressin										
0.01–0.04 units/min	–	–	–	–	–	↔	↔	↔	↔ or	–
Dobutamine										
2–10 mcg/kg per minute	+	–	+++	++	–	↔		↔	↔ or –	–
>10–20 mcg/kg per minute	++	–	++++	+++	–	↔ or –			–	–
Milrinone										
0.375–0.75 mcg/kg per minute	–	–	–	–	–	↔ or –	↔		–	–

SVR, systemic vascular resistance; PCWP, pulmonary capillary wedge pressure; MAP, mean arterial blood pressure.

measures may be treated with corticosteroids (hydrocortisone 50 mg IV every 6 hours) (5,9,14–16).

Pressure Augmentation in Subarachnoid Hemorrhage

Prophylaxis with nimodipine (Chapter 17) can be continued unless blood pressure cannot be augmented. Hemodynamic augmentation in patients with cerebral vasospasm after subarachnoid hemorrhage usually requires vasopressors and may be supplemented by inotropes if there is documented stress cardiomyopathy with a marked reduced ejection fraction on a bedside echocardiogram. Dosing depends on the persistence or resolution of clinical signs, and higher doses may be needed to see an effect. Phenylephrine is often the first line option, but norepinephrine is likely more successful clinically. Inotropes are rarely used in this setting, and none have a predictable response and are more prone to cardiac arrhythmias.

There is interest in the use of milrinone, which has both inotropic and vasodilatory properties. Milrinone has been used at a dosage of 0.75 mcg/kg per minute increasing to 1.25 mcg/kg per minute. After clinical effect, the drug can be maintained for several days with weaning in 3 subsequent days. The evidence for use of milrinone in cerebral vasospasm is uncertain, but in these high doses, reversal or marked reduction of vessel calibre is actually possible. We have used it in refractory symptomatic cerebral vasospasm but mostly after endovascular procedures with intra-arterial verapamil first (17,18).

Multiple vasopressors and inotropes can be tolerated for only a short period of time, and reduction of dose is a constant incentive. Weaning of vasopressors may be considered if the cause of shock has been found and corrected, when infection seems to be under control with antibiotics, or if myocardial infarction is excluded by serial serum troponin measurements. Weaning of vasopressors may be facilitated by the use of oral midodrine, which stimulates alpha-1 adrenergic receptors of the arteriolar and venous vasculature, leading to vasoconstriction. Often the standard starting dose is 10 mg every 8 hours, with a maximum dose of 40 mg. Midodrine resulted in a nearly 25% reduction in the duration of IV vasopressor use (19–21).

Key Pointers

1. Vasopressors increase systemic vascular resistance with little effect on cardiac output.
2. Inotropes are used when there is evidence of reduced cardiac output and reduced ejection fraction.
3. Combining inotropes and vasopressors may avoid the adverse effects of each drug at high doses.
4. Vasopressin is used when there is an inadequate response to one or two other catecholamines. It has no effect on cardiac output and heart rate.
5. Midodrine may facilitate weaning of vasopressors in selected patients.

References

1. Zafar, S.N., et al., *Presenting blood pressure in traumatic brain injury: a bimodal distribution of death.* J Trauma, 2011. **71**: 1179–1184.
2. Berry, C., et al., *Redefining hypotension in traumatic brain injury.* Injury, 2012. **43**: 1833–1837.
3. Sookplung, P., et al., *Vasopressor use and effect on blood pressure after severe adult traumatic brain injury.* Neurocrit Care, 2011. **15**: 46–54.
4. Dagal, A. and Lam, A.M. *Cerebral blood flow and the injured brain: how should we monitor and manipulate it?* Curr Opin Anaesthesiol, 2011. **24**: 131–137.
5. Meng, L., et al., *Effect of phenylephrine and ephedrine bolus treatment on cerebral oxygenation in anaesthetized patients.* Br J Anaesth, 2011. **107**: 209–217.
6. Olesen, J., *The effect of intracarotid epinephrine, norepinephrine, and angiotensin on the regional cerebral blood flow in man.* Neurology, 1972. **22**: 978–987.
7. Strandgaard, S. and Sigurdsson, S.T. *Point:Counterpoint: Sympathetic activity does/ does not influence cerebral blood flow. Counterpoint: Sympathetic nerve activity does not influence cerebral blood flow.* J Appl Physiol (1985), 2008. **105**: 1366–1368.
8. van Lieshout, J.J. and Secher, N.H. *Point:Counterpoint: Sympathetic activity does/ does not influence cerebral blood flow. Point: Sympathetic activity does influence cerebral blood flow.* J Appl Physiol (1985), 2008. **105**: 1364–1366.
9. Morelli, A., et al., *Phenylephrine versus norepinephrine for initial hemodynamic support of patients with septic shock: a randomized, controlled trial.* Crit Care, 2008. **12**: R143.
10. Vasu, T.S., et al., *Norepinephrine or dopamine for septic shock: systematic review of randomized clinical trials.* J Intens Care Med, 2012. **27**: 172–178.
11. Lollgen, H. and Drexler, H. *Use of inotropes in the critical care setting.* Crit Care Med, 1990. **18**(1 Pt 2): S56–60.
12. Stratton, L., Berlin, D.A. and Arbo, J.E. *Vasopressors and inotropes in sepsis.* Emerg Med Clin North Am, 2017. **35**: 75–91.
13. Havel, C., et al., *Vasopressors for hypotensive shock.* Cochrane Database Syst Rev, 2011. CD003709.
14. Hollenberg, S.M., *Vasoactive drugs in circulatory shock.* Am J Respir Crit Care Med, 2011. **183**: 847–855.
15. De Backer, D., et al., *Comparison of dopamine and norepinephrine in the treatment of shock.* N Engl J Med, 2010. **362**: 779–789.
16. Annane, D., et al., *Norepinephrine plus dobutamine versus epinephrine alone for management of septic shock: a randomised trial.* Lancet, 2007. **370**: 676–684.
17. Baumann, A., et al., *Seeking new approaches: milrinone in the treatment of cerebral vasospasm.* Neurocrit Care, 2012. **16**: 351–353.
18. Lannes, M., et al., *The use of milrinone in patients with delayed cerebral ischemia following subarachnoid hemorrhage: a systematic review.* Can J Neurol Sci, 2017. **44**: 152–160.
19. Anstey, M.H., et al., *Midodrine as adjunctive support for treatment of refractory hypotension in the intensive care unit: a multicenter, randomized, placebo controlled trial (the MIDAS trial).* BMC Anesthesiol, 2017. **17**: 47.
20. Hammond, D.A., Smith, M.N. and Meena, N. *Considerations on midodrine use in resolving septic shock.* Chest, 2016. **149**: 1582–1583.
21. Poveromo, L.B., Michalets, E.L. and Sutherland, S.E. *Midodrine for the weaning of vasopressor infusions.* J Clin Pharm Ther, 2016. **41**: 260–265.

Chapter 13

Antihypertensives and Antiarrhythmics

Acute brain injury can precipitate a hypertensive response, which for the most part, is the result of stress-induced, increased sympathetic activity. Furthermore, an acute increase in intracranial pressure will bring about a sharp rise in blood pressure (Cushing reflex).Treatment would seem urgent, but in any patient with hypertensive urgency, lowering the blood pressure could cause markedly reduced cerebral and renal blood flow, which is not necessarily compensated for by autoregulation (1,2).

The most common conditions associated with hypertensive emergencies are cerebral hemorrhage, acute cerebellar hemorrhage, acute pontine hemorrhage, aneurysmal subarachnoid hemorrhage, or acute stroke with associated acute medical illness (e.g., aortic dissection). Dysautonomia in encephalitis or severe Guillain-Barré syndrome may result in difficult-to-manage labile hypertension (3,4). The main challenge for the physician is to treat markedly elevated blood pressures aggressively—but not too aggressively—causing harm by unintentional and unexpected marked hypotension.

The use of intravenous (IV) antihypertensives—bolus or infusion—is ubiquitous in the neurocritical care population. The important characteristics of antihypertensive drugs are cost, onset and duration of action, and incidence of adverse effects. Costs can be prohibitive for some drugs that are new to the market or have had unexpected manufacturer price increases. The safety profile of a medication can also be a concern, such as nitroprusside and the risk of cyanide toxicity (5).

Cardiac arrhythmias are very common in patients with acute brain injury, but they are mostly short-lived, self-limiting and much less hazardous than in patients with acute cardiac disease. Many of the antiarrhythmic drugs also have antihypertensive effects, so these drug classes are best combined in one chapter. A common and usually easily treatable cardiac arrhythmia is atrial fibrillation with rapid ventricular response. Episodic bradycardia, on the other hand, rarely requires acute pharmacotherapy. Brief supraventricular or ventricular arrhythmias are often noted but improve with supplementation of potassium, calcium, or magnesium rather than antiarrhythmic drugs.

Definition of Hypertension and Blood Pressure Goals

None of the traditional-ever lowering- blood pressure targets may be applicable in patients with acute brain injury. Hypertension is vaguely understood

Table 13.1 Blood Pressure Targets in Acute Brain Injury

Diagnosis	Systolic Blood Pressure Goal
Acute ischemic stroke	≤180 mmHg
Subarachnoid hemorrhage	≤160 mmHg
Cerebral hemorrhage	≤140 mmHg
Posterior reversible encephalopathy syndrome	20% less than baseline
Eclampsia	20% less than baseline

as a blood pressure that is too high under the circumstances. A blood pressure that is too low could jeopardize collateral compensatory circulation in ischemic stroke. A blood pressure that is too high could potentially expand an intracranial hemorrhage and enlarge the territory of edema around the clot. Precise blood pressure thresholds have not been established, and goals have not been individualized to the patient's comorbidity (e.g., presence of chronic renal failure). Many blood pressure goals have evolved over the years, but although they make intuitive sense, there is no supportive evidence for any of them. Blood pressure reduction and targets, as established by consensus meetings, are shown in Table 13.1. These goals are expert opinion to provide guidance.

Blood pressure goals are different in different types of strokes. In ischemic strokes, perfusion is key, leading to institution of "permissive hypertension." In hemorrhagic stroke, pressure-linked expansion of the hematoma is the main motivation for tight close control of blood pressure, but blood pressure management should also include avoidance of marked variability of blood pressure values (6). Hypertensive surges may be linked to re-rupture of cerebral aneurysm, but other mechanisms (i.e., fibrinolysis) may be more likely (Chapter 8). Current knowledge of the benefits of blood pressure control—systolic (SBP) and diastolic (DBP)—is limited but can be summarized as follows:

- Most blood pressures can be held at SBP of 140 mmHg and DBP of 90 mmHg 24 hours after ictus
- Reducing SBP to <140 mmHg does not reduce perfusion in cerebral hemorrhage or reduce expansion (7)
- Reducing SBP to <140 mmHg may increase the risk of renal failure by 2% (8)
- Do not stop antihypertensive medications if blood pressure control is achieved, especially with beta-blockers and alpha-blockers because of the potential for serious rebound
- Do not administer thrombolysis with SBP >185 mmHg or DBP >110 mmHg
- After thrombolysis, keep SBP <180 mmHg and DBP <105 mmHg for 24 hours. Monitor blood pressure every 30 minutes for first 6 to 8 hours

Once the blood pressure is controlled, further baseline evaluation of the cause and possible secondary effects of longstanding hypertension follows (Box 13.1).

Box 13.1 Monitoring Tests with Blood Pressure Control

Electrocardiography (or echocardiography)
Chest x-ray
Sodium, potassium, creatinine, blood urea nitrogen (BUN)
Serum troponin
Urinalysis
Renal ultrasound

Current Practice of Antihypertensives

The ABCDs of antihypertensive drugs are as follows:

- Angiotensin-converting enzyme (ACE) inhibitors or angiotensin II receptor blockers (ARBs) (e.g., captopril, enalapril, lisinopril, losartan)
- Beta-blockers (e.g., atenolol, labetalol, metoprolol, propranolol)
- Calcium channel antagonists (e.g., amlodipine, clevidipine, diltiazem, nicardipine, nifedipine, verapamil)
- Diuretics (e.g., furosemide, hydrochlorothiazide) and vasodilators (e.g., hydralazine, nitroprusside) (1,2,9–15)

The general principle is to use either IV beta-blockade or direct vasodilators for initial blood pressure management. Continuous infusion with calcium-channel blockers is often the next step, but overtreatment is a possibility. First-line treatment for hypertension is IV labetalol, which blocks alpha-adrenergic, beta-1-adrenergic, and beta-2-adrenergic receptors. Cardiac output is maintained due to blockade of both alpha and beta receptors and therefore is not changed with labetalol. A commonly used second-line drug is IV nicardipine, which is effective in infusion doses of 5 to 15 mg/hr. It is an ideal drug for blood pressure reduction and does not carry the risk of causing bradydysrhythmias because it does not affect the cardiac conduction system.

Hypertension can also be paroxysmal and emerging later. These spells, also known as paroxysmal hyperactivity syndrome or sympathetic storms, are seen in the more seriously affected comatose patients and are best treated with gabapentin, which binds to voltage-gated calcium channels in the dorsal horn of the spinal cord, and with opioids such as morphine or fentanyl. Alternative treatment options are propranolol (a non-cardioselective beta-blocker), clonidine (a central-acting alpha-2-receptor agonist), dexmedetomidine (another central-acting alpha-2-receptor agonist), bromocriptine (a dopamine-D2-receptor agonist), baclofen (a $GABA_B$-receptor agonist), and benzodiazepines ($GABA_A$-receptor agonists, such as lorazepam or diazepam).

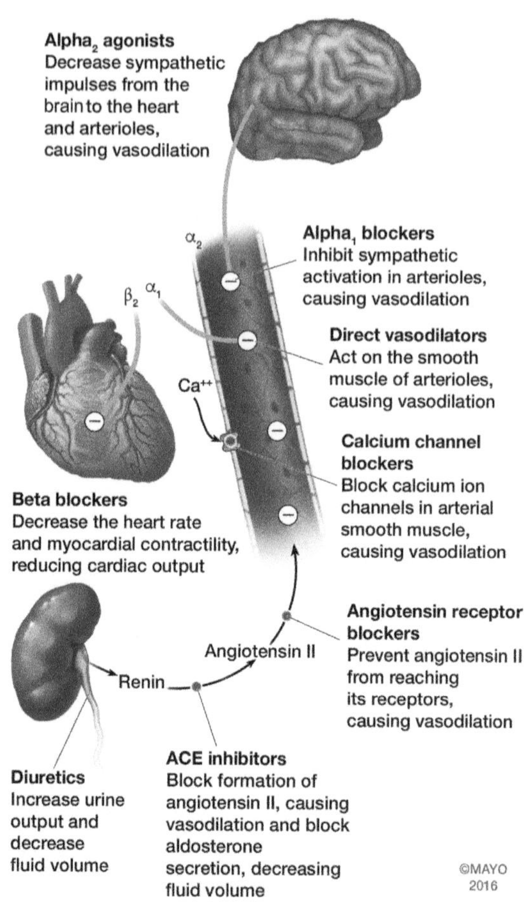

Figure 13.1 Mechanisms of major classes of antihypertensives

The main targets are shown in Figure 13.1.

A separate issue is hypertensive emergency in pregnancy in the setting of preeclampsia (16). Pregnancy precludes the use of several antihypertensive agents. All antihypertensive agents cross the placenta to some degree, but beta-blockade is considered acceptable. Antihypertensives contraindicated in pregnancy include ACE inhibitors, ARBs, and mineralocorticoid blockers. (There is a risk of growth retardation and congenital anomalies, as well as maternal hepatic toxicity.) There is a lack of data defining the efficacy of different classes of antihypertensives in pregnancy. Treatment for eclampsia is IV magnesium infusion titrated to loss of tendon reflexes and blood pressure control. This is generally achieved with an infusion of 2 g of magnesium sulfate (17).

Labetalol IV

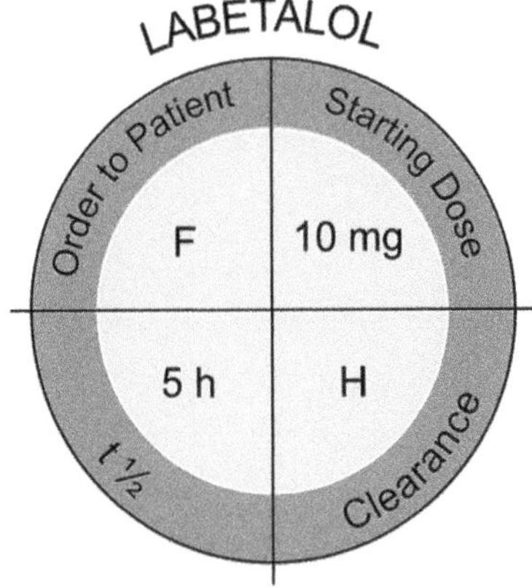

Pharmacologic Characteristics

- Combined selective alpha-1-adrenergic and nonselective beta-adrenergic blockade
- Onset: 2–5 minutes after IV administration
- Maximal effect: 2–4 hours
- Contraindications: severe bradycardia, heart block more than first-degree, cardiogenic shock, uncompensated heart failure, obstructive airway disease
- Use caution in patients with any pulmonary disease because it may cause bronchoconstriction
- Use caution in patients with hyperadrenergic states, such as pheochromocytoma or cocaine or methamphetamine intoxication, unless adequate blockade is achieved (can increase blood pressure if beta- blockade is not complete)

Dosing and Administration

- 10–20 mg IV bolus every 10 minutes (maximum cumulative 300 mg)
- IV infusion: 0.5–2 mg/min
- Change from IV to oral: 200 mg orally, then in 6–12 hours another 200–400 mg orally when the infusion is stopped

Monitoring

- Use caution in patients with liver disease: decreased first-pass metabolism leads to increased drug bioavailability
- Abrupt withdrawal may lead to rebound tachycardia, hypertension, or ischemia
- Heart rate
- Blood pressure
- Respiratory effects in patients with airway disease

Side Effects

- Vomiting
- Bronchoconstriction
- Heart block, orthostatic hypotension

Esmolol IV

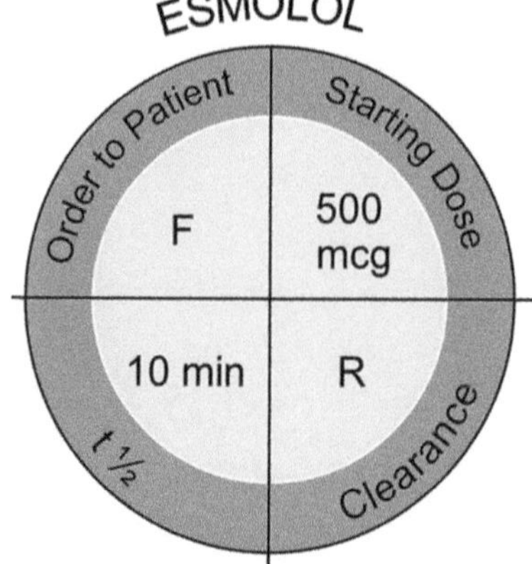

Pharmacologic Characteristics

- Largely beta-adrenergic antagonist (beta-1 selective)
- Contraindications: severe sinus bradycardia, heart block more than first-degree, diastolic heart failure, pulmonary hypertension, bronchospasm, conduction abnormalities
- No vasodilator properties
- Decreases heart rate, contractility (marked decrease), and cardiac output
- Inotropic agent, antiarrhythmic class II
- Onset: 1–5 minutes
- Peak effect: 5 minutes

Dosing and Administration

- Load: 500–1,000 mcg/kg IV over 1 minute (usually 500 mcg)
- IV infusion: 5–100 mcg/kg per minute (maximum 200 mcg/kg per minute)
- May be continued up to 48 hours
- Transition to oral dose: reduce rate by 50% 30 minutes after administering the oral agent. Consider discontinuing infusion after second oral dose has been given, and monitor blood pressure response
- No dose adjustments in patients with renal dysfunction; not removed by hemodialysis. Active metabolite is retained in patients with renal disease
- No dose adjustments in patients with hepatic dysfunction

Monitoring

- Drug interaction: combination of digoxin and calcium-channel blockers increases the risk of heart block
- Heart rate

- Blood pressure
- Renal function

Side Effects

- Hypotension (dose-related)
- Ischemia of digits
- Infusion-site reactions (including extravasation)
- Hyperkalemia
- Hypoglycemia in patients with diabetes mellitus or decreased hypoglycemia response
- Bronchospasm

Hydralazine IV

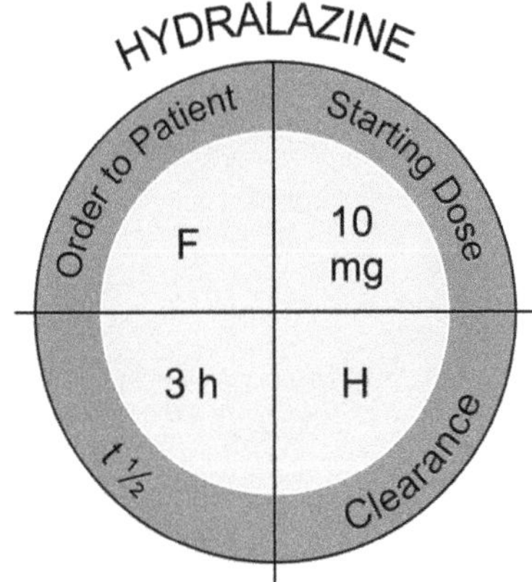

Pharmacologic Characteristics

- Direct arteriolar vasodilator with little effect on venous circulation
- Alternative choice in patients prone to bradycardia
- Safe with hypertensive urgencies associated with pregnancy (24)
- Onset of action: 5–20 minutes for IV, 20–30 minutes for oral
- Duration: 2 hours

Dosing and Administration

- 5–10 mg IV bolus followed by 5–10 mg IV every 30 minutes, maximum dose 20 mg

Monitoring

- Hypotensive response is less predictable than with other antihypertensive agents

- Complete blood count
- Gradual withdrawal of therapy to avoid rebound effects

Side Effects

- Tachycardia
- Vomiting
- Possibly worsening angina
- Agranulocytosis

Nicardipine IV

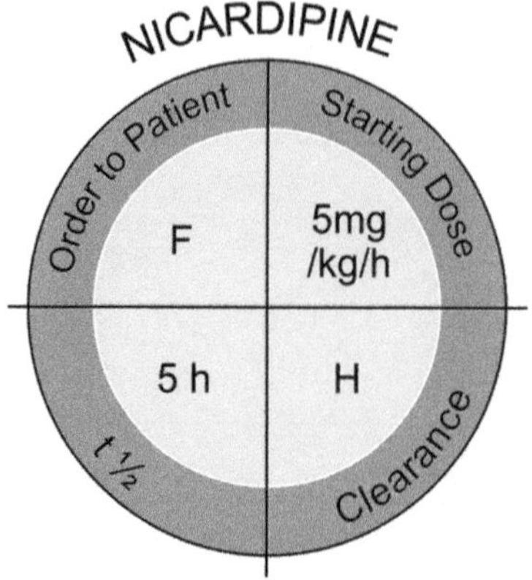

Pharmacologic Characteristics

- Dihydropyridine calcium-channel blocker with vasodilating properties
- More stable blood pressure control than intermittent IV bolus dosing
- Delayed onset of action (5–10 minutes)
- Duration: 2–6 hours

Dosing and Administration

- Infusion: start at 5 mg/hr and increase by 2.5 mg/hr every 15 minutes to achieve blood pressure control
- IV infusion maximum dose: 15 mg/hr
- Can be administered peripherally, although central access is preferred

Monitoring

- May cause significant hypotension
- Rebound common if stopped too early

Side Effects

- Hypotension
- Nausea, flushing
- Tachycardia
- Vomiting

Nitroprusside IV

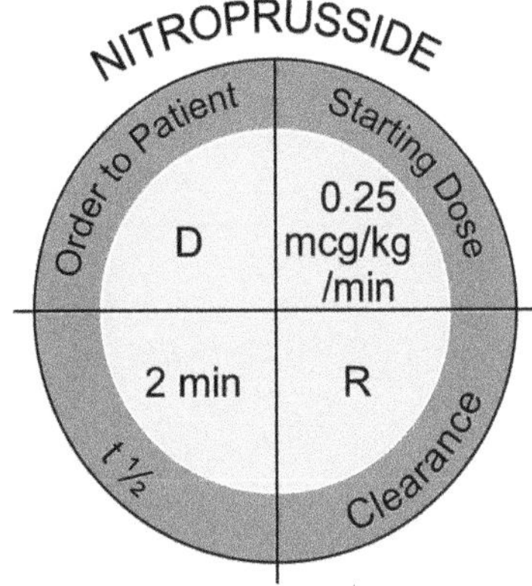

Pharmacologic Characteristics

- May be used in patients who have ingested sympathomimetic drugs and cocaine
- Avoid in acute brain injury because it may increase intracranial pressure, and there is concern about cyanide toxicity
- Often used in patients with aortic dissection in combination with beta-blocker (e.g., esmolol, labetalol)
- Cost of this medication has recently increased dramatically, making its use almost obsolete
- Onset: rapid, 1–2 minutes
- Duration: short, <10 minutes

Dosing and Administration

- IV infusion: 0.25–0.5 mcg/kg per minute, increased to effective dose of 8–10 mcg/kg per minute (higher doses should be avoided or limited to a duration of 10 minutes)

Monitoring

- Can produce a sudden or drastic decrease in blood pressure
- Dose-related decline in coronary, renal, and cerebral perfusion

Side Effects

- May result in toxic accumulation of cyanide
  - Can manifest as early as 4 hours into infusion
  - Presents as lactic acidosis
  - Risk factors for cyanide toxicity include renal or hepatic impairment, doses >2 mcg/kg per minute for 2–3 days (prolonged), or doses 10 mcg/kg per minute for >10 minutes (high dose)
  - Sodium thiosulfate infusion is used to provide sulfur donor to detoxify cyanide
- Angina
- Ataxia
- Seizures
- Stroke

Clevidipine IV

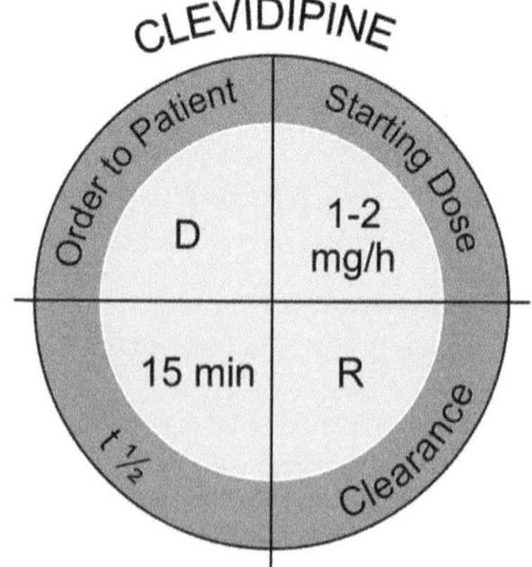

Pharmacologic Characteristics

- Third-generation calcium-channel blocker
- Rapid onset, <1 minute
- No effect on cardiac filling pressure
- Some reflexive tachycardia
- Contraindicated in patients with severe aortic stenosis (risk of severe hypotension)
- Very short half-life (15 minutes) compared to others and possible quick rebound after discontinuation
- Expensive

Dosing and Administration

- IV infusion of 1–2 mg/hr (maximum dose of 21 mg/hr)
- Double the dose every 90 seconds to achieve blood pressure control

- Dedicated line is needed for administration
- Can be administered peripherally

Monitoring

- Replace bottle every 12 hours
- Provides 2 kcal/ml from fat; calories should be counted toward daily nutrition allotments
- Limited experience with usage duration of >72 hours
- Allergies to eggs or soy (used in the emulsion)

Side Effects

- Nausea
- Dyslipidemia (lipid emulsion vehicle)

Amlodipine PO

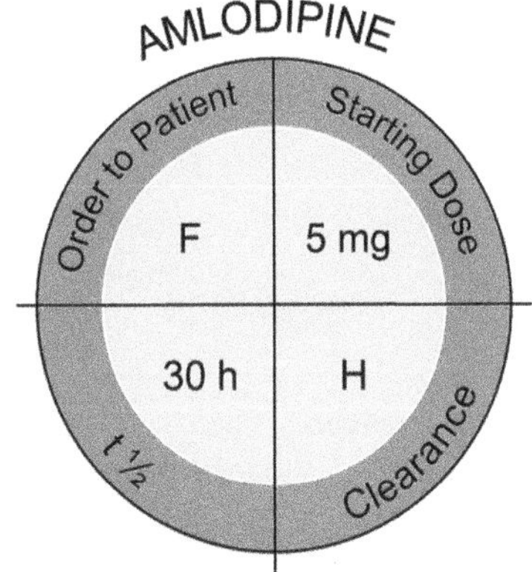

Pharmacologic Characteristics

- Calcium-channel blocker
- Vasodilator of peripheral arteries
- Blood pressure reduction at 24–48 hours (slower onset)
- Onset: 30–50 minutes; peak effect: 6–9 hours (single dose)

Dosing and Administration

- Initial dose: 5 mg/day
- Maximum dose: 10 mg once daily (range 2.5–10 mg once daily)
- Titrate every 7–14 days with a starting dose of 2.5 mg once daily

Monitoring

- No dose adjustment in patients with renal impairment
- When used with simvastatin, the maximum dose of simvastatin should not exceed 20 mg/day due to increased risk of myalgia and rhabdomyolysis (inhibited simvastatin metabolism due to CYP3A4)

- Concomitant ingestion of grapefruit juice can increase amlodipine levels, increasing risk for hypotension

Side Effects

- Peripheral edema (most common side effect; can occur within 2–3 weeks)
- Pulmonary edema (use caution in heart failure patients)
- Increased risk for angina pectoris

Lisinopril PO

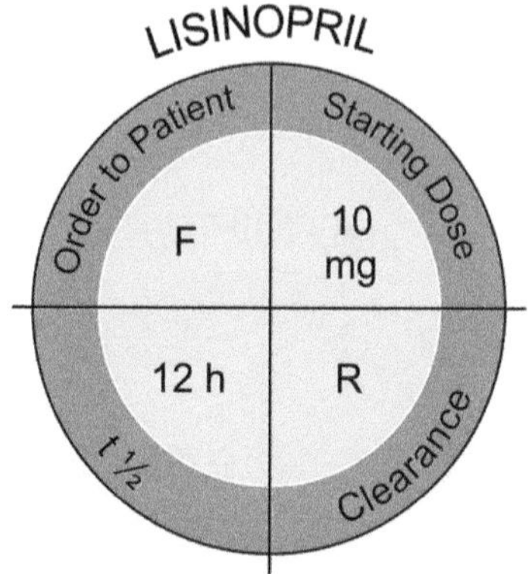

Pharmacologic Characteristics

- ACE inhibitor and potent vasodilator (prevents conversion of angiotensin I to angiotensin II, causing an increase in plasma renin levels and a reduction in aldosterone secretion)
- Recommended first-line agent to improve kidney function in patients with hypertension and chronic kidney disease (regardless of race or diabetes)
- Contraindications: angioedema with other ACE inhibitors, idiopathic or hereditary angioedema, pregnancy (teratogenic), or plasma exchange (causes unopposed bradykinin release, resulting in profound decreases in blood pressure)
- Onset: 7 hours; duration: 24 hours

Dosing and Administration

- 10 mg orally once daily; target dose 40 mg
- 5 mg orally once daily if patient is maintained on a diuretic
- Doses up to 80 mg/day have been used with a significant increase in blood pressure response
- In patients with moderate renal dysfunction (creatinine clearance [CrCl] 10–30 ml/min), start at 5 mg daily
- In patients with severe renal dysfunction (CrCl < 10 ml/min), start at 2.5 mg/day

- In patients undergoing hemodialysis, start at 2.5 mg/day
- No dose adjustments needed in patients with hepatic dysfunction

Monitoring

- Electrolytes (e.g., potassium)
- Blood pressure
- Change in renal function, serum creatinine

Side Effects

- Acute renal failure
- Angioedema
- Dizziness
- Cough
- Hyperkalemia
- Cholestatic jaundice

Losartan PO

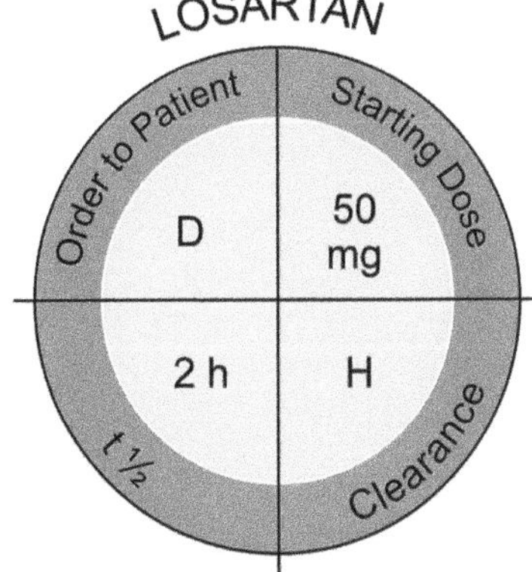

Pharmacologic Characteristics

- ARB: blocks vasoconstrictive properties of angiotensin II on the receptor, thus allowing vasodilation
- Elevated levels of renin, angiotensin I, and angiotensin II
- Similar efficacy in lowering blood pressure as ACE inhibitors
- Not recommended for blood pressure management in blacks
- Slow onset: adjust dose weekly; full effects may not be seen for up to 3 weeks

Dosing and Administration

- Initial: 50 mg orally once daily; range 25–100 mg/day
- Start at 25 mg orally once daily with diuretics
- May need to be administered twice daily to achieve adequate blood pressure control (better steady-state maintenance)

- No dosage adjustments needed in patients with renal dysfunction
- Reduce dose to 25 mg once daily in patients with hepatic dysfunction

Monitoring

- Blood pressure
- Renal function, serum creatinine
- Electrolytes (e.g., potassium)

Side Effects

- Cough (lower incidence than seen with ACE inhibitors)
- Hypotension
- Hyperkalemia
- Angioedema
- Renal failure

Enalaprilat IV

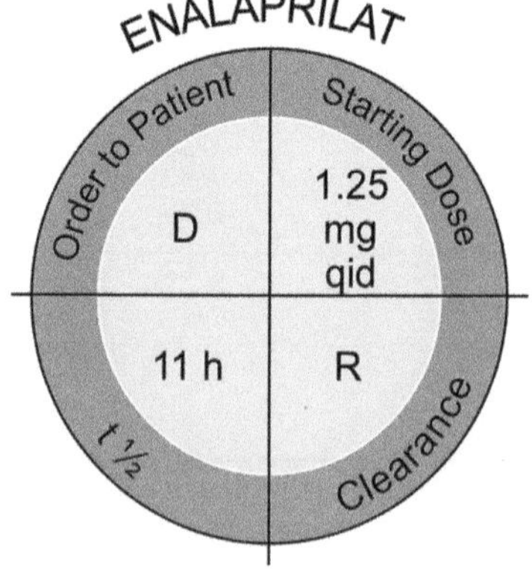

Pharmacologic Characteristics

- Active ester formulation of the ACE inhibitor enalapril
- Vasodilator
- Onset: 15 minutes
- Peak effect up to 4 hours after dose

Dosing and Administration

- Initial dose: 1.25 mg bolus IV
- Maximum: 5 mg every 6 hours IV
- IV to oral dosing (enalaprilat to enalapril) conversion: 1.25 mg IV every 6 hours = 5 mg orally once daily

Monitoring

- Blood pressure lability

- Renal function
- Electrolytes

Side Effects

- Hypotensive effect is dependent on plasma volume and renin activity
- Hypovolemic patients with high renin plasma activity have greater hypotensive response
- Cough
- Angioedema
- Hyperkalemia
- Worsening renal function

Verapamil PO

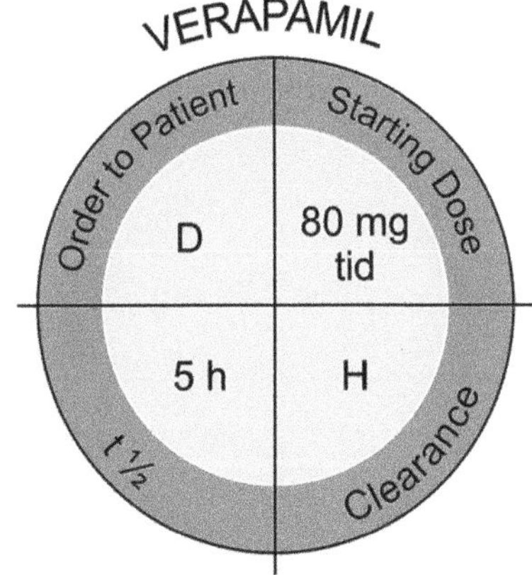

Pharmacologic Characteristics

- Preferred for hypertension control in patients with chronic kidney disease
- Calcium-channel-receptor blocker with ionotropic and antiarrhythmic properties
- Reduces signal conduction through the atrioventricular node
- Increases myocardial oxygen supply and reduces demand
- Minimal vasodilator properties (when compared to other calcium-channel blockers)
- Onset: 30 minutes; peak effect: 1–2 hours

Dosing and Administration

- 80–120 mg orally three times daily
- Maximal dose: 360 mg/day
- Do not crush extended-release products.
- Reduce dose in patients with liver cirrhosis
- Half-life is prolonged in patients with hepatic dysfunction

Monitoring

- Monitor for electrocardiographic (EKG) changes
- Avoid use in patients with heart failure (lack of benefit), left ventricular dysfunction, second- or third-degree block
- Can increase intracranial pressure in patients with supratentorial brain tumors

Side Effects

- Conduction abnormality causing first-degree atrioventricular block with sinus bradycardia
- Headache
- Constipation
- Increased transaminase levels

Hydrochlorothiazide (HCTZ) PO

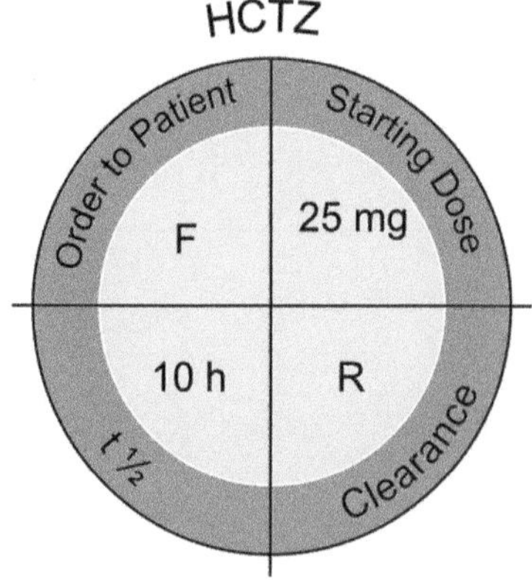

Pharmacologic Characteristics

- Thiazide diuretic
- Contraindicated in patients with sulfonamide-derived drug allergies
- Ineffective in patients with CrCl < 30 ml/min unless given in combination with a loop diuretic

Dosing and Administration

- 12.5–25 mg once daily orally; increase to maximum dose of 50 mg/day
- No dose adjustment is necessary in patients with renal impairment but contraindicated in anuria

Monitoring

- More electrolyte abnormalities are seen with higher doses (doses >50 mg/day)
- Blood pressure response
- Fluid balance, weight

Side Effects

- Hypotension
- Hypercalcemia, hyperglycemia, hyperuricemia
- Hypokalemia, hyponatremia, hypomagnesemia
- Hypersensitivity reaction
- Hemolytic anemia
- Thrombocytopenia, leukopenia
- Photosensitivity

Clonidine PO

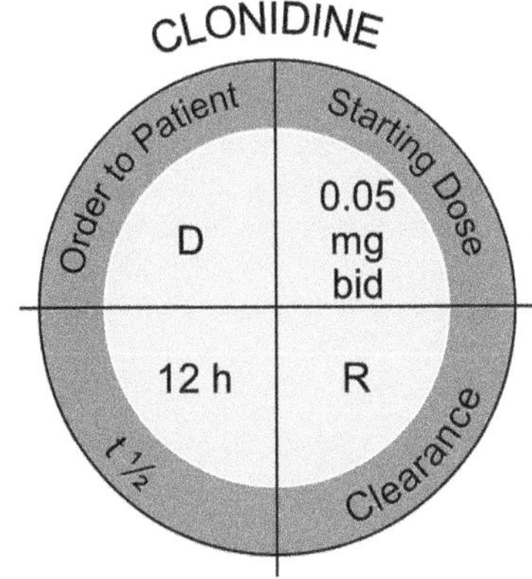

Pharmacologic Characteristics

- Central-acting alpha-2 agonist
- Has benefit in treatment of sympathetic storming by reducing sympathetic outflow from the central nervous system
- Decreases peripheral resistance, renal vascular resistance, blood pressure, and heart rate
- Onset: 30–60 minutes; peak: 2–4 hours
- Transdermal patch: onset after 2–3 days (not intended for acute blood pressure control)

Dosing and Administration

- 0.1 mg twice daily orally, to maximum 2.4 mg/day in divided doses
- Prolonged elimination in patients with renal dysfunction

Monitoring

- Marked rebound effect if discontinued abruptly
- Change patch weekly
- Blood pressure, heart rate

Side Effects

- Marked bradycardia
- Hypotension
- Rebound hypertension

Control of Blood Pressure After Urgent Control

Transitioning to an oral drug occurs after the neurologic injury has stabilized and hypertension has been controlled. Oral administration often involves a combination of antihypertensives, and several can be considered. Generally, the first-line antihypertensive is a thiazide diuretic, a calcium-channel blocker, an ACE inhibitor, or an ARB, but it is best to avoid combinations of ACE inhibitors and ARBs. For blacks, ACE inhibitors and ARBs are much less effective and calcium-channel blockers or thiazide diuretics are recommended for initial management (18).

The use of antihypertensive drugs to prevent recurrence of stroke is currently based on best evidence obtained from a meta-analysis of eight randomized trials (19). There is consensus that a combination of an ACE inhibitor and a long-acting calcium-channel blocker is preferred. The ACCOMPLISH trial (20) argued for the use of amlodipine with benazepril. In elderly patients, a low-dose thiazide, ACE inhibitor, or long-acting calcium-channel blocker is preferred.

Antiarrhythmic Drugs

The most common arrhythmias in the neurosciences ICU are sinus tachycardia or sinus bradycardia, atrial fibrillation (or flutter) with rapid ventricular response, paroxysmal supraventricular tachycardia, and, rarely, ventricular tachycardia and torsades de pointes (21) (Table 13.2). Cardiac arrhythmias

Table 13.2 Cardiac Arrhythmias in the Neurosciences ICU

• Drug-induced arrhythmias	• Levofloxacin • Fosphenytoin • Nicardipine • Quetiapine • Ondansetron
• Electrolyte abnormalities	• Hypomagnesemia • Hypokalemia • Hypocalcemia
• Acute pulmonary embolus	
• Acute myocardial ischemia	
• Posterior fossa surgery	
• Brainstem compression/shift	
• Aneurysmal subarachnoid hemorrhage	
• Marked vasovagal response often due to vomiting	

Table 13.3 Antiarrhythmic Drugs	
Arrhythmia	**Commonly used therapy**
Sinus tachycardia	Metoprolol
Atrial fibrillation and rapid ventricular rate	Metoprolol (22,23) Diltiazem Amiodarone
Paroxysmal supraventricular tachycardia	Verapamil
Ventricular tachycardia	Magnesium sulfate (21) Amiodarone
Sinus bradycardia	Atropine

are often attributed to a "central effect" (the acute brain lesion), but the possibility of electrolyte abnormalities, drug effects, or structural myocardial disease should be explored.

The maximum heart rate decreases with age, and tachycardia may result in increased oxygen demand. The maximum tolerable heart rate is 210 – age (in years), and this is a reasonable target. Anti-arrhythmic drugs for each of these conditions are shown in Table 13.3.

Diltiazem IV

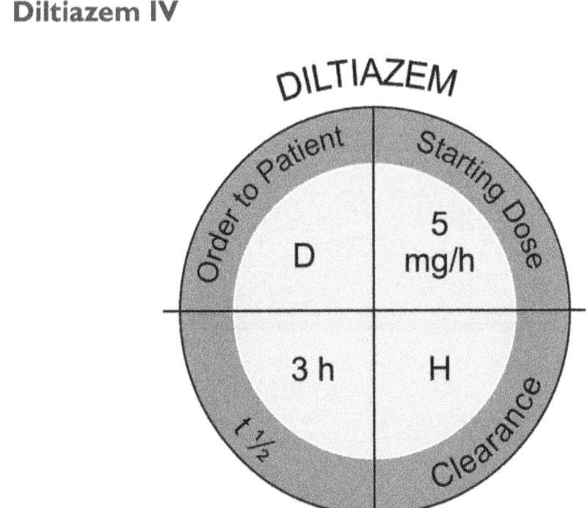

Pharmacologic Characteristics

- Moderate vasodilation
- Decrease in cardiac contractility, sinoatrial node automaticity, and atrioventricular node conduction
- Specifically for rate control in atrial fibrillation, or atrial flutter (heart rate >120 beats per minute)
- Onset (IV): immediate, 3 minutes

Dosing and Administration

- Loading dose 0.25 mg/kg (~20 mg) over 2 minutes IV; repeat dose after 15 minutes to 0.35 mg/kg if no control
- Infusion dose: 5–15 mg/hr
- IV to oral transition [rate (mg/hr) × 3 + 3] × 10
  - 3 mg/hr: 120 mg/day orally
  - 5 mg/hr: 180 mg/day orally
  - 7 mg/hr: 240 mg/day orally
  - 11 mg/hr: 360 mg/day orally
- Hepatically metabolized; may require dose adjustments in patients with liver dysfunction

Monitoring

- Duration of IV use >24 hours: possibility of decreased drug clearance, prolonged half-life, and increased diltiazem or metabolite concentrations
- Not removed by intermittent dialysis
- EKG
- Blood pressure, heart rate
- Liver function tests (periodically)

Side Effects

- Bradycardia
- Hypotension

Amiodarone IV

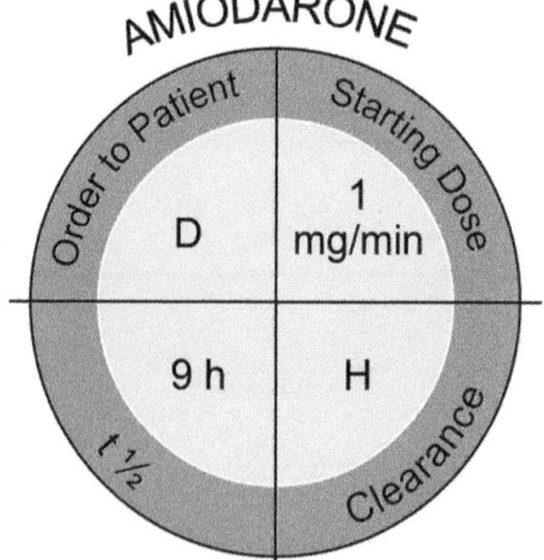

Pharmacologic Characteristics

- Blocks sodium channels (class I antiarrhythmic property)
- Blocks myocardial potassium and calcium channels (class II antiarrhythmic property)

- To treat ventricular tachycardia and rate control in atrial fibrillation
- Lengthens cardiac action potential (class III antiarrhythmic property)
- Some negative ionotropic effects (class IV antiarrhythmic property)
- Extensively metabolized by the liver via CYP enzymes
- Prolonged half-life: 53 days (after chronic administration), 9 hours (after single IV dose)

Dosing and Administration

- 150 mg IV load, given over 10 minutes
- 1 mg/min infusion (6 hours), followed by 0.5 mg/min infusion in remaining 18 hours
- Oral dose: 800 mg, when blood pressure control achieved but lower dose later (aiming at 200–400 mg daily)

Monitoring

- Liver function tests
- Thyroid function (long-term use)
- Drug–drug interactions (potent inhibitor of CYP3A4, 1A2, 2C9, and 2D6)
- Electrolytes (magnesium and potassium)
- EKG
- Heart rate and blood pressure
- Baseline chest x-ray

Side Effects

- Interstitial pneumonitis
- Phlebitis
- QT prolongation
- Hypothyroidism
- Hepatotoxicity

Metoprolol IV

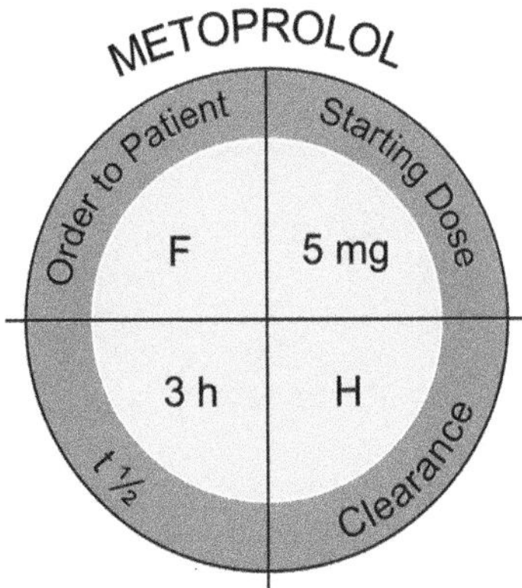

Pharmacologic Characteristics

- Selective beta-1-receptor blocker (blocks binding catecholamines to beta-1 receptor located on cardiac smooth muscles)
- Inhibits adrenergic stimulation and slows conduction through the atrioventricular node
- For rate control in sinus tachycardia and atrial fibrillation

Dosing and Administration

- 2.5–5 mg IV bolus over 2 minutes; may repeat up to maximum 15 mg
- 25 mg orally twice a day; titrate up to 100 mg orally twice a day (maximal dose is 150 mg three times a day)
- 1:2.5 ratio for IV to oral conversion (e.g., 5 mg IV every 6 hours = 25 mg orally twice daily)
- Half-life prolonged in patients with hepatic dysfunction
- No dosage adjustments in patients with renal impairment

Monitoring

- Liver function tests; adjust with abnormal values
- Heart rate, blood pressure
- EKG

Side Effects

- Hypotension
- Bradycardia
- Bronchospasm (at high doses)
- Hyperkalemia (slight increase)
- Prolonged hypoglycemia response (in type I diabetics)

Atropine IV

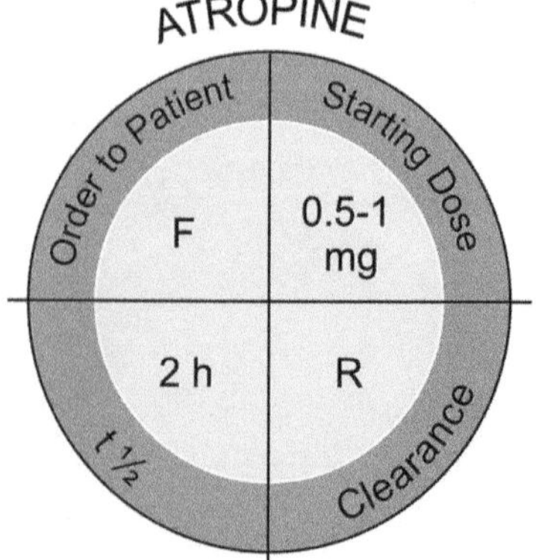

Pharmacologic Characteristics

- Anticholinergic drug; antagonizes the muscarine-like activity of acetylcholine

- For acute symptomatic bradycardia (e.g., hypotension, syncope, atrioventricular block)

Dosing and Administration

- 0.5 mg IV every 3–5 minutes to maximum total dose of 3 mg

Monitoring

- Tachycardia
- Use caution in patients with significant renal insufficiency

Side Effects

- Somnolence
- Anticholinergic effects of mydriasis, flushing
- Urinary retention in patients with prostatic hypertrophy
- Fever, dry mouth, decreased bowel sounds

Key Pointers

1. The preferred first-line treatment of hypertension in acute brain injury is IV labetalol or IV nicardipine.
2. Most blood pressures can be targeted at SBP of 140 mmHg and DBP of 90 mmHg for 24 hours.
3. After thrombolysis, keep SBP <180 mmHg and DBP <105 mmHg for at least 24 hours.
4. Most common arrhythmia is atrial fibrillation with rapid ventricular rate and is treated with IV metoprolol, IV diltiazem, or IV amiodarone.
5. IV atropine is needed only for symptomatic bradycardia.

References

1. Papadopoulos, D.P., et al., *Cardiovascular hypertensive emergencies.* Curr Hypertens Rep, 2015. **17**: 5.
2. Ipek, E., Oktay, A.A. and Krim, S.R. *Hypertensive crisis: an update on clinical approach and management.* Curr Opin Cardiol, 2017. **32**: 397–406.
3. Ropper, A.H. and Wijdicks, E.F. *Blood pressure fluctuations in the dysautonomia of Guillain-Barre syndrome.* Arch Neurol, 1990. **47**: 706–708.
4. Shannon, J.R., et al., *Sympathetically mediated hypertension in autonomic failure.* Circulation, 2000. **101**: 2710–2715.
5. Pollack, C.V., et al., *Clevidipine, an intravenous dihydropyridine calcium channel blocker, is safe and effective for the treatment of patients with acute severe hypertension.* Ann Emerg Med, 2009. **53**: 329–338.
6. Lattanzi, S., et al., *Blood pressure variability and clinical outcome in patients with acute intracerebral hemorrhage.* J Stroke Cerebrovasc Dis, 2015. **24**: 1493–1499.
7. Butcher, K.S., et al., *The Intracerebral Hemorrhage Acutely Decreasing Arterial Pressure Trial.* Stroke, 2013. **44**: 620–626.
8. Qureshi, A.I., et al., *Intensive blood-pressure lowering in patients with acute cerebral hemorrhage.* N Engl J Med, 2016. **375**: 1033–1043.

9. Cohn, J.N., McInnes, G.T. and Shepherd, A.M. *Direct-acting vasodilators.* J Clin Hypertens (Greenwich), 2011. **13**: 690–692.

10. Elliott, W.J. and Ram, C.V. *Calcium channel blockers.* J Clin Hypertens (Greenwich), 2011. **13**: 687–689.

11. Epstein, M. and Calhoun, D.A. *Aldosterone blockers (mineralocorticoid receptor antagonism) and potassium-sparing diuretics.* J Clin Hypertens (Greenwich), 2011. **13**: 644–648.

12. Frishman, W.H. and Saunders, E. *Beta-adrenergic blockers.* J Clin Hypertens (Greenwich), 2011. **13**: 649–653.

13. Grimm, R.H., Jr. and Flack, J.M. *Alpha 1 adrenoreceptor antagonists.* J Clin Hypertens (Greenwich), 2011. **13**: 654–657.

14. Izzo, J.L., Jr. and Weir, M.R. *Angiotensin-converting enzyme inhibitors.* J Clin Hypertens (Greenwich), 2011. **13**: 667–675.

15. Taylor, A.A., Siragy, H. and Nesbitt, S. *Angiotensin receptor blockers: pharmacology, efficacy, and safety.* J Clin Hypertens (Greenwich), 2011. **13**: 677–686.

16. Olson-Chen, C. and Seligman, N.S. *Hypertensive emergencies in pregnancy.* Crit Care Clin, 2016. **32**: 29–41.

17. ElFarra, J., Bean, C. and Martin, Jr., J.N. *Management of hypertensive crisis for the obstetrician/gynecologist.* Obstet Gynecol Clin North Am, 2016. **43**: 623–637.

18. James, P.A., et al., *2014 evidence-based guideline for the management of high blood pressure in adults: report from the panel members appointed to the Eighth Joint National Committee (JNC 8).* JAMA, 2014. **311**: 507–520.

19. Lee, M., et al., *Renin-angiotensin system modulators modestly reduce vascular risk in persons with prior stroke.* Stroke, 2012. **43**: 113–119.

20. Jamerson, K., et al., *Benazepril plus amlodipine or hydrochlorothiazide for hypertension in high-risk patients.* N Engl J Med, 2008. **359**: 2417–2428.

21. Hsia, H.H., *Ventricular tachycardias.* Card Electrophysiol Clin, 2016. **8**: 75–78.

22. Khoo, C.W. and Lip, G.Y.H. *Acute management of atrial fibrillation.* Chest, 2009. **135**: 849–859.

23. Hassan, O.F., Al Suwaidi J., and Salam, A.M. *Anti-arrhythmic agents in the treatment of atrial fibrillation.* J Atr Fibrillation, 2013. **6**: 864.

24. Sharma C, Soni A, Gupta A, et al Hydralazine vs nifedipine for acute hypertensive emergency in pregnancy: a randomized controlled trial.Am J Obstet Gynecol. 2017. pii: S0002-9378(17)30965-1

Chapter 14

Fluid Therapy

Although technically not a drug, intravenous (IV) fluids and the far more consequential fluid resuscitation are common therapeutic interventions in patients with critical illness. Surveys of current practices have shown that crystalloids are preferred by intensivists. There are good reasons for the growing consternation with current fluid resuscitation practices, with many intensivists arguing for a more restrictive approach. Excessive fluid therapy may cause fluid overload with pulmonary edema, putting demand on the cardiac system ("fluid creep"). Fluid overload might promote infection due to an altered immune system and may interfere with coagulation; in particular, crystalloids may promote a hypercoagulable state. Equally concerning is that hemodilution is often responsible for unnecessary blood transfusions. A more recently identified concern is that the infusion of large amounts of saline may lead to hyperchloremic acidosis in critically ill patients, which might have an impact on coagulation and renal function. With all these warnings, fluid management has become a complicated therapeutic intervention.

Regulation of Fluid Status

Next to the intracellular volume, body water is found in the extracellular space, divided into the interstitial and intravascular volumes. Complex mechanisms that control homeostasis maintain two-thirds of body water in this extracellular space. The movement of body water across these compartments is largely determined by osmotic forces. Solutes that cannot freely cross the cell membrane may produce an osmotic gradient and thus influence the distribution of body water between compartments. This active osmotic state (usually between intracellular and extracellular fluids separated by a cell membrane) is called *tonicity.* Sodium is a typical example of a solute that cannot move freely across the cellular membrane and therefore increases tonicity. The primary determinant of plasma osmolality is plasma sodium concentration, which is thus a major factor in fluid shifts across the compartments.

Hypovolemia triggers at least three physiologic pathways: antidiuretic hormone (ADH), renin, and norepinephrine, all of which enhance sodium reabsorption. At the collecting duct, ADH increases water and sodium reabsorption by binding to its receptor and activating the water channel protein aquaporin. In the proximal tubule cells, sodium reabsorption is increased by the activation of renin-angiotensin II. Aldosterone also is stimulated, increasing reabsorption of sodium at the distal tubule and collection duct. Norepinephrine and epinephrine decrease the glomerular filtration rate and enhance sodium reabsorption at the proximal tubule.

Hypervolemia, in contrast, stimulates sodium excretion through natriuretic peptides and suppression of the vasopressor hormones. The natriuretic peptides suppress sympathetic tone and the renin angiotensin II–aldosterone axis, and block the renal effects of ADH. Atrial natriuretic peptide inhibits thirst and the appetite for salt.

General Principles of Fluid Management

Fluid management in acute brain injury requires maintenance of an adequate intravascular fluid volume, which, in turn, maintains hemodynamics and vital signs. This is best achieved with the use of isotonic fluids. Normal saline (0.9% sodium chloride) is widely used because it maintains serum osmolality and is a common choice for fluid bolus administration during resuscitation.

The most important goal when deciding which maintenance fluid to administer is to approximate insensible losses from lungs and skin and to compensate for excessive diuresis or fluid loss from fever (Fig. 14.1). Insensible fluid loss is often underestimated.

Daily fluid requirements are shown in Box 14.1. Gastrointestinal losses average 250 ml/day, and the increased evaporation associated with fever ranges widely and can amount to 500 ml per degree Celsius. Diarrhea associated with gut feeding may result in additional, largely imperceptible losses. Sweating can be profuse in patients with traumatic brain injury, typically occurring in association with tachycardia, hyperthermia, and tachypnea (paroxysmal sympathetic hyperactivity) (1).

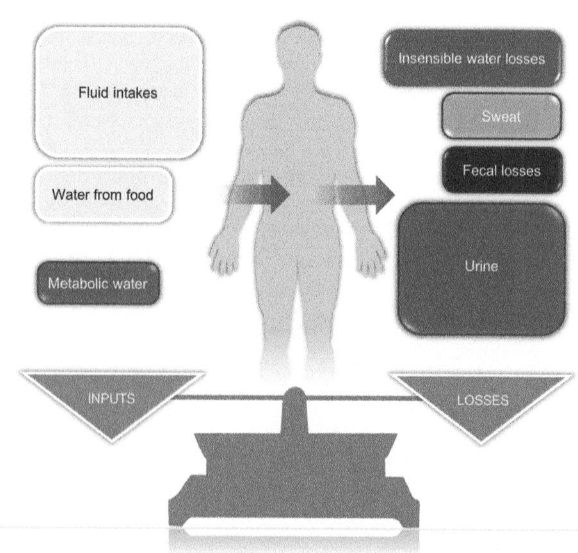

Figure 14.1 Fluid intake and fluid losses

Box 14.1 Daily Fluid Requirement

- 30–40 ml/kg per day
- Maintain urine output ≥0.5 ml/kg per hour
- Match urinary output
- With fever, increase of 500 ml per degree Celsius
- 1.5% NaCl with trending hyponatremia
- 0.45% NaCl with trending hypernatremia

Fluids and Administration

Crystalloids are solutions in which sodium is the major osmotically active particle (e.g., isotonic saline, lactated Ringer's solution, hypertonic saline). 0.9% sodium chloride is slightly hypertonic to plasma (308 mOsm/kg vs. plasma osmolality of 289 mOsm/kg). The distribution of this fluid when administered will follow the normal rule of proportions; thus, only 250 ml of every liter will remain in the intravascular compartment.

Colloids work by changing the intravascular plasma colloid osmotic pressure, which normally is in balance with the interstitial colloid osmotic pressure. Colloid solutions change the whole blood rheology because the large molecules cannot pass through the capillary membrane and attract water. With colloids, the volume administered intravascularly does not distribute, and 250 ml iso-osmotic colloids (5% albumin) results in an approximately similar change in volume. Hyperosmotic solutions (25% albumin) will draw far more into the intravascular system and will pull fluid from the brain into the vasculature; in contrast, hypotonic fluids will permeate the blood–brain barrier and pull fluid into the brain, potentially worsening cerebral edema. Albumin 5% expands intravascular volume by only 15 ml of water per gram, but albumin 25% expands intravascular volume five times more than the infused volume. This difference is explained by a much higher colloid osmotic pressure, which is the major determinant of fluid distribution. The effect of both types of albumin lasts at least 24 hours. Still, most of the total body albumin moves into the extravascular compartment.

To summarize: Crystalloids distribute over the fluid volumes proportionally, assuming a 1:3 distribution; thus, a 1-L infusion results in 250 ml in the intravascular space and 750 ml in the interstitial space but lasts not more than an hour or so. Colloids are fluids with macromolecules that are dissolved in saline over other salt solutions to increase the plasma oncotic pressure and thus remain in a vascular compartment longer, up to 16 hours. Distribution over the fluid compartments is reversed to 3:1; thus, a 1-L infusion will retain 750 ml in the intravascular space. Moreover, the volume-expanding effect of albumin when compared to crystalloid is 1 versus 1.5 L (1,2). Hypertonic saline solutions are basically volume expanders, and 250 ml will attract 1,750 ml from the interstitial space. When 250 ml of 7.5% sodium chloride is administered, the intravascular volume will increase three- to fourfold due to its osmotic effect of drawing in water (Fig. 14.2).

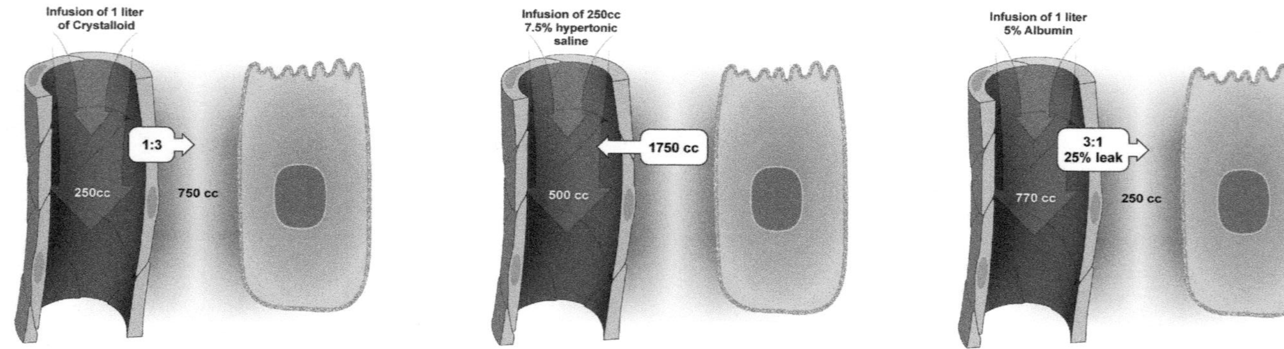

Figure 14.2 Distribution of crystalloids and colloids (isotonic and hypotonic saline) over compartments

Box 14.2 Infusion Rate of Fluids Using Different Techniques

- Gravity flow not more than 125 ml/min IV
- Pressure-infusion bag, IV flow rate is three times faster
- Manual squeezing, IV flow rate is doubled
- Intraosseous flow rates are variable; may reach pressure bag rates (3,4)

Most importantly, the clinician should remember that after aggressive fluid resuscitation, the interstitial space has increased and the 3:1 ratio may have doubled. This implies that over time, fluids stay in the intervascular space to a lesser degree, and they lose the effectiveness to expand the intravascular volume.

Fluids are administered with usually two large-bore IV access catheters (16-gauge) and are obtained emergently; If veins cannot be cannulated and fluid administration is urgently required, use of an intraosseous tibial drill is considered. (The network of venous sinusoids in the tibia does not collapse during hypotension or hypovolemia and allows a gravity-driven flow rate of up to 4 ml/min.)

Once venous access is secured, a 500-ml IV fluid bag is started at a rate of 70 to 100 ml/hr, depending on the need for further fluid resuscitation. Rate-increasing techniques (Box 14.2) should be used if fluid administration does not appear to have a measurable effect.

Several fluid solutions are available in the hospital setting, and their pharmacologic characteristics and side effects are shown in Table 14.1. The clinician should remember that IV drugs are administered with saline or sucrose vehicles, and the volume may amount to considerable quantities in patient receiving multiple drugs. Some examples are shown in Table 14.2.

Table 14.1 Fluid Solutions

	0.9% Sodium Chloride	Ringer's Lactate	10% Dextran-70	5% Albumin	25% Albumin
Osmolality (mOsm/L)	285–310	250–270	280–325	290	310
Half-life	0.5 hour	0.5 hour	48 hours	20 days	20 days
Side effects	Risk for hyperchloremic acidosis Dilutional coagulopathy	Risk for hyperkalemia Endothelial dysfunction	Anaphylaxis Coagulopathy	Anaphylaxis Fluid overload Increased mortality in patients with tramatic brain injury	Anaphylaxis Fluid overload
Duration of expansion	1–4 hours	1–4 hours	6 hours	12–24 hours	12–24 hours
Sodium (mmol/L)	154	130	154	130–160	130–160
Chloride (mmol/L)	154	109	154	130–160	130–160

Table 14.2 Fluids Associated with IV Drug Administration

Drug	Infusion Volume
Cefazolin	1 g, 50 ml
Cefepime	1 g, 50 ml
Famotidine	20 and 40 mg, 50 ml
Levetiracetam	All doses, 100 ml
Pantoprazole	40 mg, 100 ml
Potassium chloride	10 mEq/100 ml
Valproic acid	All doses, 50 ml
Vancomycin	<1,750 mg, 250 ml; >1,750 mg, 500 ml
Piperacillin/tazobactam	2.25 g, 50 ml; 3.375 g, 50 ml; 4.5 g, 100 ml

Types of fluids

Ringer's Lactate

Pharmacologic Characteristics

- Osmolality: 250–275 mOsm/L
- Relative hypotonic
- Plasma half-life: 1–4 hours
- Contains more lactate, more potassium, but less sodium than 0.9% NaCl

Dosing and Administration

- 250–500 ml initial replacement, over 30 minutes

Monitoring

- Abdominal ultrasound
- Lactate and potassium levels
- Chest x-ray

Side Effects

- Increased risk of hypervolemia
- Increased risk of hyponatremia
- Increased risk of metabolic alkalosis (lactate increases pH) with multiple infusions
- Hyperkalemia

Crystalloids

Pharmacologic Characteristics

- Normal saline (0.9% NaCl) osmolality 285–310 mOsm/L
- Isotonic (5)
- Plasma half-life: 1–4 hours

Dosing and Administration

- Preferred maintenance fluid in neurocritical care patients
- 250–500 ml initial replacement, over 30 minutes

Monitoring

- Abdominal ultrasound
- Electrolytes (sodium and chloride)
- Chest x-ray

Side Effects

- Large volumes cause hyperchloremic metabolic acidosis
- May cause hypernatremia due to delayed excretion of salt and water load
- High chloride load could reduce renal function (by inducing renal artery vasoconstriction)

Colloids

Pharmacologic Characteristics

- Expands intravascular volume five times more than infused volume
- Duration of expansion: 12 hours
- Albumin 5%
  - Plasma half-life: 16–24 hours
  - Osmolality: 290 mOsm/L
  - Administer at a rate no faster than 2–4 ml/min when the patient is euvolemic, 5–10 ml/min in a patient with hypoproteinemia
  - Preferred option for pure fluid deficit correction
- Albumin 25%
  - Plasma half-life: 16–24 hours
  - Osmolality: 310 mOsm/L
  - Administer at a rate no faster than 1 ml/min when the patient is euvolemic, 2–3 ml/min in a patient with hypoproteinemia
  - Preferred option when oncotic or osmotic effects are desired
  - Can be administered with furosemide

Dosing and Administration

- 250 ml; may repeat
- More than 500 ml is seldom administered for resuscitation

Monitoring

- Abdominal ultrasound
- Electrolytes
- Hemodynamic properties
- Urine output/fluid balance
- Chest x-ray

Side Effects

- Increased mortality in traumatic brain injury (6)
- Associated with increased intracranial pressure (7)
- Increased fluid overload and transfusion-associated circulatory overload (TACO)
- All colloids increase the risk for allergic reactions
- Potential for transmittable diseases

Dextrans

Pharmacologic Characteristics

- Dextran-70 10%
- Osmolality: 280–235 mOsm/L
- Plasma half-life: 4–6 hours

Dosing and Administration

- 500 ml, but no more than 20 ml/kg IV during first 24 hours

Monitoring

- Abdominal ultrasound
- Electrolytes
- Chest x-ray
- Blood pressure and heart rate
- Renal function
- Urine output/fluid balance

Side Effects

- Anaphylactoid reactions
- Interferes with blood cross-matching

Fluid Management Principles in the Neurosciences ICU

- Critically ill patients are more prone to disturbances in intravascular volume, electrolyte shifts/balances, and osmotic changes from neuroendocrine changes (8)
- Avoid hypotonicity
- There is no role for dextrose-based solutions in patients with acute neurologic disorders unless a severe hypernatremia needs correction. Large volumes of dextrose-containing solutions may worsen hyperglycemia. (Hyperglycemia and anaerobic cerebral glucose metabolism result in toxic accumulation of lactate and intracellular acidosis, which in turn, may set off lipid peroxidation and free radical formation.)
- Hypertonic solutions (starting with 3% NaCl and higher) need a central access to prevent severe phlebitis, which may occur with only a single bolus

- Subarachnoid hemorrhage
  - Euvolemia is the main goal to prevent cerebral vasospasm with isotonic solutions; avoid hypotonic or hypertonic fluids
  - Hypovolemia is associated with more symptomatic cerebral vasospasm
  - Hypervolemia is associated with poor functional outcomes and more cardiovascular side effects (9)
  - With persistent negative fluid balance, start fludrocortisone (10)
- Ischemic stroke
  - Give isotonic fluids and avoid hypovolemia
  - Avoid dextrose containing fluids
  - Daily fluid management of 30 ml/kg body weight (11)
- Traumatic brain injury
  - Give isotonic fluids
  - Conflicting evidence exists for albumin use; the general consensus is to avoid it
  - Ringer's lactate may show promise, with improved control of intracranial pressure, a better electrolyte profile, and decreased fluid intake with potential metabolic benefits (12)

Volume Depletion and Acute Resuscitation

Clinical signs of volume depletion, such as reduced skin turgor and dry skin, are far from reliable. Progressive oliguria (to less than 20 ml per hour), mild tachycardia, and "soft" blood pressures are some of the more common subtle signs.

Hypovolemia can be associated with increased serum creatinine and blood urea nitrogen (BUN) values, hypernatremia, hyperkalemia or hypokalemia, and metabolic alkalosis. The urine is relatively concentrated, with an osmolality often exceeding 450 mOsm/kg.

The BUN/serum creatinine ratio is approximately 10:1. In hypovolemia, there is a decrease in urea excretion (prerenal azotemia) and the BUN/serum creatinine ratio increases to greater than 20:1. The serum creatinine concentration will increase when hypovolemia reduces the glomerular filtration rate.

Often a 500-ml bolus of normal saline will improve parameters (16). Hyperhydration with unbalanced crystalloids can result in "salt water drowning." Excessive fluid loading may contribute to multisystem injury (gut edema, liver congestion, renal parenchymal edema). Extravascular lung water increase may lead to acute respiratory distress syndrome. Best parameter is mean arterial blood pressure (MAP). If there is evidence of sepsis, the current surviving sepsis campaign suggest 30ml/kg of IV crystalloid in the first 3 hours, but this recommendation has created a controversy (17,18).

The following actions are recommended:

- Crystalloids (13)
- 500 ml normal saline or 250 ml 5% albumin over 30 minutes (14,15)
- Elevate legs at 45 degrees (Trendelenburg position)
- Restrict fluid resuscitation (<3,000 ml/day)
- In a younger adult, aim for MAP of 55 mmHg
- In an older adult, aim for MAP of 65 mmHg

- Urine output is a good guide; 40 ml/hr is adequate
- No further fluids after improvement of oliguria and normalization of serum lactate levels
- The concept of "permissive hypotension" has emerged in trauma resuscitation. Many trauma resuscitation protocols include acceptance of a MAP between 50 and 65 mmHg
- Another new approach in trauma resuscitation is so-called balance transfusion, in which red blood cells and fresh-frozen plasma are provided in a ratio of 1 unit of red blood cells to 1 unit of fresh-frozen plasma

Fluid Overload and Prevention

Fluid overload is best defined as "fluid-in minus fluid-out" divided by admission weight multiplied by 100. Clinically, fluid overload may increase admission weight by 10% or result in clinically new pitting edema, crackles, and anasarca. An increase of intravascular volume by 20% could lead to pulmonary edema.

The following actions are recommended:

- Start vasopressor administration if hypotension persists after a crystalloid infusion of 30 ml/kg.
- A normal serum lactate level is the endpoint of fluid resuscitation.
- The passive leg-raising test can be used to predict fluid responsiveness in non-ventilated patients (14,15).
- Ultrasound can be used to measure pulse variation, stroke volume variation, and respiratory variation in the inferior vena cava.
- Restrict fluids in hemodynamically stable patients or initiate diuresis when the patient has been off vasopressors for 12 hours.
- Consider changing the dialysis plan if needed to achieve net negative fluid balances.

Key Pointers

1. Two large-bore IV access lines (16-gauge) are needed in any patient with acute brain injury.
2. Avoid hypovolemia in patients with acute brain injury (poor cerebral blood flow and oxygenation).
3. Administration of a large volume of crystalloid results in hyperchloremia and metabolic acidosis.
4. Euvolemia is the goal in most patients with an acute brain injury.
5. Synthetic colloids may be harmful in patients with traumatic brain injury.

References

1. Meyfroidt, G., Baguley, I.J. and Menon, D.K. *Paroxysmal sympathetic hyperactivity: the storm after acute brain injury.* Lancet Neurol, 2017. **16**: 721–729.
2. Frazee, E. and Kashani, K. *Fluid management for critically ill patients: a review of the current state of fluid therapy in the intensive care unit.* Kidney Dis (Basel), 2016. **2**: 64–71.

3. Petitpas, F., et al., *Use of intra-osseous access in adults: a systematic review.* Crit Care, 2016. **20**: 102.
4. White, S.J., Hamilton, W.A. and Veronesi, J.F. *A comparison of field techniques used to pressure-infuse intravenous fluids.* Prehosp Disaster Med, 1991. **6**: 429–434.
5. Kumar, G.W., E. and Stephens, R. *Intravenous fluid therapy.* Trends Anaesth Critical Care, 2014. **4**: 55–59.
6. Gantner, D., Moore, E.M. and Cooper, D.J. *Intravenous fluids in traumatic brain injury: what's the solution?* Curr Opin Crit Care, 2014. **20**: 385–359.
7. Cooper, D.J., et al., *Albumin resuscitation for traumatic brain injury: is intracranial hypertension the cause of increased mortality?* J Neurotrauma, 2013. **30**: 512–518.
8. van der Jagt, M., *Fluid management of the neurological patient: a concise review.* Crit Care, 2016. **20**: 126.
9. Martini, R.P., et al., *The association between fluid balance and outcomes after subarachnoid hemorrhage.* Neurocrit Care, 2012. **17**: 191–198.
10. Diringer, M.N., et al., *Critical care management of patients following aneurysmal subarachnoid hemorrhage: recommendations from the Neurocritical Care Society's Multidisciplinary Consensus Conference.* Neurocrit Care, 2011. **15**: 211–240.
11. Jauch, E.C., et al., *Guidelines for the early management of patients with acute ischemic stroke: a guideline for healthcare professionals from the American Heart Association/American Stroke Association.* Stroke, 2013. **44**: 870–947.
12. Ichai, C., et al., *Half-molar sodium lactate infusion to prevent intracranial hypertensive episodes in severe traumatic brain injured patients: a randomized controlled trial.* Intensive Care Med, 2013. **39**: 1413–1422.
13. Annane, D., et al., *Effects of fluid resuscitation with colloids vs crystalloids on mortality in critically ill patients presenting with hypovolemic shock: the CRISTAL randomized trial.* JAMA, 2013. **310**: 1809–1817.
14. Monnet, X., et al., *Passive leg-raising and end-expiratory occlusion tests perform better than pulse pressure variation in patients with low respiratory system compliance.* Crit Care Med, 2012. **40**: 152–157.
15. Monnet, X. and Teboul, J.L. *Passive leg raising: five rules, not a drop of fluid!* Crit Care, 2015. **19**: 18.
16. Hammond, N.E., Taylor, C., Finfer, S. et al. *Patterns of intravenous fluid resuscitation use in adult intensive care patients between 2007 and 2014: An international cross-sectional study.* PLoS One, 2017. **12**: e0176292.
17. Marik, P.E. and Malbrain, M.L.N.G. *The SEP-1 quality mandate may be harmful: How to drown a patient with 30 mL per kg fluid!* Anaesthesiol Intensive Ther, 2017. **49**: 323–328.
18. De Backer, D. and Dorman, T. *Surviving sepsis guidelines: a continuous move toward better care of patients with sepsis.* JAMA, 2017. **317**: 807–808.

Chapter 15

Drugs to Correct Electrolyte Disorders

Critically ill patients develop minor electrolyte imbalances, and for hospitalists and intensivists replacement orders are everyday chores (1–4). Changes in serum sodium values are very common in patients with acute neurocritical illness, and these derangements are important to recognize not only because the patient's level of consciousness may surreptitiously change but because they may cause seizures when there is a steep decline. Rapid correction of sodium levels may also lead to secondary injury (e.g., rapid osmotic shifts causing acute demyelination) (5). In hyponatremia, the patient's volume status must be taken into account (6,7). Cerebral salt wasting (hypovolemic hyponatremia) is more common in certain central nervous system disorders than the syndrome of inappropriate antidiuretic hormone secretion (SIADH; normovolemic hyponatremia). At the other extreme, hypernatremia is less frequently encountered and is most commonly due to diabetes insipidus and osmotic diuretics (5–7). Seizures may be a clinical manifestation of electrolyte disorders with hyponatremia, hypocalcemia, and hypomagnesemia most considered (8).

Common Electrolyte Replacements

Potassium

Potassium depletion is associated with diuretic agents, vomiting, and diarrhea related to gastrointestinal feeding. Hypokalemia may be a result of profound sweating, and skin losses may be substantial in patients with paroxysmal sympathetic hyperactivity (e.g., traumatic brain injury). When the serum potassium level decreases (<3 mmol/L), total body potassium stores most likely are significantly depleted, and electrocardiographic (EKG) changes are seen. Severe hypokalemia produces not only EKG abnormalities (prominent U waves, ST-segment changes, dampened T wave) but also atrial and ventricular arrhythmias. Muscle weakness with hypokalemia is seldom noted in patients admitted to the neurosciences intensive care unit (ICU) and can only be expected when the serum potassium level is less than 2 mmol/L.

Hyperkalemia (defined as a serum potassium level >5.5 mmol/L) is common in general ICUs because a large number of the patients have renal or adrenal dysfunction and receive multiple medications that have an impact on potassium levels (12). Hypoadrenalism is the most common adrenal disorder resulting in hyperkalemia. Rhabdomyolysis may cause hyperkalemia, but it is rarely severe enough to warrant treatment unless acute renal failure emerges and contributes (Chapter 19) (13).

Magnesium

Hypomagnesemia is also fairly common in neurosciences ICU, although it is rarely severe enough to become symptomatic (i.e., myoclonus, postural tremor, seizures) (9). A deficit is commonly seen in patients with chronic alcohol use disorder, but it may also be caused by prolonged use of antimicrobials (i.e., amphotericin), parenteral nutrition, and acute renal disorders. Normally, magnesium depletion results in marked reduction of magnesium excretion by the kidney, but renal magnesium wasting can occur with diuretics and aminoglycosides. It is expected in patients with diarrhea associated with nasogastric feeding, hypocalcemia, or refractory hypokalemia. Potassium-sparing diuretics might be necessary in patients who have hypomagnesemia associated with a thiazide or loop diuretic.

Phosphate

Phosphate metabolism is disturbed in patients with profound vomiting and sepsis, and with the use of some of the antiepileptic drugs, but any critical illness may deplete phosphate and calcium stores (10,11). Hypophosphatemia can occur as part of a refeeding syndrome (e.g., percutaneous endoscopic gastrostomy tube placement in underfed patients with advanced amyotrophic lateral sclerosis or prolonged nothing-by-mouth (nil per os) status in surgical or stroke patients). Patients with prolonged vomiting and malnourished alcohol or drug addicts are also at major risk of refeeding syndrome; in fact, any patient with no substantial feeding for a week is at risk. Renal loss of phosphate due to frequent use of mannitol can be implicated in some patients with hypophosphatemia. In asymptomatic patients, treatment is indicated when the serum phosphate level reaches 2.0 mg/dL or lower. Oral phosphate supplements contain 250 mg of elemental phosphate per tablet and should suffice. An aggressive intravenous approach is needed only in patients who receive nutritional support.

Replacement therapy in symptomatic derangements is shown in Table 15.1.

Disorders of Sodium and Water Homeostasis

Knowing its flaws, it is useful to try to assess volume status and to try to classify the derangements in hypervolemia, euvolemia or hypovolemia.

Management of severe hyponatremia and hypernatremia is much more complex and requires knowledge about fluid composition and the effects of mineralocorticoids and vasopressor analogs (14). Hyponatremia occurs if water increases more than sodium and if there is no change to sodium content; therefore, excessive free water intake (electrolyte-free, that is) can lead to excessive hyponatremia. Acute adrenal failure can lead to hyponatremia and is possible with rapid withdrawal of chronic corticosteroid use. Postoperative neurosurgical patients tend to develop dilutional hyponatremia as a result of the administration of hypotonic fluids.

Generally, hyponatremia may be associated with normal or increased osmolality. Normal serum osmolality with hyponatremia (pseudo-hyponatremia) may indicate severe hyperlipidemia (14). Cerebral salt wasting is a common occurrence in patients admitted to the neurosciences ICU (18,19,20).

Table 15.1 Replacement Therapy in Severe Electrolyte Abnormalities Other Than Sodium Disorders

Electrolyte Abnormality	Cause	Consequences	Treatment
Hypomagnesemia	Alcohol use disorder. Gastrointestinal and renal loss, amphotericin	Cardiac arrhythmias, muscle weakness	1–2 g of magnesium sulfate in 20 mL of normal saline over 1 hour (8,9)
Hypermagnesemia	Renal failure, antacids, enemas, exogenous supplementation	Muscle weakness, hypotension, asystole (extreme)	1–2 g of calcium gluconate IV over 15 minutes
Hypocalcemia	Critical illness, hypoparathyroidism, fat-deficient diet, hyperphosphatemia, acute pancreatitis	Cardiac arrhythmias, tetany, seizures, laryngospasm	1–2 g calcium gluconate IV over 15 minutes; then 6 g calcium gluconate in 500 ml normal saline with infusion 4–6 hours (8,10)
Hypercalcemia	Diabetes insipidus, malignancy, hyperparathyroidism; exogenous supplementation	Seizures, coma, cardiac arrhythmias	Hydration, 0.9% NaCl, 500 ml/hr
Hypophosphatemia	Parenteral nutrition, alcohol use disorder, renal failure, refeeding syndrome	Congestive cardiomyopathy, respiratory failure, rhabdomyolysis	Potassium phosphate, 0.08 mmol/kg IV in 500 ml of 0.45% saline over 6 hours (11)
Hyperphosphatemia	Renal failure, phosphate enemas, exogenous supplementation	Similar to those with hypocalcemia	Phosphate binders, 1 g of calcium orally three times a day (11)
Hypokalemia	Vomiting, prolonged starvation, gastrointestinal loss, diuretic use	Ventricular fibrillation, quadriplegia, glucose intolerance	KCl 10 mEq/hr IV infusion (20 mEq/hr with cardiac monitoring)
Hyperkalemia	Crush injury, hemolysis, renal failure, laboratory error	Cardiac arrest, cardiac conduction abnormalities, muscle weakness	1 g of calcium gluconate IV over 5 minutes (12,13), insulin with dextrose, diuretics, beta-2 agonists

Table 15.2 Potential Causes of Hyponatremia in the Neurosciences ICU

Hypovolemia	Normovolemia or Hypervolemia
• Diuretics (thiazide, loop)	• Syndrome of inappropriate antidiuretic hormone secretion
• Addison's disease (acute corticosteroid withdrawal)	• Acute renal failure
• Gastrointestinal and skin losses	• Congestive heart failure
• Dietary sodium restriction (with excess hypotonic fluid intake)	• Hepatic failure
• Cerebral salt wasting	• Medications (e.g., NSAIDs, morphine, selective serotonin reuptake inhibitors, carbamazepine)

Hyponatremia

- Clinical manifestations are expected only with rapidly declining sodium values (<125 mmol/L).
- Severe hyponatremia typically manifests with acute confusion, followed by stupor and generalized tonic–clonic seizures. Coma may occur when sodium values fall below 110 mmol/L.
- Mortality in hyponatremic patients with a serum sodium level of 125 mmol/L or less on admission is approximately 30%. Mortality increases further at levels of 115 mmol/L or less. It is a telltale sign of major illness.
- A rare syndrome of postoperative hyponatremia in premenopausal women with cerebral edema and respiratory arrest with fatal outcome has been described.
- Postoperative severe hyponatremia has also been documented in patients with transurethral prostatectomy, usually associated with bladder irrigation. This condition however has been rarely associated with cerebral edema.
- In subarachnoid hemorrhage (SAH), volume status is more important than hyponatremia per se (20). Volume resuscitation is achieved with 0.9% sodium chloride or 5% albumin alone. If the fluid balance remains negative in SAH, fludrocortisone, 0.2 mg orally twice daily, is effective.
- Treatment of severe symptomatic hyponatremia can be associated with rapid overshoot, resulting in hypernatremia. This is associated with osmotic demyelination syndromes (central pontine myelonolysis [CPM] or extrapontine myelinolysis [EPM]).
- The clinical manifestations of CPM can be diverse, but pseudobulbar palsy, facial weakness, inability to swallow or speak, and quadriplegia are prominent. Lesions in the base of the pons may also be trident- or bat-shaped because horizontal tracts are preferentially involved and vertical tracts are spared.
- In EPM, magnetic resonance imaging may reveal bilateral thalamic involvement of the lateral and centromedian nucleus.
- Treatment of asymptomatic hyponatremia is focused on correcting the volume derangement alone.

Table 15.3 Treatment of Symptomatic Hyponatremia

Volume Contraction	Volume Dilution
• 0.9% NaCl (or 1.5%) infusion	• Calculate need to normalize serum sodium by using 3% NaCl (513 mmol/L) in the formula: $\frac{513 - \text{current serum Na}}{0.5 \times \text{body weight (kg)} + 1}$ to provide total mmol/L.
• Fludrocortisone acetate, 0.4 mg/day orally, in divided doses	• Rate: raise serum sodium 1 mmol/L per hour

- Treatment of cerebral salt wasting should include free water restriction and fluid replacement with isotonic or hypertonic saline fluids. Fluid restriction is discouraged.
- Treatment of SIADH is restriction of free water, and that alone slowly corrects hyponatremia.
- A strategy to correct acutely severe hyponatremia is shown in Table 15.3.
- A strategy to avoid overcorrection of hyponatremia is shown in Box 15.1.

Hypernatremia

- The causes of hypernatremia are shown in Table 15.4.
- Consequently, patients unable to communicate thirst are at highest risk.
- Hypernatremia is common, although thirst protects against the development of a steep increase. The causes are shown in Table 15.3 (15).
- Elderly patients with an altered sense of thirst or gastrointestinal losses are at risk of hypernatremia.
- Marked hypotension and volume depletion are common, and patients become drowsy or stuporous. Consciousness further

Box 15.1 Strategy to Avoid Overcorrection of Severe Hyponatremia [14]

- Correct sodium by 6 mmol/L in 6 hours.
- An increase in serum sodium concentration by 4–6 mmol/L could prevent dangerous shifts from cerebral edema.
- Start with 30 mL/hr of 3% sodium chloride infusion.
- Avoid any hypertonic saline bolus.
- With overcorrection of severe hyponatremia, start additional 5% dextrose in water (D5W) in individual doses of 6 ml/kg body weight, given over 1–2 hours.
- Administer desmopressin 2–4 mcg/day IV in divided doses.
- Be much more careful in patients with alcoholic liver disease or malnutrition, who are at high risk of demyelination syndromes.

Table 15.4 Causes of Hypernatremia in the Neurosciences ICU	
Hypovolemia	**Normovolemia or Hypervolemia**
Gastrointestinal loss	Hypertonic sodium solutions
Diuretics (e.g., mannitol)	Corticosteroid excess
Diabetes insipidus	
Increased insensible fluid loss	

declines after a period of delirium; this is due to hypertonic dehydration of the brain.

- Generalized tonic–clonic seizures are unusual, even in patients with marked increases in sodium levels (>160 mmol/L).
- Loss of proportionally more water than salt causes hypernatremia in most patients if water is not replenished.
- Hypernatremia is often iatrogenic due to osmotic diuresis, insufficient sodium-to-water intake, or large amounts of IV sodium infusion.
- Overzealous infusion of fluids may potentially cause brain edema, but this is rare.
- Treatment of severe hypernatremia depends on rapidity of rise of sodium (Table 15.5).
- Hypernatremia with diabetes insipidus is characterized by hypotonic urine (osmolality <300 mOsm/kg or specific gravity <1.010) and polyuria (>30 mL/kg per day).
- Calculating the free water deficit is useful when treating patients with diabetes insipidus. The formula for this calculation is:

$$\text{Free water deficit} = \text{Normal TBW} - \text{Current TBW},$$

where TBW = total body water.

Table 15.5 Treatment of Symptomatic Hypernatremia (15)	
Pure Water Loss or Hypotonic Hypernatremia	**Hypertonic Hypernatremia**
Calculate need to normalize serum sodium by using 5% dextrose in the formula: $\frac{0 - \text{current plasma Na}}{0.5 \times \text{body weight} + 1}$ or 0.45% NaCl in the formula: $\frac{77 - \text{current plasma Na}}{0.5 \times \text{body weight} + 1}$ to provide total mmol/L.	Furosemide 40–80 mg IV Switch to electrolyte-free water infusion (i.e., 5% dextrose in water).
• Rate: reduce serum sodium 10 mmol/L in 24 hours	
• Desmopressin, 2–4 mcg IV in 2 divided doses	

Box 15.2 Protocol to Treat Mild Diabetes Insipidus

- Applies to stable hypernatremia (<150 mmol/L).
- Monitor polyuria and match with fluid intake.
- Consider flushes of free water (250 ml) through nasogastric tube.
- Monitor body weight, urine specific gravity.
- Minimize excessive IV fluids containing sodium chloride.

- Normal TBW is 60% of lean body weight (in kilograms) in men and 50% in women:

Current TBW = normal TBW × (140 / current serum sodium level).

- To calculate the amount of replacement fluid volume needed:

Replacement fluid volume (in liters) = Free water deficit × (1/1 − X)

where

X = replacement fluid sodium concentration − isotonic fluid sodium concentration.

- Treatment of hypernatremia associated with diabetes insipidus is shown in Boxes 15.2 and 15.3.

Drugs to Manage Sodium Disorders

Vaptans are contraindicated in anuria (no benefit) and in hypovolemic hyponatremia. They are mostly used in difficult-to-manage euvolemic or hypervolemic hyponatremia when serum sodium levels are 125 mmol/L or less (e.g., in patients with advanced cardiac failure). Tolvaptan rapidly increases serum sodium and urine output. It is used in chronic forms of hyponatremia and should not be used for acute symptomatic hyponatremia due to its potential for rapid rise within 24 hours after administration. Experience in the neurosciences ICU is limited, and risks are not well known.

Box 15.3 Rising or Severe Hypernatremia in Diabetes Insipidus

- Start desmopressin 0.5–1 mcg IV, and repeat if inadequate response (maximum 4 mcg/day in divided doses).
- Start 0.45% sodium chloride or 5% dextrose in water infusion, and calculate infusion rate (see text).
- Monitor serum sodium every 2–4 hours.
- Monitor urine specific gravity.

Conivaptan IV

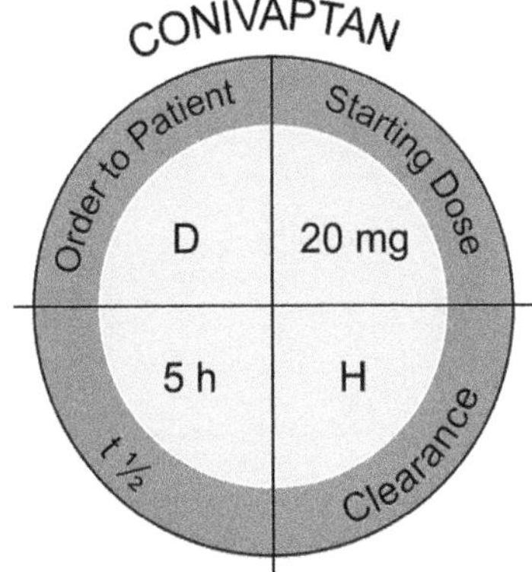

Pharmacologic Characteristics

- Arginine vasopressin receptor antagonist
- Promotes excretion of free water, resulting in increased urine output and decreased urine osmolality
- Used to treat euvolemic or hypervolemic hyponatremia
- Use with caution in patients with hypervolemic hyponatremia
- Not recommended when the creatinine clearance (CrCl) is <30 ml/min
- Use is contraindicated with potent CYP3A4 inhibitors (e.g., ketoconazole, itraconazole, rotinavir, clarithromycin)

Dosing and Administration

- Bolus of 20 mg infused over 30 minutes, followed by a continuous infusion of 20 mg over 24 hours for 2–4 days
- No dosage adjustments in patients with mild hepatic disease; decrease bolus and infusion doses to 10 mg in those with moderate to severe liver disease

Monitoring

- Hepatic function
- Urine output
- Fluid status
- Electrolytes
- Blood pressure

Side Effects

- Orthostatic hypotension
- Hypokalemia
- Headache
- Nausea, vomiting, constipation, diarrhea
- Increased risk of osmotic demyelination syndrome (if sodium is corrected >12 mmol/L in 24 hours)

Tolvaptan PO

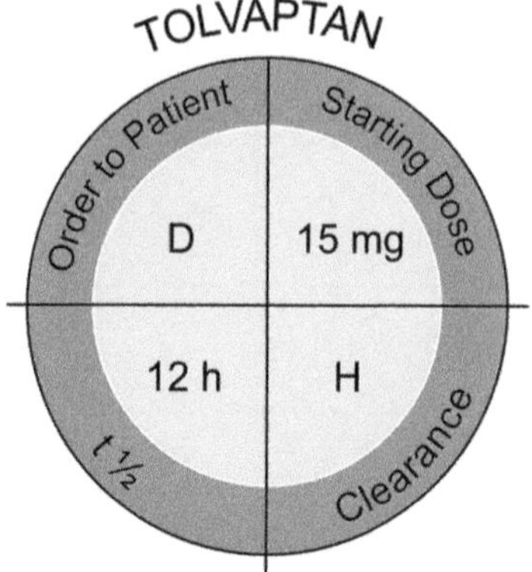

Pharmacologic Characteristics

- Arginine vasopressin receptor antagonist
- Promotes free water excretion, resulting in increased urine output and decreased urine osmolality
- Used to treat euvolemic or hypervolemic hyponatremia

Dosing and Administration

- 15 mg orally once daily; may increase to 30 mg/day after 24 hours
- Maximum 60 mg orally once daily
- Avoid fluid restriction during the first 24 hours
- Maximum use is limited to 30 days due to the risk of hepatotoxicity
- No dosage adjustments are needed in patients with in renal dysfunction, but use of tolvaptan has not been studied in patients with a CrCl <10 ml/min
- Reduce the dose if given concurrently with potent CYP3A4 inhibitors

Monitoring

- Hepatic function
- Urine output
- Fluid status
- Electrolytes
- Blood pressure
- Uric acid levels

Side Effects

- Hepatotoxicity
- Increased thirst
- Nausea

- Polyuria
- Constipation, anorexia
- Fever
- Gout
- Hyperkalemia

Fludrocortisone PO

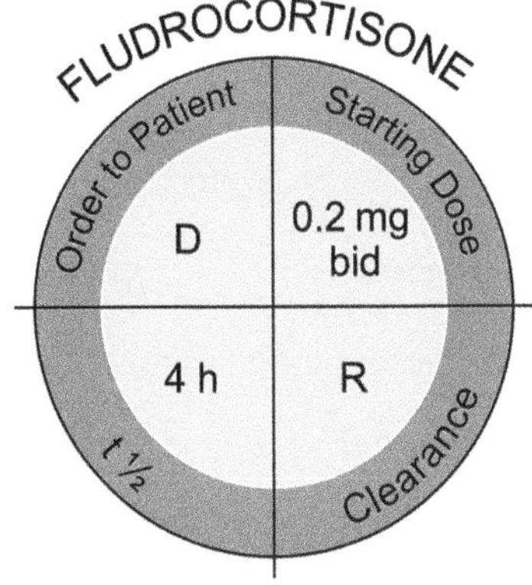

Pharmacologic Characteristics

- Very potent mineralocorticoid with glucocorticoid properties
- Promotes sodium reabsorption and potassium excretion from distal tubules
- Hepatic metabolism

Dosing and Administration

- 0.1–0.4 mg/day orally in divided doses twice a day (16,17)
- No adjustments are needed in patients with hepatic or renal dysfunction

Monitoring

- Fluid balance
- Electrolytes
- Blood glucose
- Blood pressure

Side Effects

- Transient hypokalemia; may require supplemental replacement
- Gastrointestinal upset
- Mild adrenal suppression

Desmopressin PO

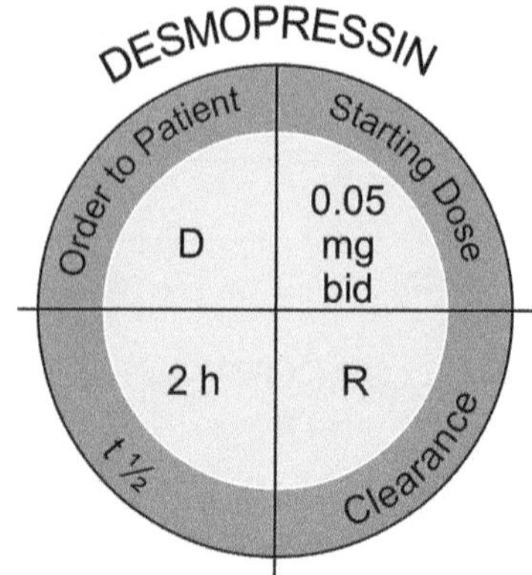

Pharmacologic Characteristics

- Vasopressin analog
- Increases cAMP levels in renal tubular cells, increases water permeability
- Ineffective in treatment of nephrogenic diabetes insipidus

Dosing and Administration

- 0.05 mg orally twice a day (range 0.1–1.2 mg/day, divided two or three times a day)
- 2–4 mcg/day, divided twice a day, given IV or subcutaneously
- 10–40 mcg/day intranasally, divided one to three times a day (10-mcg dose = 0.1 ml volume)
- No dosage adjustments are needed in patients with hepatic dysfunction
- Injectable and oral administration not recommended when CrCl < 50 ml/min

Monitoring

- Fluid status, monitor for polydipsia
- Decreasing urinary output and increasing urine osmolality
- Drug–drug interactions with other drugs known to cause hyponatremia

Side Effects

- Hyponatremia (overshoot)
- Seizures (from hyponatremia)
- Hypertension
- Worsening heart failure
- Thrombotic events (rare)

Sodium Chloride ("Salt") Tablets

Pharmacologic Characteristics

- 1 g NaCl = 17.1 mEq NaCl
- Little effect unless the patient has a pure sodium deficit (and not a TBW deficit)

Monitoring

- Electrolytes
- Fluid status

Side Effects

- Thirst, with subsequent increase in free water intake

Key Pointers

1. Cerebral salt wasting is most common and is best treated with saline replacement and fludrocortisone.
2. Magnesium, potassium, and calcium deficits require monitoring but are easy to correct.
3. Refeeding syndrome (severe hypophosphatemia) may occur in undernourished patients.
4. Diabetes insipidus can be managed with fluid replacement and desmopressin.
5. Osmotic demyelination syndrome is rare but can be seen with a very rapid rise in sodium levels (>2 mmol/hr).

References

1. Diringer, M., *Neurologic manifestations of major electrolyte abnormalities.* Handb Clin Neurol, 2017. **141**: 705–713.
2. French, S., Subauste, J. and Geraci, S. *Calcium abnormalities in hospitalized patients.* South Med J, 2012. **105**: 231–237.
3. Piper, G.L. and Kaplan, L.J. *Fluid and electrolyte management for the surgical patient.* Surg Clin North Am, 2012. **92**: 189–205.
4. Urso, C., Brucculeri, S. and Caimi, G. *Acid-base and electrolyte abnormalities in heart failure: pathophysiology and implications.* Heart Fail Rev, 2015. **20**: 493–503.
5. Narins, R.G., *Therapy of hyponatremia: does haste make waste?* N Engl J Med, 1986. **314**: 1573–1575.
6. Schrier, R.W., *Pathogenesis of sodium and water retention in high-output and low-output cardiac failure, nephrotic syndrome, cirrhosis, and pregnancy (2).* N Engl J Med, 1988. **319**: 1127–1134.
7. Schrier, R.W., *Pathogenesis of sodium and water retention in high-output and low-output cardiac failure, nephrotic syndrome, cirrhosis, and pregnancy.* N Engl J Med, 1988. **319**: 1065–1072.
8. Nardone, R., Brigo, F. and Trinka, E. *Acute symptomatic seizures caused by electrolyte disturbances.* J Clin Neurol, 2016. **12**: 21–33.

9. Rubeiz, G.J., et al., *Association of hypomagnesemia and mortality in acutely ill medical patients.* Crit Care Med, 1993. **21**: 203–209.
10. Cooper, M.S. and Gittoes, N.J. *Diagnosis and management of hypocalcaemia.* BMJ, 2008. **336**: 1298–1302.
11. Shiber, J.R. and Mattu, A. *Serum phosphate abnormalities in the emergency department.* J Emerg Med, 2002. **23**: 395–400.
12. Crawford, A.H., *Hyperkalemia: recognition and management of a critical electrolyte disturbance.* J Infus Nurs, 2014. **37**: 167–175.
13. Packham, D.K. and Kosiborod, M. *Potential new agents for the management of hyperkalemia.* Am J Cardiovasc Drugs, 2016. **16**: 19–31.
14. Sterns, R.H., *Disorders of plasma sodium—causes, consequences, and correction.* N Engl J Med, 2015. **372**: 55–65.
15. Adrogué, H.J. and Madias, N.E. *Hypernatremia.* N Engl J Med, 2000. **342**: 1493–1499.
16. Hasan, D., et al., *Effect of fludrocortisone acetate in patients with subarachnoid hemorrhage.* Stroke, 1989. **20**: 1156–1161.
17. Human, T., et al., *Treatment of hyponatremia in patients with acute neurological injury.* Neurocrit Care, 2017. **27**: 242–248.
18. Yee, A.H., Burns, J.D. and E.F.M. *Wijdicks. Cerebral salt wasting: pathophysiology, diagnosis, and treatment.* Neurosurg Clin N Am, 2010. **21**: 339–352.
19. Rabinstein, A.A. and E.F.M. Wijdicks. *Hyponatremia in critically ill neurological patients.* Neurologist, 2003. **9**: 290–300.
20. Wijdicks, E.F.M., Vermeulen, M., J.A. ten Haaf, et al. *Volume depletion and natriuresis in patients with a ruptured intracranial aneurysm.* Ann Neurol, 1985. **18**: 211–216.

Chapter 16

Antidotes with Overdose

Overdoses of illicit drugs can be seen in conjunction with traumatic brain injury and anoxic-ischemic injury—in fact, the illegal drug is often the main culprit in the acute brain injury. To appreciate the effects of coexisting illicit drugs, a detailed history is needed. Denial of drug use by family members can be assumed, and urine drug testing is far from perfect. Serum and urine toxicology samples should be analyzed (and stored for potential later use).

Over a million patients reporting to emergency departments have drug poisoning; of these, one in four are admitted (1,2). In the United States and elsewhere, there is a rapidly escalating "fentanyl epidemic," mostly as a result of street drugs that can be fairly easily obtained. Novel synthetic opioid intoxications are presenting themselves (13). In these fentanyl overdoses, the presentation in the emergency department or intensive care unit is often the result of respiratory arrest and devastating anoxic brain injury.

Alcohol intoxication remains common in patients seen during the nighttime hours. Most of it is self-limiting, but the central nervous system–depressing intoxication signs may merge with clinical signs of an acute brain injury, particularly if brain trauma is not obvious. It is a common clinical error to overemphasize the effects of alcohol and underemphasize the traumatic brain injury. In any overdose, supportive care and prevention of secondary complications remain crucially important, and a poisoned patient may require specific therapy (3–7). In appropriate circumstances, this should include contact with a regional poison center in the United States (1-800-222-1222).

Toxins and Major Laboratory Abnormalities

Early clues about which toxin should be considered may come from careful scrutiny of laboratory abnormalities. They may not be specific for the drug and may have been caused by sudden changes in hemodynamic stability. The electrolyte abnormalities and acid–base abnormalities seen with certain drugs and toxins are shown in Table 16.1.

Table 16.1 Drugs and Toxins Causing Laboratory Abnormalities (8)

Metabolic acidosis	Methanol, ethylene glycol, propylene glycol, paraldehyde, isoniazid or salicylate poisoning, cyanide and hydrogen sulfate poisoning
Respiratory alkalosis	Salicylates
Osmolar gap	Methanol and ethylene glycol
Hypoglycemia	Insulin, sulfonylureas, beta-blockers
Hyperglycemia	Corticosteroids, second-generation antipsychotics
Hyponatremia	Ecstasy, carbamazepine, oxcarbazepine, selective serotonin antagonists
Hyperammonemia	Valproic acid

Neurology of Drug Overdose

A summary of neurologic manifestations and complications appears in Table 16.2 and Table 16.3. Many manifestations pertain to abnormal eye findings and changes in muscle tone. Extrapyramidal findings are uncommon but point to cocaine and neuroleptic agents, including the atypical antipsychotics.

Table 16.2 Drugs and Neurologic Complications

Class	Neurologic Manifestations	Late Concerns
Amphetamines	Mydriasis, paranoia, hallucinations, delirium, focal signs (cerebral hemorrhage)	Cerebral infarcts (vasculopathy)
Cocaine	Seizures, dystonia, chorea, migraine, coma, subarachnoid hemorrhage, rhabdomyolysis	Anoxic-ischemic brain injury, cerebral infarction, aneurysmal rupture
Barbiturates	Coma, hypoxic-ischemic encephalopathy	Persistent vegetative state, cerebral infarct
Hallucinogens	Colored geometric images, catalepsy, mydriasis, insomnia, coma	Ischemic stroke, cognitive decline
Opioids	Coma to euphoria, miotic pupils (but normal findings on eye exam do not exclude opioid intoxication), seizures	Persistent vegetative state from anoxic-ischemic brain injury

Table 16.3 Neurologic Findings with Toxins	
Eye Findings	
Miosis	Opioids (heroin), organophosphates, clonidine
Mydriasis	Tricyclic antidepressants, Ecstasy
Horizontal nystagmus	Ethanol, antiepileptic drugs, ketamine, phencyclidine
Vertical nystagmus	Opioids
Motor Findings	
Flaccidity	Benzodiazepines, baclofen
Rigidity	Neuroleptic agents, carbon monoxide, hypoglycemics

First Treatment Considerations

The first principle of detoxification is to prevent further absorption of the toxic substance. Gastrointestinal decontamination, enhancing elimination of the toxins, and extracorporeal removal of the toxins are the main options but are less specific, and simple in concept. In some types of intoxications, antidotes are available, but most patients do not need one or cannot have one. Antidotes are agents that reverse the toxic effect (e.g., naloxone), sometimes in a spectacular way (e.g., awakening from coma), or controls the consequences of the toxicity, which is sometimes lifesaving (e.g., improving hemodynamics). Often, however, the benefit of antidotes is questionable due to their time-dependent effect and potential serious adverse effects such as seizures (9). Moreover, their benefit over supportive care is unclear (10). A new approach is to use intravenous (IV) lipid emulsions, which shift lipophilic drugs into the vascular compartments. The principles of detoxification are shown in Table 16.4.

Table 16.4 Principles of Detoxification

Principle	Effect	Examples
Gastric Decontamination	Enhanced elimination	Barbiturates, carbamazepine
Hemodialysis	Active removal	Salicylate, lithium
Urine Alkalization	Increased elimination	Salicylates, barbiturates
Antidotes	Reduce effect, increase metabolism, or prevent toxic metabolism	Flumazenil, naloxone
Emulsions	Remove lipophilic drugs	Tricyclic antidepressants, calcium-channel blockers, beta-blockers

Gastrointestinal decontamination is originally referred to as induction of early emesis. When a patient is seen within 1 hour after ingestion, administration of ipecac syrup 30 ml followed by 300 ml of water causes vomiting within 30 minutes. However, this method has largely been abandoned because it carries a substantial risk of aspiration. Gastric lavage is a more useful approach for intubated patients. This method involves flushing the stomach with 200 ml of warm tap water to attempt to remove ingested tablets. Activated charcoal (1 g/kg body weight) is another commonly used method. A cathartic usually is co-administered, and the absorbent is able to bind many drugs. Use of charcoal, in a single dose or multiple doses, is predicated on ingestion of a potentially life-threatening toxin and is used preferably in patients who ingested the substance less than 1 hour previously. Alcohol and lithium are not absorbed by activated charcoal.

Bowel irrigation involves the use of a polyethylene glycol electrolyte solution or potassium chloride, 1 to 2 L per hour. It is primarily reserved for use in "body packers", who are transporting illicit drugs and have become intoxicated when the shielded carrier ruptures.

Elimination of toxins can also be facilitated using forced diuresis and increase of urinary pH. This method is mostly used in patients who have ingested salicylates or phenobarbital. Forced diuresis involves increasing the urine flow rate from 3 to 6 ml/kg per hour using isotonic fluids or diuretics. An increase in urinary pH (7 or more) is achieved with the use of IV sodium bicarbonate, 1 to 2 mEq/kg every 3 to 4 hours. Hypokalemia, an expected consequence of this intervention, should be treated by adding potassium chloride to the bicarbonate infusion.

Commonly Used Agents for Detoxification

Gastrointestinal Decontamination

- Activated charcoal (25–100 g) only within 1 hour of ingestion
  - Most toxins are already absorbed, but this method can be used with large overdoses
  - Option in DOAC related cerebral hemorrhage (Chapter 7)
  - Commonly considered with acetaminophen ingestion
  - Consider use for ingestions of amlodipine, carbamazepine, dapsone, phenobarbital, theophylline, verapamil SR, or quinine
  - Low risk and easily administered; use suspension formulation
  - Co-administration with sorbitol or other cathartics is not recommended
  - Administer IV antiemetics to minimize the risk of vomiting with its use
  - Ensure that bowel sounds are present prior to administering

- Gastric lavage (300 ml warm water via large-bore orogastric tube)
- Whole-bowel irrigation (polyethylene glycol via nasogastric tube)
- Cathartics (1–2 ml/kg sorbitol, 70% solution; or 250 ml magnesium citrate, 10% solution)

Emulsions

- The presumed principle is that IV lipid emulsion shifts lipophilic drugs into the vascular compartments
- Indicated in any patient with severe toxicity due to ingestion of a lipophilic drug, such as antiemetics (11), tricyclic antidepressants, calcium-channel blockers
- 1–1.5 ml/kg IV of a 20% lipid emulsion over 1 minute followed by a continuous infusion of 0.25 ml/kg per minute for 60 minutes

Major Toxidromes

Traditionally, intoxications have been divided into toxidromes (a mashup of "toxins" and "syndromes"). These include opioid, sedative-hypnotic, anticholinergic, cholinergic, and sympathomimetic toxidromes. Clinicians will also need to rule out co-ingestion of other pharmacologically active substances. Very few toxins have specific neurologic manifestations—the proverbial "coma—seizures—death."

Opioid Toxidrome

Several substances (e.g., hydrocodone, hydromorphone, oxycodone, methadone, fentanyl, heroin) cause an opioid toxidrome. The urine toxicology screen may be falsely positive (e.g quinolones such as levofloxacin) and not always useful. Several black market opioids contain adulterants. It is important to search for an opioid transdermal patch and remove it.

Clinical Features

- Miosis to pinpoint pupils is a classic clinical feature
- Miosis rarely occurs with tramadol or meperidine ingestions
- Miosis may be absent if there is concurrent toxicity with sympathomimetic or anticholinergic agents
- Decreased respiratory rate (<10 per minute) and tidal volumes
- Decreased arousal to deep unresponsive coma
- Decreased autonomic activity with bradycardia, hypotension (from histamine release), and hypothermia
- Bowel sounds are hypoactive or silent
- Tramadol and meperidine may cause seizures and also serotonin syndrome when selective serotonin reuptake inhibitors (SSRIs) or other serotonergic agents have been co-ingested

Antidote Administration

- Naloxone IV antagonizes opioid effects by competing for opiate receptor sites in the central nervous system.

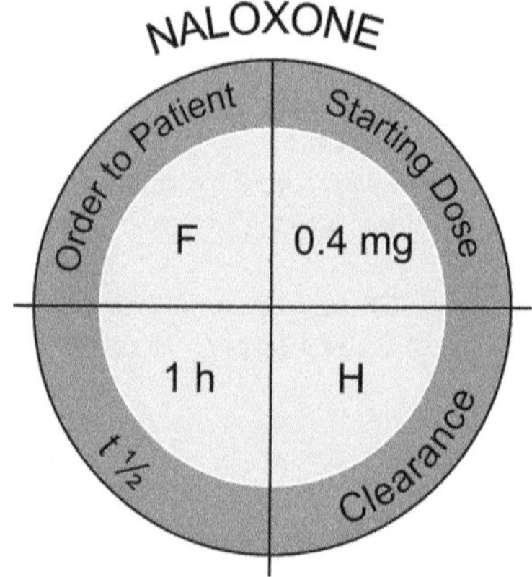

- The goal of naloxone administration is to produce adequate ventilation, not full return of consciousness.
- Administer 0.4 mg naloxone IV (initially).
- For apneic patients, repeating up to 10 mg.
- If no response after 10 mg, reconsider diagnosis.
- Naloxone can be administered intranasally, subcutaneously, or intramuscularly if there is a delay in obtaining IV access; however, these alternate routes are associated with a slower onset, delayed effect, and slower absorption.
- Hemodialysis is less effective in opioid toxicity because of the large volume distribution of many of the opioids.

Concerns

- Acute respiratory distress syndrome (complication of morphine, heroin, or methadone toxicity) can be a result of iatrogenic reversal of opioid toxicity
- Methadone overdose is long-acting and is associated with QT prolongation and torsades de pointes. It requires multiple doses of naloxone
- Monitor for electrolyte abnormalities (hypocalcemia, hypokalemia, hypomagnesemia)
- Buprenorphine may be resistant to typical doses of naloxone. Consider naloxone infusion
- Loperamide: QRS and QT prolongation on the electrocardiogram (EKG); may lead to wide complex tachycardia

Sedative-Hypnotic Toxidrome

This toxidrome includes several benzodiazepine substances such as alprazolam, diazepam, and lorazepam. Symptoms depend on the number of pills taken and are less common with isolated oral ingestions.

Clinical Features

- Hypothermia, hypotension, bradycardia, depressed respiratory rate
- Slurred speech, ataxia, depressed consciousness
- May present with severe flaccidity of all limbs
- High likelihood of co-ingestion with alcohol

Antidote Administration

- Flumazenil IV is a nonspecific competitive antagonist to benzodiazepine receptors

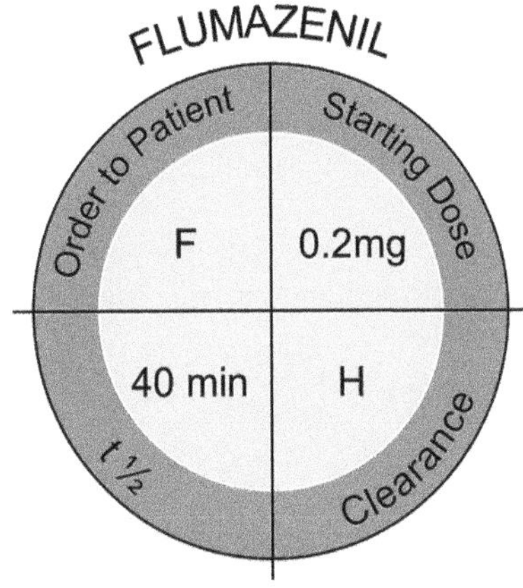

- Administer 0.2 mg flumazenil IV initially
- Repeated dose: 0.2 mg IV at 1-minute intervals (maximum dose 1 mg) until desired effect is seen. In case of resedation, the maximum dose is 3 mg in 1 hour
- Peak effect: 6–10 minutes; duration ~1 hour
- Does not consistently reverse apnea from benzodiazepine overdose
- The effects of toxicity depend on the pharmacology of the benzodiazepine involved (half-life, metabolites, and lipophilicity)
- Gastrointestinal decontamination with charcoal is usually of no benefit

Concerns

- Benzodiazepine-like agents such as zolpidem can produce similar effects.
- Baclofen can cause an effect similar to benzodiazepine toxicity.
- Flumazenil use is controversial in setting of overdose because it may precipitate withdrawal seizures. Benzodiazepine reversal may result in a single seizure, more often following a combined benzodiazepine and tricyclic antidepressant overdose (and other agents that have seizure-inducing effects).
- Consider propylene glycol toxicity in the case of an overdose from parenteral diazepam and lorazepam. Risks include skin necrosis or extravasation, hemolysis, cardiac dysrhythmias, hypotension, lactic acidosis, and seizures.

Sympathomimetic Toxidrome

Cocaine and methamphetamine are examples of substances that can induce a sympathomimetic toxidrome. The dose of these agents varies significantly and is patient-initiated. It may be necessary to inquire about recently increased usage. Symptomatic treatment and supportive care is the hallmark of management.

Clinical Features

- Widely dilated pupils nearly obscuring the iris
- Tachycardia (dose-dependent), hypertension, hyperthermia (from peripheral vasoconstriction), tachypnea, diaphoresis
- Increased myocardial oxygen demand
- Supraventricular and ventricular arrhythmias
- Agitation, psychosis

Antidote Administration

- Phentolamine IV 5–10 mg every 5–15 minutes to counteract alpha-adrenergic effects (from norepinephrine release)

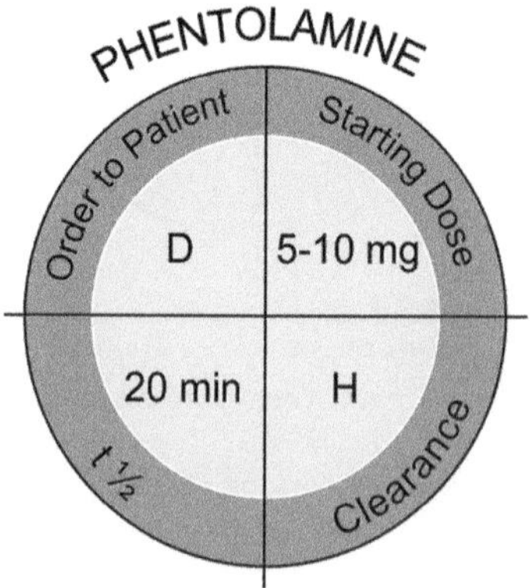

- Sedation with lorazepam 4 mg IV or diazepam 10 mg IV
- Droperidol 2.5–5 mg or haloperidol 10 mg IV to combat acute psychotic agitation from glutamine, norepinephrine, serotonin, and dopamine release
- Seizures can be treated with lorazepam but are rare and rarely recurrent
- Most antipyretics are ineffective. Treatment of hyperthermia requires cooling devices, sedation, and neuromuscular paralysis
- Correct metabolic acidosis with sodium bicarbonate 50 to 150 mEq IV
- Activated charcoal is rarely indicated

Concerns

- Levamisole (cocaine adulterant, immunomodulator): causes agranulocytosis, leukoencephalopathy, cutaneous vasculitis

- Avoid using succinylcholine for paralysis if rhabdomyolysis is suspected
- Avoid administering beta-1 selective blockers for hypertension (results in unopposed alpha-adrenergic stimulation); mixed agents like labetalol are preferred
- Risk of intracranial hemorrhage
- Risk of acute bowel infarction
- Risk of acute ST-elevation myocardial infarction

Anticholinergic Toxidrome

This toxidrome involves tricyclic antidepressants, antihistamines, and antipsychotics. Serum drug levels will not be helpful or readily available to determine acute toxicity.

Clinical Features

- Anticholinergic toxidrome is also described as "red as a beet" (cutaneous facial exfoliation), "dry as a bone" (anhidrosis), "hot as a hare" (hyperthermia), "blind as a bat" (non-reactive mydriasis), "mad as a hatter" (delirium), and "full as a flask" (urinary retention)
- Visual hallucinations and carphologia (picking at imaginary objects)
- Tachycardia (early, reliable clinical sign)
- Decreased or absent bowel sounds

Antidote Administration

- Physostigmine IV binds reversibly to inhibits acetylcholinesterase in the peripheral nervous system and central nervous system to overcome acetylcholine blockade at the neuromuscular junction

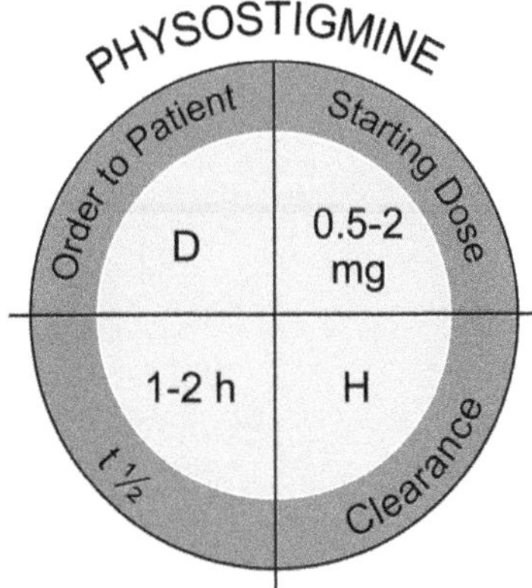

- Physostigmine may be superior to benzodiazepines in managing agitation and delirium in this setting

- Physostigmine 0.5–2 mg IV, slow IV push (1 mg/min); can repeat dose every 30 minutes until response
- Do not use physostigmine if toxicity other than pure anticholinergics

Concerns

- EKG will detect prolonged QRS and arrhythmias (overdose with tricyclic antidepressants).
- Agitation and seizures are treated with benzodiazepines.
- Avoid phenothiazines (e.g., promethazine, prochlorperazine) or butyrophenones (e.g., haloperidol) for sedation, since they have anticholinergic effects.

Cholinergic Syndrome

This syndrome involves organophosphates and carbamates. The onset and duration depend on the agent involved; oral and respiratory exposure effects are seen before the effects of dermal exposure. Risk factors are exposure to highly fat-soluble organophosphates. Avoid forced emesis because it increases the risk of aspiration and seizures.

Clinical Features

- SLUDGE: salivation, lacrimation, urinary incontinence, defecation, gastric cramps, emesis
- DUMBELS: defecation, urination, miosis, bronchorrhea/bronchospasm/bradycardia, emesis, lacrimation, salivation
- Muscle weakness, from nicotinic effects (due to depolarizing effects of succinylcholine): neck flexion weakness, proximal muscle weakness, and rapidly emerging respiratory failure

Antidote Administration

- Atropine, 1–2 mg IV. Double the dose after 2–3 minutes. For severe toxicity, use 2–5 mg

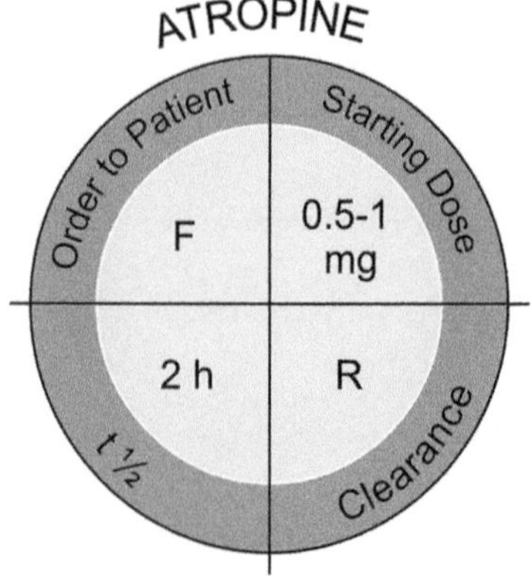

- Pralidoxime, 1–2 g IV, either infused or via slow IV push

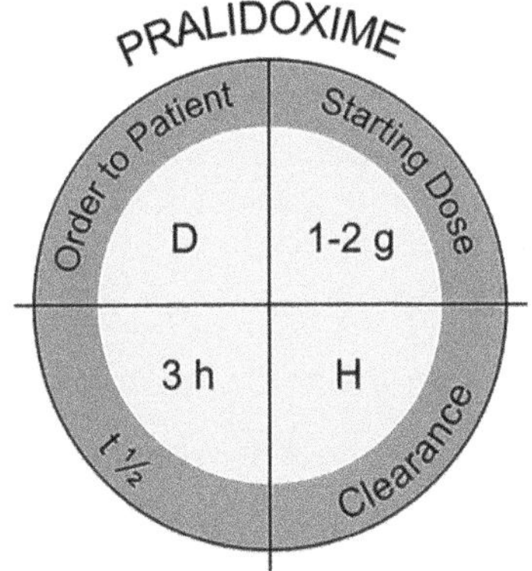

  - Binds to nicotinic receptors (atropine does not)
  - Beneficial in neuromuscular junction dysfunction
  - Requires concurrent atropine doses (transient oxime-induced acetylcholine inhibition)
  - Prolonged half-life in poisonings: 3–4 hours
- Diazepam 10–20 mg IV for seizures. Phenytoin has no effect on organophosphate-induced seizures

Concerns

- Heart block, prolonged QT interval; greater risk in elderly or those with severe toxicity
- Bradycardia and hypotension are usually present in moderate to severe toxicities
- Tachycardia and hypertension may occur due to direct sympathomimetic stimulation. There is a risk of acute myocardial infarction
- Acute renal failure with rhabdomyolysis

Toxic Dysautonomias

Presentation of the serotonin syndrome is virtually the same as that of neuroleptic malignant syndrome (NMS), with marked dysautonomic features. In addition to agitation, delirium, hallucinations, and manic behavior, the syndrome includes hyperthermia, diaphoresis, diarrhea, lacrimation, shivering, but most characteristically profound myoclonus. Clonus can be elicited but is not commonly spontaneously present. Rigidity is uniformly present and most pronounced in the legs. Success has been reported with cyproheptadine, but resolution takes days after discontinuation of the responsible SSRI (and possible additional use of opioids). NMS is severe and immediately life-threatening (12). Drugs to consider as the cause of NMS are haloperidol, fluphenazine, chlorpromazine, clozapine, risperidone, olanzapine, metoclopramide, droperidol, and promethazine (all antagonize Dopamine -2 receptors to varying degrees). Antipsychotic drugs used for bipolar disorder, schizoaffective disorders, and psychotic depression can also be drugs of abuse and have a high proclivity for toxicity. Typically overdose occurs with neuroleptic agents, but atypical antipsychotics (e.g., quetiapine) may produce similar syndromes. Table 16.5 shows the most typical antidotes for these syndromes.

Table 16.5 Antidotes for Serotonin Syndrome and Neuroleptic Malignant Syndrome

Antidotes	Dose	Indication
Cyproheptadine PO 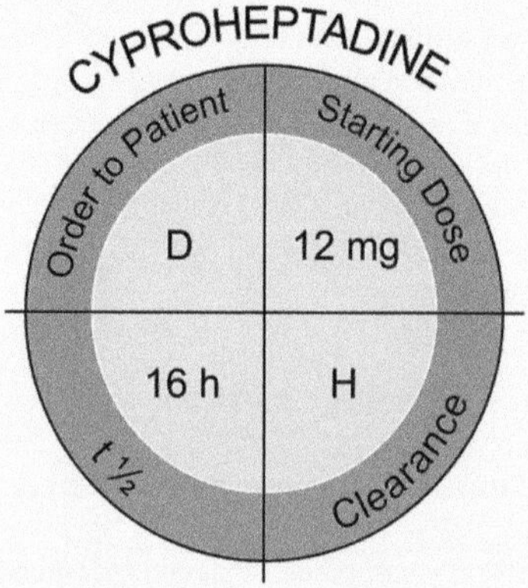 CYPROHEPTADINE Order to Patient: D Starting Dose: 12 mg t 1/2: 16 h Clearance: H	12 mg orally once, then 2 mg every 2 hours (or 4–8 mg every 6 hours)	Selective serotonin reuptake inhibitors, atypical antipsychotics
Dantrolene IV 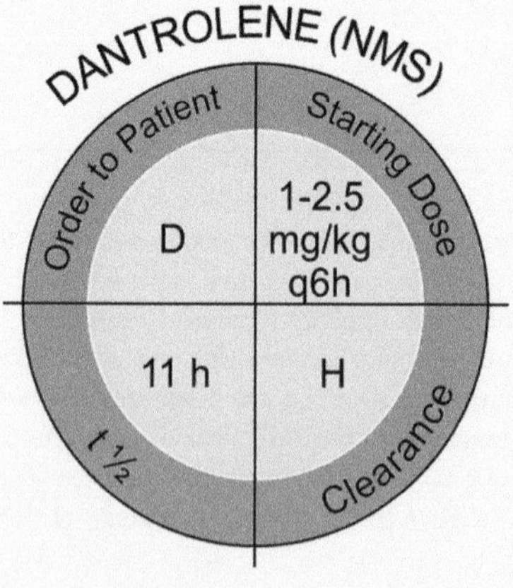 DANTROLENE (NMS) Order to Patient: D Starting Dose: 1-2.5 mg/kg q6h t 1/2: 11 h Clearance: H	1–2.5 mg/kg IV every 6 hours for 2 days (total dose 10 mg/kg), then change to oral administration	Neuroleptic malignant syndrome or malignant hyperthermia

Key Pointers

1. The general approach is to provide supportive care and to use antidotes only if vital organs are involved.
2. A combination of neurologic findings and changes in vital signs may lead to identification of a toxidrome.
3. An acute cholinergic syndrome requires an urgent combination of drugs (pralidoxime and atropine); an acute anticholinergic syndrome can be treated with physostigmine.
4. An opioid toxidrome can be treated with naloxone.
5. A sympathomimetic toxidrome and sedative-hypnotic toxidrome may be treated without any antidotes; the patient is observed, supported and treated symptomatically.

References

1. Albert, M., McCaig, L.F. and Uddin, S. *Emergency Department Visits for Drug Poisoning: United States, 2008–2011*, N.C.f.H. Statistics, Editor. 2015: Hyattsville, MD.
2. Warner, M., et al., *Drug Poisoning Deaths in the United States, 1980–2008*, N.C.f.H. Statistics, Editor. 2011: Hyattsville, MD.
3. Dart, R.C., *Medical Toxicology*. 3rd ed. 2003, Philadelphia, PA: Lippincott Williams & Wilkins.
4. Erickson, T.B., Thompson, T.M. and Lu, J.J. *The approach to the patient with an unknown overdose*. Emerg Med Clin North Am, 2007. **25**: 249–281.
5. Frithsen, I.L. and Simpson, Jr., W.M. *Recognition and management of acute medication poisoning*. Am Fam Physician, 2010. **81**: 316–323.
6. Roberts, E. and Gooch, M.D. *Pharmacologic strategies for treatment of poisonings*. Nurs Clin North Am, 2016. **51**: 57–68.
7. Olson, K.R., et al., eds. *Poisoning and Drug Overdose*. 7th ed. 2017, Lange Publishing: Columbus, OH.
8. Edlow, J.A., et al., *Diagnosis of reversible causes of coma*. Lancet, 2014. **384**: 2064–2076.
9. Chen, H.Y., Albertson, T.E. and Olson, K.R. *Treatment of drug-induced seizures*. Br J Clin Pharmacol, 2016. **81**: 412–419.
10. Buckley, N.A., et al., *Who gets antidotes? Choosing the chosen few*. Br J Clin Pharmacol, 2016. **81**: 402–407.
11. Weisberg, L.S., *Management of severe hyperkalemia*. Crit Care Med, 2008. **36**: 3246–3251.
12. Pileggi, D.J. and Cook, A.M. *Neuroleptic malignant syndrome*. Ann Pharmacother, 2016. **50**: 973–981.
13. Schneir, A., Metushi, I.G. Sloane, C. et al. *Near death from a novel synthetic opioid labeled U-47700: emergence of a new opioid class*. Clin Toxicol (Phila), 2017. **55**: 51–54.

Chapter 17

Drugs Used to Prevent Complications

Acute immobilization with anticipated prolonged bed rest and tubes and catheters require the use of prophylactic drugs. Many prophylactic measures relate to failure to move limbs (spinal cord injury), failure to breathe adequately (mechanical ventilation bundles), and placement of intravenous (IV) catheters (infection precautions). In the neurosciences ICU one preventive measure stands out. Prevention of cerebral vasospasm is essential in the management of patients with aneurysmal subarachnoid hemorrhage; unfortunately after many clinical trials oral nimodipine is the only drug proven to prevent later cerebral infarction after a ruptured aneurysm.

Prevention of Deep Venous Thrombosis

Subcutaneous (SQ) heparin or low-molecular-weight heparin (LMWH) is frequently used in immobilized patients to prevent venous thromboembolism (VTE) and pulmonary embolus. This is achieved with administration of heparin (5,000 units three times a day) or enoxaparin (40 mg once daily). Use of anticoagulants for treatment are discussed in Chapter 7.

Heparin (Prophylactic) SQ

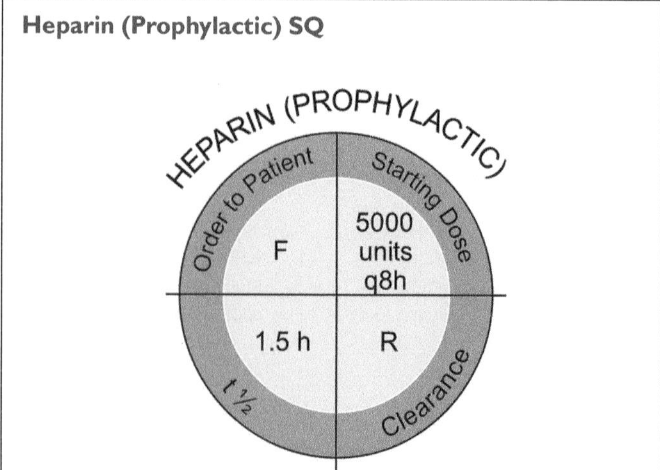

Pharmacologic Characteristics

- Synthesized from either bovine or porcine intestines
- Indirectly binds to antithrombin, resulting in a conformational change that prevents the activation of fibrinogen to fibrin
- Affects the intrinsic pathway of the clotting cascade
- Unfractionated heparin (UFH) inhibits factor Xa better than LMWH
- Rapid onset of action

Dosing and Administration

- 5,000 units SQ three times a day
- 7,500 units SQ three times daily in patients with body mass index (BMI) >40 or weight >140 kg
- Initiate therapy:
  - 48 hours after cerebral hemorrhage
  - 24 hours after craniotomy
  - 24 hours after IV alteplase
  - 12 hours after traumatic brain injury (after documentation of stable cerebral contusions, if any)
  - 3 hours in any stable resuscitated non-surgical neurocritically ill patient

Monitoring

- Combined with intermittent calf compression devices
- Ultrasound of legs (optional)
- Ultrasound of arms with central venous catheter (optional)
- Baseline liver function tests and coagulation parameters (to assess for underlying liver disease)
- Baseline complete blood count with hemoglobin and platelet count
- Platelet count
- Abnormal bruising or bleeding

Side Effects

- Dermatologic reactions (skin necrosis and allergies) less likely with UFH than with LMWH
- Heparin-induced thrombocytopenia antibodies incidence is 0.5–5%
- Hyperkalemia (rare)
- Osteoporosis with long-term administration (>6 months)

Enoxaparin (Prophylactic) SQ

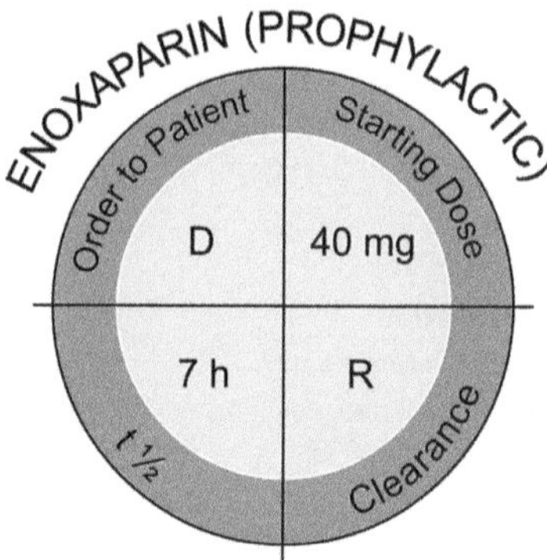

Pharmacologic Characteristics

- Derived from UFH
- Low molecular weight: 4,000–5,000 Daltons (compared to UFH ~15,000 Daltons)
- Factor Xa inhibitor with some activity against antithrombin III
- Slightly more effective in preventing venous thromboembolic events than UFH
- Greater bioavailability than UFH. Alternative is Daltaparin 5000 units/day SQ but cannot be used in patients with renal dysfunction

Dosing and Administration

- 40 mg/day SQ
- In patients with BMI >40, increasing the dose by 30% may be appropriate, but ideal dose is not known
- In patients with creatinine clearance (CrCl) <30 ml/min, reduce enoxaparin dose to 30 mg/day

Monitoring

- Measure anti-Xa level when drug is at steady state and 4 hours after last dose administered (for therapeutic dosing)
- Monitor activity with anti-Xa levels in renal disease or obesity
- Baseline complete blood count
- Baseline coagulation studies and liver function tests
- Renal function indices
- Platelet count

Side Effects

- Heparin-induced thrombocytopenia (<1%; lower incidence than with UFH)
- Increased risk of bleeding events with CrCl <30 ml/min
- Hypersensitivity (angioedema, pruritus, urticaria, hyperkalemia)
- Vesiculobullous rash and ischemic skin necrosis
- Major bleeding that cannot be adequately reversed with protamine
- Transient increase in liver function tests

Fondaparinux SQ

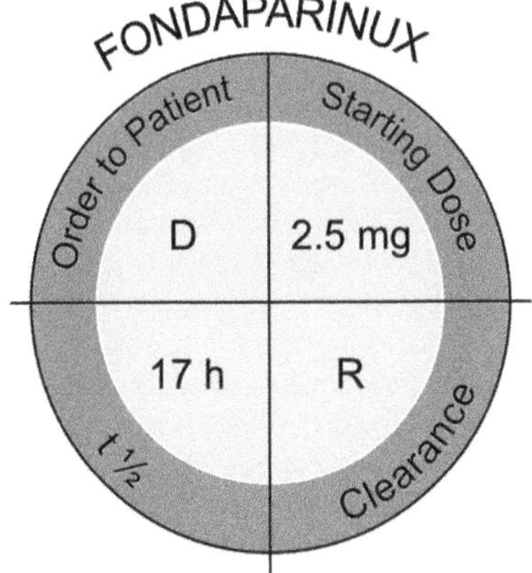

Pharmacologic Characteristics

- Synthetic pentasaccharide factor Xa inhibitor
- Antithrombin-mediated inhibition of factor Xa; inhibits thrombin formation and clot propagation
- For heparin-induced thrombocytopenia
- Probably as effective as LWMH in preventing VTE

Dosing and Administration

- 2.5 mg SQ once daily
- Avoid in patients with CrCl <30 ml/min; decrease dose to 1.5 mg SQ once daily for CrCl 30–50 ml/min
- No dosage adjustments are needed in patients with mild to moderate hepatic dysfunction; not studied in those with severe hepatic dysfunction

Monitoring

- Renal function
- Baseline and periodic complete cell count
- Platelet count
- Signs of bleeding
- Prothrombin time (PT) and activated partial thromboplastin time (aPTT) do not measure degree of anticoagulation
- Anti-Xa levels at 3 hours after administration: 0.39–0.5 mg/L (therapeutic range for prophylaxis)

Side Effects

- Thrombocytopenia (uncommon)
- Bleeding risk increases with age >75 years, decreased renal function, and weight <50 kg

Prevention of Hyperglycemia

In critically ill patients, the major risk factors for hyperglycemia are increased cortisol levels, increased catecholamines, glucagon, growth hormone, gluconeogenesis, or glycogenolysis. Insulin resistance is seen in more than 80% of critically ill patients. Hyperglycemia is associated with poor outcomes, increased mortality rates, prolonged hospitalization and intensive care unit stays, nosocomial infections, and increased ventilator-dependent days (1). In addition, there are worse neurologic outcomes and higher intracranial pressure values in traumatic brain injury patients. Moreover, ischemic damage is mitigated with lower glucose levels (in acute strokes), and there is reduced benefit of recanalization after stroke and reduced salvageable penumbral tissue when the patient is hyperglycemic. It has been demonstrated that hyperglycemia causes increased permeability of the blood–brain barrier. The target goal of serum glucose should be 140 to 180 mg/dl, avoiding the more liberal goal of 180 to 200 mg/dl.

On the other hand, there is increased mortality with intensive insulin therapy (serum glucose 80–110 mg/dl) and a higher incidence of hypoglycemia (1). Hyperglycemia in nondiabetic patients may need even more aggressive control, but precise targets are not known (2). Some basic recommendations are:

- Insulin sliding scale: individualized based on prior insulin use
- Short-acting, regular insulin 250 units in 250 ml of 0.45% sodium chloride at 1–5 units per hour if glucose exceeds 200 mg/dl
- Infuse insulin into existing IV line with compatible IV solution
- Avoid IV fluids containing dextrose solutions when trying to normalize hyperglycemia
- Point-of-care glucose testing hourly while on infusion
- With every 20-mg/dl change (<180 mg/dl), reduce infusion rate by 1–2 units per hour
- With every 50-mg/dl change (>200 mg/dl), increase infusion rate by 2 units per hour
- Severe hyperglycemia (>800 mg/dl) requires potassium supplementation of IV fluids and bicarbonate (Box 17.1)
- Severe hypoglycemia (<40 mg/dl) occurs in up to 20% of patients on IV insulin therapy and in up to 30% when defined as a glucose level <60 mg/dl

Prevention of Stress Ulcers

The best prevention of stress ulcers is early enteral nutrition with a prokinetic agent (3,4). Enteral nutrition may be as beneficial as drugs in preventing stress ulcers.

Box 17.1 Management of Acute Severe Hyperglycemia

- Rehydrate up to 5 L in diabetic ketoacidosis (DKA) and up to 10 L in hyperosmolar hyperglycemic state (HHS), usually 15–20 ml/kg per hour
- IV fluids 0.9% NaCl with hyponatremia (Na <135 mmol/L); 0.45% NaCl with hypernatremia or 0.9% NaCl at rate of 250–500 ml/hr after initial hydration
- Add dextrose to IV fluids when serum glucose is at 200 mg/dl in DKA, 250–300 mg/dl in HHS
- Potassium, 20–40 mEq hourly with values 3.3–5.3, added to maintenance IV fluids
- Dilute bicarbonate ($NaHCO_3$), 100 mEq in 400 ml, infuse for 2 hours when pH <6.9; use is controversial
- IV insulin therapy if serum potassium is >3.2 mmol/L

Drug Options

- Histamine-2 receptor blockers (H2RBs) antagonize histamine-2 receptors on the parietal cells to decrease gastric acid secretion. Examples are famotidine, ranitidine, and cimetidine.
- Proton pump inhibitors (PPIs) block acid secretion by irreversibly binding to and inhibiting the hydrogen-potassium ATPase pump on the parietal cell. Examples are lansoprazole, pantoprazole, esomeprazole, and omeprazole.
- Sucralfate coats and protects the stomach lining and is well tolerated except for small risk of aluminum toxicity (use caution in patients with renal disease).
- PPIs and H2RBs increase the risk of ventilator-associated pneumonia, *Clostridium difficile* infections (higher pH allows for bacterial growth in the stomach). PPIs pose a greater risk than H2RBs in this setting.

Indications for Stress Ulcer Prophylaxis

- Coagulopathy, platelet count <50,000/m^3, International Normalized Ratio (INR) >1.5, PT >2 times control
- Mechanical ventilation for >48 hours
- History of gastrointestinal ulceration or recent bleeding (<1 year)
- Traumatic brain or spinal cord injury
- Two or more of the following:
  - Sepsis >1 week
  - Occult gastrointestinal bleeding for a week
  - Corticosteroid use

Famotidine PO/IV

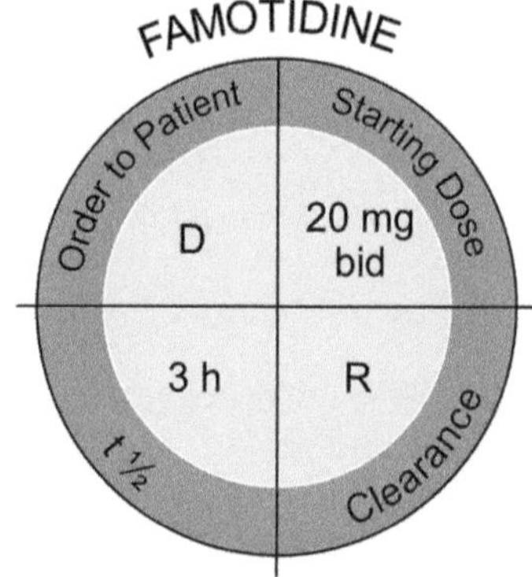

Pharmacologic Characteristics

- H2RB
- Duration: 10–12 hours

Dosing and Administration

- 20 mg orally or IV twice daily
- IV push over 2 minutes
- 20 mg once daily with CrCl <50 ml/min

Monitoring

- Renal function
- Signs of bleeding
- Hematocrit, platelets
- Liver function tests

Side Effects

- Acute confusional state
  - Reversible
  - Increased risk with age >50 years
  - Increased risk with hepatic or renal dysfunction
- Electrocardiographic (EKG) changes (with concomitant renal dysfunction)
- Thrombocytopenia

Ranitidine PO

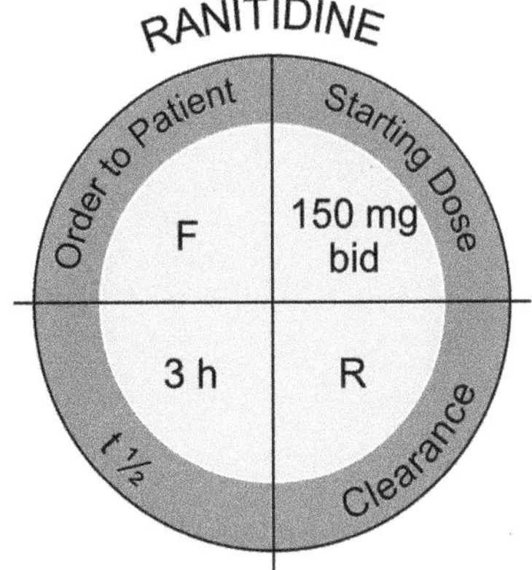

Pharmacologic Characteristics

- H2RB
- Duration: 6–8 hours

Dosing and Administration

- 150 mg orally twice daily; 50 mg IV every 6–8 hours
- IV push over 2 minutes
- If CrCl is <50 ml/min, decrease dose to 150 mg once daily orally or 50 mg every 24 hours IV

Monitoring

- Renal function
- Signs of bleeding
- Liver function tests

Side Effects

- Confusion
- Agranulocytosis
- Transient elevation in liver function test results
- Bradycardia (with rapid IV administration)
- Thrombocytopenia

Cimetidine PO

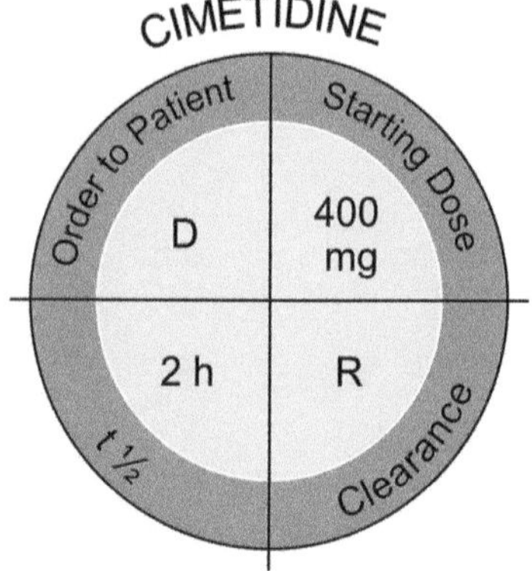

Pharmacologic Characteristics

- H2RB
- Has fallen out of favor due to adverse events (more than famotidine and ranitidine)
- Duration: 24 hours

Dosing and Administration

- 400 mg orally once daily
- 200 mg orally once daily if CrCl is <50 ml/min

Monitoring

- Renal function
- Signs of gastrointestinal bleeding
- Liver function

Side Effects

- Confusion
- Agranulocytosis
- Elevated liver function test results

Pantoprazole PO or IV

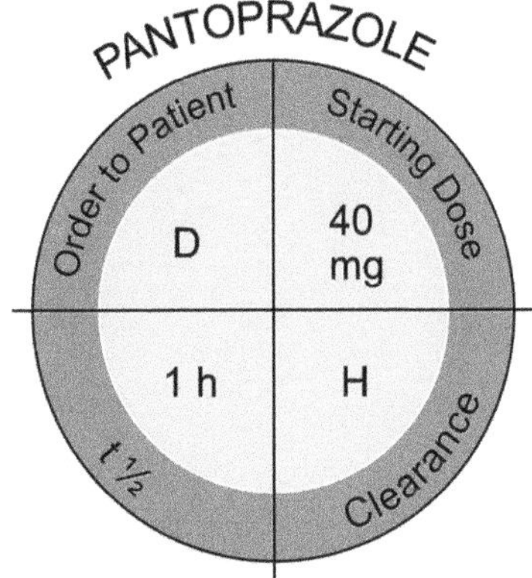

Pharmacologic Characteristics

- PPI
- Irreversibly inhibits hydrogen/potassium ATPase pump on parietal cells to decrease gastric pH
- Onset: 2.5 hours (oral), 15–30 minutes (IV)
- Duration: 7 days (oral), 24 hours (IV)

Dosing and Administration

- 40 mg once daily orally or IV
- Flush IV line before and after administration; give over 2 minutes slow push or 15-minute infusion
- Tablets should be swallowed whole; oral packet can be administered via enteral tube
- No dosage adjustments are needed in patients with renal or hepatic disease

Monitoring

- Signs of bleeding
- Gastrointestinal upset
- Electrolytes
- Hematocrit, platelets

Side Effects

- Headache
- Dizziness
- Nausea, vomiting, diarrhea
- Leukopenia, thrombocytopenia
- Interstitial nephritis
- *Clostridium difficile*-associated diarrhea
- Hypomagnesemia (rare)
- Vitamin B12 deficiency (prolonged use)

Omeprazole PO

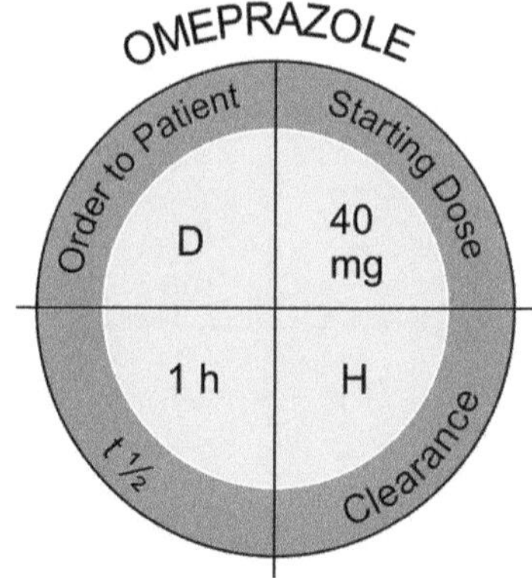

Pharmacologic Characteristics

- PPI
- Irreversibly inhibits hydrogen/potassium ATPase pump on parietal cells to decrease gastric pH
- Onset: <2 hours
- Duration: up to 72 hours

Dosing and Administration

- 20–40 mg once daily orally
- Decrease dose to 10 mg once daily for maintenance of healing ulcer in patients with hepatic impairment. There is an ~2–3 fold increase in half-life in patients with mild to severe hepatic dysfunction
- Capsule and tablet should be swallowed whole. Omeprazole is also available in suspension form for administration via enteral tube
- No dosage adjustments needed in patients with renal dysfunction
- May decrease antiplatelet activity of clopidogrel by inhibiting activation

Monitoring

- Gastrointestinal irritation
- Serum magnesium

Side Effects

- Headache
- Abdominal pain
- Nausea and vomiting, diarrhea
- Systemic lupus erythematosus (new onset or exacerbations)
- Interstitial nephritis
- *Clostridium difficile*-associated diarrhea
- Hypomagnesemia (rare)
- Vitamin B12 deficiency (prolonged use)

Lansoprazole PO

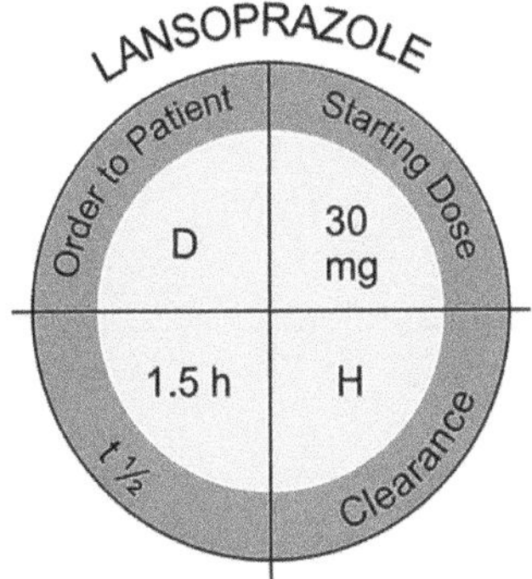

Pharmacologic Characteristics

- PPI
- Irreversibly inhibits hydrogen/potassium ATPase pump on parietal cells to decrease gastric pH
- Onset: 2 hours
- Duration: 24 hours

Dosing and Administration

- 30 mg once daily
- Capsules may be opened and contents sprinkled on applesauce. Suspension is available for enteral access
- Swallow oral disintegrating tablets whole. Allow to dissolve on tongue
- Morning administration is preferred for greater control of acid production
- No dosage adjustments are needed in patients with renal impairment
- No dosage adjustments are needed in patients with mild to moderate hepatic impairment; bioavailability is increased but no dosage adjustments are suggested

Monitoring

- Complete blood count
- Liver function
- Renal function

Side Effects

- Headache
- Abdominal pain
- Diarrhea
- Systemic lupus erythematosus (new onset or exacerbations)
- Interstitial nephritis
- *Clostridium difficile*-associated diarrhea
- Hypomagnesemia (rare)
- Vitamin B12 deficiency (prolonged use)

Sucralfate PO

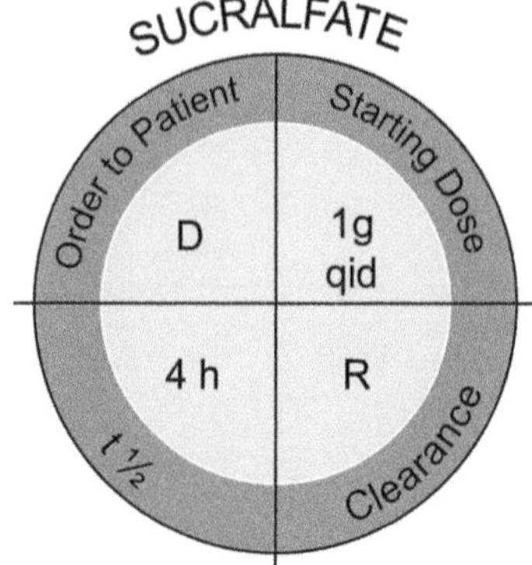

Pharmacologic Characteristics

- Contains aluminum salt (watch for accumulation in patients with renal dysfunction)
- Forms viscous coating that acts on the surface to protect the gastric lining of the stomach
- Duration of action: up to 6 hours
- Minimally absorbed

Dosing and Administration

- 1 g orally every 6 hours, on an empty stomach with water
- Separate administration from other medications by 2 hours

Monitoring

- Renal function

Side Effects

- Constipation
- Less risk for pneumonia than H2RB (25)

Prevention of Infections

A number of infections are anticipated. Prophylactic use of antibiotics is not warranted and does not improve outcomes, but empiric antibiotic treatment should be started in the presence of warning signs such as chest infiltrate, leukocytosis, or fever. Recent clinical trials on the preventive use of antibiotics in patients with stroke did not show improved outcomes (5,6).

Prevention of Ventilator-Associated Pneumonia

Ventilator-associated pneumonia is defined as a pneumonia that occurs more than 48 hours after intubation; it is expected to occur in 10% to 20% of ventilated patients (7). Raising the head of the bed 30 to 45 degrees to avoid aspiration together with subglottic aspiration may reduce the risk. Moreover,

Table 17.1 Empiric Antibiotics in Pneumonia	
Unknown organism	Piperacillin-tazobactam 4.5 g IV q6h OR cefepime or ceftazidime 2 g IV q8h
Gram-positive	Vancomycin, third-generation cephalosporin, fluoroquinolone, linezolid
Gram-negative	Third- or fourth-generation cephalosporin, fluoroquinolone

oral decontamination with chlorhexidine reduces the risk by decreasing colonization (8). Early tracheostomy reduces the risk if the period of ventilation is expected to exceed 48 hours. There is an increased risk with PPI or H2RB therapy (higher gastric pH allows for organism growth) (9,10). Empiric regimens should cover *Staphylococcus aureus* and other Gram-negative bacilli, and the clinicians should initiate anaerobic coverage if aspiration is suspected. Cases of nosocomial pneumonia with fungi are rare. The need for antimicrobials targeted toward methicillin-resistant *Staphylococcus aureus* (MRSA) and *Pseudomonas* species is determined based on the patient's risk factors.

The risks for multi-drug–resistant organisms need to be considered, such as IV antibiotic use in the past 90 days, presence of septic shock, acute respiratory distress syndrome, more than 4 days of hospitalization, and renal replacement therapy. Vancomycin or linezolid should be initiated if pneumonia is suspected to be caused by MRSA. The choice of appropriate empiric antibiotics (Table 17.1) against likely organisms should be based on local surveillance patterns. The clinician should review culture sensitivities and resistance patterns locally. Narrowing of the antibiotic regimen should be based on culture data (11).

Prevention of Urinary Tract Infections

Approximately 3% to 10% of catheterized patients develop bacteriuria. The best prevention is aseptic insertion of the catheter (11). Generally, an antibiotic-coated catheter or antimicrobial prophylaxis has no effect. Risk factors for catheter-associated urinary tract infections (CAUTI) include female sex, advanced age, history of diabetes, colonization of catheter bag, errors in catheter care, and aggressive perianal care (12).

The presence of an indwelling urinary catheter increases the risk of urinary tract infections. CAUTI criteria include catheters in place for 48 hours or more, positive urine culture, fever, and suprapubic or flank pain. Spinal cord injury patients may not complain of flank pain. Other nonspecific signs might include fever, abdominal pain, and new-onset delirium. For purposes of analysis, a midstream specimen is preferable to an indwelling-catheter sample or the free catch method.

The clinician should determine whether the infection represents colonization or asymptomatic bacteria or active infection. Asymptomatic bacteriuria should not be treated (except in pregnant or renal transplant patients). The duration of treatment should be 2 weeks (i.e., complicated urinary tract infection) based on local resistance patterns. Third-generation cephalosporins are commonly used as first-line agents due to growing resistance to sulfamethoxazole-trimethoprim and fluoroquinolone antibiotics (13) (Box 17.2).

Box 17.2 Catheter-Associated Urinary Tract Infection (CAUTI)
Ceftriaxone, 1 g IV daily *or* Cefotaxime, 1 g IV every 8 hours *or* Ciprofloxacin 400 mg IV every 12 hours (500 mg orally twice daily) *or* Levofloxacin 500 mg orally or IV daily

Prevention of Vascular Access Infections

It is common practice to try to prevent central line-associated bloodstream infections (CLABSI) and catheter-related bloodstream infections (CRBSI) (14,15). Intraluminal infection is associated with manipulation of the catheter hub or infusion of contaminated fluids (16,17). The use of total parenteral nutrition infusion increases the risk of CRBSI (18–21). Coagulase-negative staphylococci are the most common sources of catheter-related infections, most of which are resistant to methicillin. Daily reassessment of the need for the line, with removal if possible, reduces the risk of bloodstream infection (22,23). Generally, the use of chlorhexidine bathing and chlorhexidine dressings reduces the risk. Antibiotic choices are shown in Box 17.3.

Prevention of Ventriculitis

The risk for infection from a ventriculostomy increases after 5 to 7 days. Antibiotic prophylaxis has not been proven to prevent ventriculitis, although many neurosurgeons have used antibiotic-impregnated catheters (24).

Prevention

- Should target Gram-positive organisms (skin organisms)
- Albeit of uncertain benefit, many neurosurgeons still prefer prophylaxis with cefazolin 1 g every 8 hours (2 g every 8 hours if the patient's weight is >80 kg); dose reduction in patients with renal impairment
- First-generation cephalosporins are active against most Gram-positive organisms, but not MRSA or enterococci

Treatment

- Treatment of infection requires removal of the device and empiric therapy with vancomycin plus either a fourth-generation cephalosporin

Box 17.3 Central Line-Associated Bloodstream Infection (CLABSI)	
Vancomycin, dosed to goal trough 10–15 mcg/ml	*And* Cefepime, 2 g IV every 12 hours

Table 17.2 Shunt Infection/Nosocomial Meningitis	
Vancomycin, dosed to goal trough 15–20 mcg/ml	*And* one of the following:
	• Cefepime, 2 g IV every 8 hours
	• Ceftazidime, 2 g IV every 8 hours
	• Meropenem, 2 g IV every 8 hours

or carbapenem active against *Pseudomonas* species (Table 17.2). Some guidelines provide regimens of intraventricular vancomycin, aminoglycosides, and polymyxins, but these are not proven to eradicate difficult-to-control infections (4)

Prevention of Constipation

Constipation occurs in 25% to 50% of older adults and is often multifactorial. Risk factors include female gender, immobility, medications, poor nutrition, and decreased hydration. Patients with spinal cord injury, Parkinson's disease, paraplegia, multiple sclerosis, and autonomic neuropathy are at highest risk. Multiple drugs can be implicated, including antiepileptic drugs, anticholinergic medications, and opioid analgesics. Treatment options include laxatives (bulk-forming, stimulant, or osmotic) and stool softeners. Senna and docusate sodium are often used together.

Senna PO

Pharmacologic Characteristics

- Stimulant laxative, anthraquinone class
- Increases rate of colonic transit, inhibits water and electrolyte secretion, stimulates peristalsis

Dosing and Administration

- 8.8-mg tablets, 2 tablets once daily, usually at bedtime
- Maximum of 4 tablets daily

Monitoring

- Relief of constipation
- Electrolytes if persistent diarrhea

Side Effects

- Stomach pain
- Diarrhea
- Abdominal cramps

Docusate Sodium PO

Pharmacologic Characteristics

- Effective for stool softening, to alleviate constipation when in combination with a laxative
- Anionic surfactant used to stimulate intestinal fluid secretion and penetration of fluid into stool

Dosing and Administration

- 50–200 mg/day orally, either once daily or divided twice daily

Monitoring

- Abdominal pain
- Relief of constipation

Side Effects

- Abdominal pain
- Nausea
- Diarrhea

Bisacodyl PO/PR

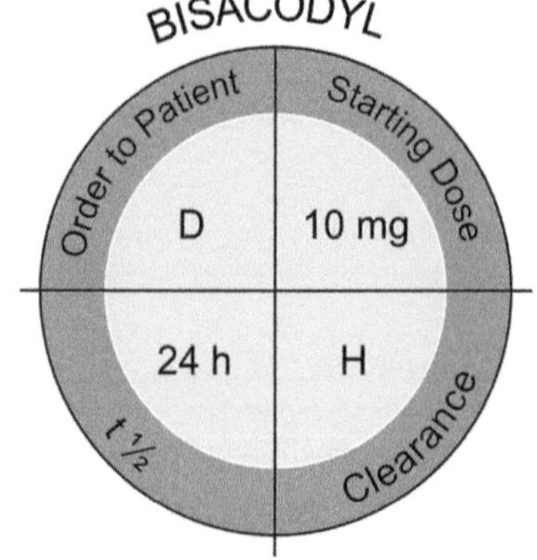

Pharmacologic Characteristics

- Stimulant laxative; causes strong but brief increases in peristaltic movements
- Stimulates parasympathetic reflexes, which results in peristalsis
- May be more effective in spinal cord injury

Dosing and Administration

- 10–15 mg nightly, up to 30 mg (orally); 10 mg rectally
- Tablets should be swallowed whole
- Results are typically seen 15–60 minutes after administration (rectally) or 6–12 hours after oral administration
- Avoid in patients with bowel obstruction

- Avoid milk products within 1 hour of taking tablets; milk degrades the enteric coating of the tablets, increasing the risk of gastric irritation

Monitoring

- Abdominal pain
- Significant change in bowel patterns

Side Effects

- Abdominal pain
- Nausea and vomiting
- Diarrhea
- Cramps

Prevention of Cerebral Vasospasm

Multiple clinical trials have been conducted, but nimodipine has remained the only effective drug in preventing symptomatic cerebral vasospasm after aneurysmal subarachnoid hemorrhage. The evidence for its use in traumatic subarachnoid hemorrhage is less clear. Nimodipine may cause hypotension and then is discontinued. Underuse of nimodipine may exist. (Intra-arterial management for symptomatic cerebral vasospasm is operator-dependent although many interventionalists would use verapamil or nicardipine.)

Nimodipine PO

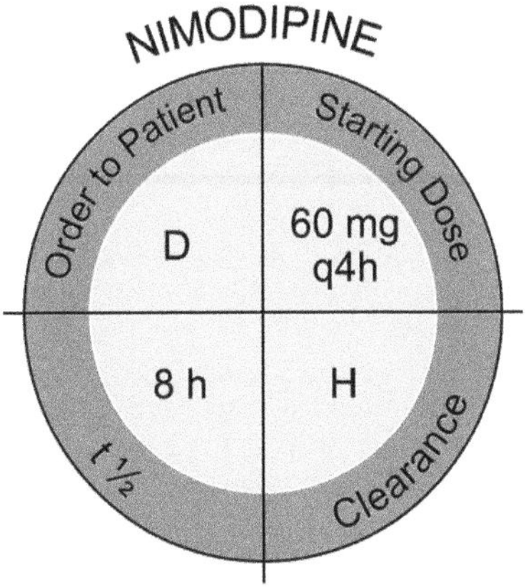

Pharmacologic Characteristics

- Dihydropyridine L-type calcium-channel antagonist
- No measurable effect on cerebral artery caliber
- Concomitant use of CYP3A4 inhibitors (increased risk of hypotension)

Dosing and Administration

- 60 mg orally every 4 hours
- 30 mg orally every 2 hours if transient marked hypotension
- Continue for 21 days and discontinue if no aneurysm is found

Monitoring

- Blood pressure
- Transaminases

Side Effects

- Hypotension (far more common than appreciated)
- Diarrhea
- Nausea

Key Pointers

1. Prophylaxis with UFH or LMWH is needed in all patients with acute brain injury without contraindications
2. Stress ulcer prophylaxis is indicated for high-risk patients, but not all patients in the ICU
3. Before prescribing antibiotics for urinary tract infections, an accurate diagnosis is required, not just the presence of bacteriuria.
4. Prevention of constipation is important using a bowel regimen
5. Nimodipine proven effective is for prevention of symptomatic cerebral vasospasm. Hypotension is a common reason for holding medication.

References

1. Finfer, S., et al., *NICE-Sugar Study Investigators: Intensive versus conventional glucose control in critically ill patients.* N Engl J Med, 2009. **360**: 1283–1297.
2. Krinsley, J.S., et al., *Glucose control, diabetes status, and mortality in critically ill patients: the continuum from intensive care unit admission to hospital discharge.* Mayo Clin Proc, 2017. **92**: 1019–1029.
3. *ASHP Therapeutic Guidelines on Stress Ulcer Prophylaxis. ASHP Commission on Therapeutics and approved by the ASHP Board of Directors on November 14, 1998.* Am J Health Syst Pharm, 1999. **56**: 347–379.
4. Tunkel, A.R., et al., *2017 Infectious Diseases Society of America's Clinical Practice Guidelines for Healthcare-Associated Ventriculitis and Meningitis.* Clin Infect Dis, 2017 [E-pub before print].
5. Ulm, L., et al., *The Randomized Controlled STRAWINSKI Trial: Procalcitonin-guided antibiotic therapy after stroke.* Front Neurol, 2017. **8**: 153.
6. Westendorp, W.F., et al., *The Preventive Antibiotics in Stroke Study (PASS): a pragmatic randomised open-label masked endpoint clinical trial.* Lancet, 2015. **385**: 1519–1526.
7. Dettenkofer, M., et al., *Surveillance of nosocomial infections in a neurology intensive care unit.* J Neurol, 2001. **248**: 959–964.
8. Klompas, M., et al., *Strategies to prevent ventilator-associated pneumonia in acute care hospitals: 2014 update.* Infect Control Hosp Epidemiol, 2014. **35**: 915–936.

9. Kalil, A.C., et al., *Management of adults with hospital-acquired and ventilator-associated pneumonia: 2016 Clinical Practice Guidelines by the Infectious Diseases Society of America and the American Thoracic Society.* Clin Infect Dis, 2016. **63**: e61–e111.

10. Safdar, N., Crnich, C.J. and Maki, D.G. *The pathogenesis of ventilator-associated pneumonia: its relevance to developing effective strategies for prevention.* Respir Care, 2005. **50**: 725–739; discussion 739–741.

11. Wilson, J.W. and Estes, L.L. *Mayo Clinic Antimicrobial Therapy Quick Guide.* 2011, New York: Oxford University Press.

12. Hooton, T.M., et al., *Diagnosis, prevention, and treatment of catheter-associated urinary tract infection in adults: 2009 International Clinical Practice Guidelines from the Infectious Diseases Society of America.* Clin Infect Dis, 2010. **50**: 625–663.

13. Nicolle, L.E., *Catheter-related urinary tract infection.* Drugs Aging, 2005. **22**: 627–639.

14. Safdar, N., et al., *Chlorhexidine-impregnated dressing for prevention of catheter-related bloodstream infection: a meta-analysis.* Crit Care Med, 2014. **42**: 1703–1713.

15. Simmons, S., Bryson, C. and Porter, S. *"Scrub the hub": cleaning duration and reduction in bacterial load on central venous catheters.* Crit Care Nurs Q, 2011. **34**: 31–35.

16. Chopra, V., et al., *The risk of bloodstream infection associated with peripherally inserted central catheters compared with central venous catheters in adults: a systematic review and meta-analysis.* Infect Control Hosp Epidemiol, 2013. **34**: 908–918.

17. Crnich, C.J. and Maki, D.G. *The promise of novel technology for the prevention of intravascular device-related bloodstream infection. I. Pathogenesis and short-term devices.* Clin Infect Dis, 2002. **34**: 1232–1242.

18. Dissanaike, S., et al., *The risk for bloodstream infections is associated with increased parenteral caloric intake in patients receiving parenteral nutrition.* Crit Care, 2007. **11**: R114.

19. Mermel, L.A., et al., *Clinical practice guidelines for the diagnosis and management of intravascular catheter-related infection: 2009 update by the Infectious Diseases Society of America.* Clin Infect Dis, 2009. **49**: 1–45.

20. O'Grady, N.P., et al., *Guidelines for the prevention of intravascular catheter-related infections.* Am J Infect Control, 2011. **39**: S1–34.

21. O'Horo, J.C., et al., *Arterial catheters as a source of bloodstream infection: a systematic review and meta-analysis.* Crit Care Med, 2014. **42**: 1334–1339.

22. O'Horo, J.C., et al., *The efficacy of daily bathing with chlorhexidine for reducing healthcare-associated bloodstream infections: a meta-analysis.* Infect Control Hosp Epidemiol, 2012. **33**: 257–267.

23. Pronovost, P., et al., *An intervention to decrease catheter-related bloodstream infections in the ICU.* N Engl J Med, 2006. **355**: 2725–2732.

24. Lozier, A.P., et al., *Ventriculostomy-related infections: a critical review of the literature.* Neurosurgery, 2002. **51**: 170–181.

25. Alquraini, M., Alshamsi, F. M.H. Møller, et al. *Sucralfate versus histamine 2 receptor antagonists for stress ulcer prophylaxis in adult critically ill patients: A meta-analysis and trial sequential analysis of randomized trials.* Crit Care, 2017. **40**: 21–30.

Chapter 18

Drugs Used to Treat Withdrawal Syndromes

Withdrawal syndromes are undeniably serious and may require extensive pharmacotherapy. The safety of the patient must be balanced against the risks and side effects of the medications administered to control the agitation.

Prior alcoholism accounts for the overwhelming proportion of patients with withdrawal syndromes. There has been a significant increase in alcohol use over the years, including young adults, and nearly half of them will experience withdrawal symptoms. Of these, ~10% of cases will be severe and will need multiple medications to manage symptoms (1). The drugs used to treat alcohol withdrawal syndrome (AWS) include benzodiazepines, dexmedetomidine, and propofol. Other drugs that can be used are carbamazepine, valproate, phenobarbital and baclofen. Gabapentin is effective for mild forms of AWS. Antipsychotics (e.g., haloperidol, quetiapine) have been used to manage severe hallucinosis and delirium; however, they are not as preferable because of the risk of QT prolongation on electrocardiography (and possible torsades de pointes).

Other serious withdrawal syndromes are neurology-specific, such as baclofen withdrawal, which is usually due to pump malfunction. Withdrawal syndromes, such as those associated with nicotine withdrawal, are seemingly trivial but could lead to agitation and tachycardia (2,3).

Alcohol Withdrawal Syndrome

The symptoms of AWS depend on the time of the last drink and could occur as early as 24 hours. In many cases, there is a significant increase in drinking in the weeks before abstinence. AWS has been characterized in the fifth edition of the American Psychiatric Association's *Diagnostic and Statistical Manual of Mental Disorders* (DSM-5; Box 18.1), but some patients have extreme presentations. Often, agitation is far more subtle and difficult to recognize. AWS is defined as the development of tremors, irritability, anxiety, or agitation with eventually profound dysautonomia or hyperactivity marked by hypertension, tachycardia, fever (rising to 39°C), and diaphoresis (4). Auditory hallucinations occur in 80% of patients and often are perceived as the voices of relatives or drinking companions. A single, generalized tonic–clonic seizure may be the first presenting sign of withdrawal in 20% of the more severe cases and may be followed by more events. In many patients, poor sleep, nocturnal dread, and nightmares may antedate classic symptoms of alcohol

Box 18.1 ***Diagnostic and Statistical Manual of Mental Disorders* (DSM-5) Diagnostic Criteria for Alcohol Withdrawal (2)**

A. Cessation of (or reduction in) alcohol use that has been heavy and prolonged
B. Two (or more) of the following, developing within several hours to a few days after criterion A
   - Autonomic hyperactivity
   - Increased hand tremor
   - Insomnia
   - Nausea or vomiting
   - Transient visual, tactile, or auditory hallucinations or illusions
   - Psychomotor agitation
   - Anxiety
   - Generalized tonic–clonic seizures

withdrawal delirium. An estimated 15% to 30% of intensive care unit (ICU) patients have an alcohol addiction and are at risk of developing AWS (5).

Alcohol withdrawal symptoms peak 3 days after the last drink and will subside in 7 days. The mechanism is caused by stimulation of GABA receptors and the inhibition of *N*-methyl-D-aspartate (NMDA) activity.

The Clinical Institute Withdrawal Assessment (CIWA) scale has been universally accepted to assist in nursing care. The syndrome becomes rapidly severe when agitation and dysautonomia are present along with delirium tremens (2,6,7). When at-risk patients are assessed using a CIWA protocol (Boxes 18.1 and 18.2), each component is graded for severity. Reliable cutoff values are not known; multiple medications can be used when two or more symptoms are present. This poses some difficulty in the neurosciences ICU because some of these symptoms may be due to acute brain injury.

Box 18.2 Clinical Institute Withdrawal Assessment of Alcohol Scale, Revised (CIWA-Ar)

- Nausea or vomiting
- Tremor
- Headache
- Paroxysmal sweats
- Anxiety
- Agitation, insomnia
- Tactile disturbances
- Auditory disturbances
- Visual hallucinations
- Orientation

Initial Approach to Drugs for Alcohol Withdrawal

In any patient with alcohol withdrawal, thiamine therapy is required and should be part of the CIWA order set. The commonly used "100 mg dose" has little justification, and thiamine doses of 200-500 mg IV every 8 hours for 3-5 days depending on an estimation of nutritional status should be considered. Diazepam or lorazepam is usually the first agent administered before escalating to dexmedetomidine (8). Benzodiazepines can be used to reduce the incidence of withdrawal-associated seizures (9). Clinical use of carbamazepine, levetiracetam, and valproic acid is not proven to prevent seizures in more severe cases. If a patient is admitted with seizures, carbamazepine has potential benefit in controlling alcohol withdrawal seizures, but it has no significant effect on delirium tremens. Clonidine can be used to reduce symptoms of withdrawal but is not recommended. One alternative (to be used only as a last resort) is to give enteral ethanol via nasogastric tube every 4 to 6 hours, but few hospital practice committees have allowed this intervention. It is best to avoid the use of haloperidol due to hypotension and QT prolongation; haloperidol lowers the seizure threshold and thus may only be considered to manage severe hallucinations (2).

Lorazepam IV

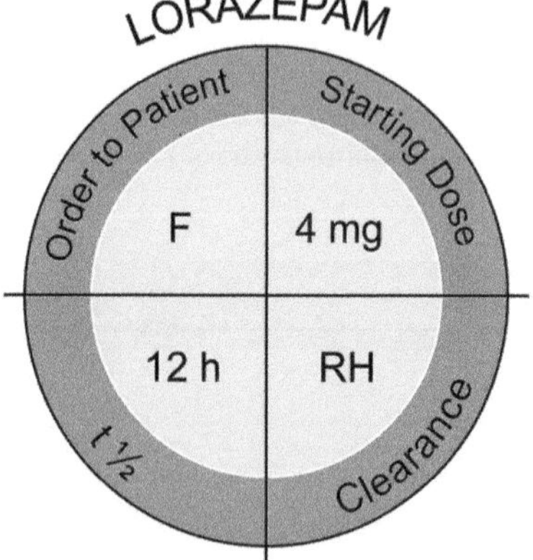

- 2–4 mg given intravenously (IV) as needed; no active metabolite; commonly used as part of the CIWA for Alcohol revised (CIWA-Ar) protocol in many institutions

Diazepam IV

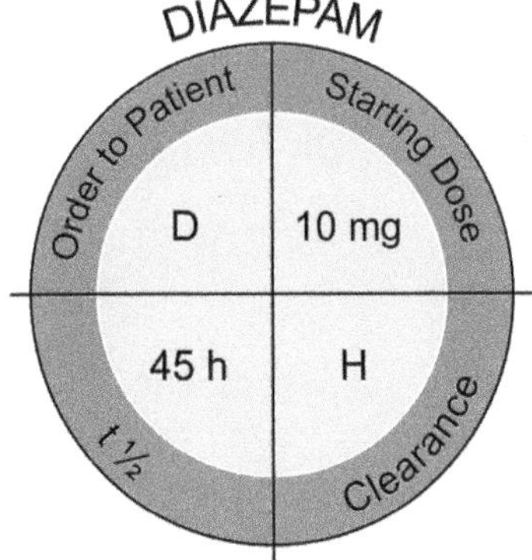

- Gradual escalation from 10 mg to a maximum of 120 mg/day
- Diazepam is preferred because of its active metabolite and lower risk of withdrawal or seizures compared to shorter-acting agents without active metabolites. Diazepam also provides smoother withdrawal from alcohol than agents with shorter half-lives
- Benzodiazepines with shorter half-lives and no active metabolites (e.g., alprazolam, lorazepam, oxazepam) may be preferred in the elderly and in patients with hepatic disease

Carbamazepine PO

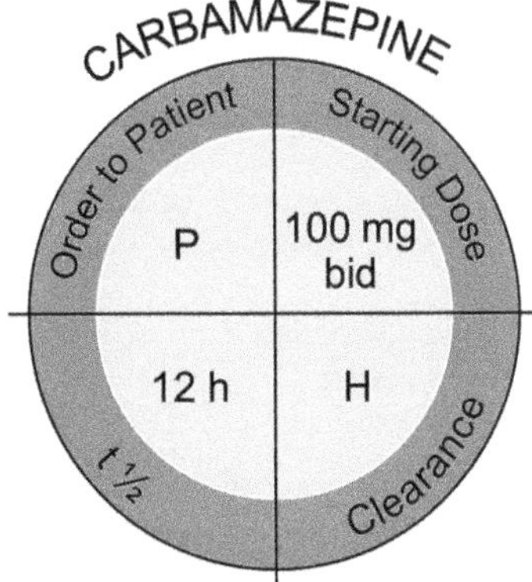

- 200 mg orally twice daily
- Preferred antiepileptic drug if seizures have occurred (10,11)

Approach to Refractory Withdrawal Delirium

Dexmedetomidine IV

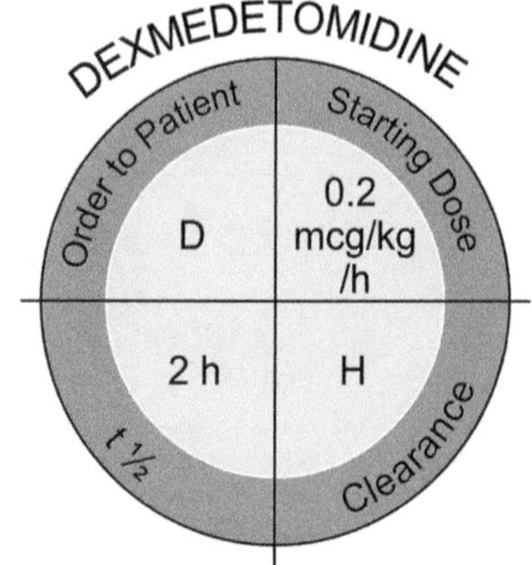

Pharmacologic Characteristics

- Dexmedetomidine is a selective alpha-2 agonist and also results in sedation, analgesia, and anxiolysis
- Dexmedetomidine compares favorably to benzodiazepines and reduces lorazepam use (12)
- Minimal effect on respiratory depression, thus attractive for patients without respiratory compromise (non-ventilated) (13)
- Onset (for sedation): 5–10 minutes

Dosing and Administration

- Start infusion at 0.2 mcg/kg per hour (14)
- Higher dose and longer duration, up to 1.5 mcg/kg per hour, has been used but is associated with a higher risk of bradycardia
- No dosage adjustment is needed in patients with renal or hepatic disease, but clearance is markedly prolonged in those with severe hepatic dysfunction
- Recommended maximum duration of use is 24 hours, though this maximum is often exceeded

Monitoring

- If bradycardia occurs with a loading dose of dexmedetomidine, stop the infusion
- Hypotension is related to the loading dose, and the infusion may be resumed at half the previous rate
- Richmond Agitation-Sedation Scale (RASS) score
- Respiratory rate

Side Effects

- Bradyarrhythmias
- Hypotension

Propofol IV

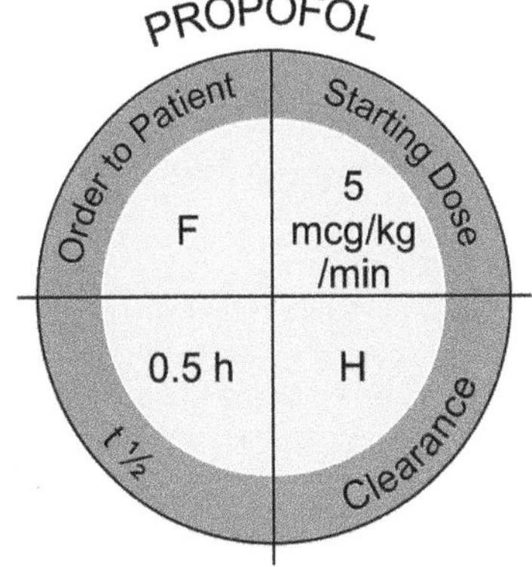

Pharmacologic Characteristics

- Amnesic, anxiolytic, anticonvulsant, and muscle relaxant properties
- Highly lipophilic, crosses the blood–brain barrier rapidly for immediate drug response
- Contains egg phospholipids, so avoid in patients who are allergic to eggs
- No significant advantage over benzodiazepines or dexmedetomidine (15)
- Use propofol when the patient is already intubated, when there is a concern for seizures, when the patient is unresponsive to benzodiazepines, when refractory delirium tremens is present, or when the patient is not a candidate for other adjunctive therapies
- Used in patients with benzodiazepine-resistant withdrawal (due to downregulation and decreased sensitivity of GABA receptors, leading to ineffectiveness of benzodiazepines)

Dosing and Administration

- Dosing 5–100 mcg/kg per minute; higher infusion rates for chronic alcoholism
- No dosage adjustments are needed in patients with in renal or hepatic dysfunction

Monitoring

- Decreased use of benzodiazepines and antipsychotics
- Blood pressure
- Triglycerides

Side Effects

- Risk of propofol related infusion syndrome with longer duration of use and higher doses (more prevalent in younger population)
- Hypotension
- Hypertriglyceridemia

Barbiturates

Pharmacologic Characteristics

- As effective as benzodiazepines (16–19)
- Useful in the ICU setting when large doses of benzodiazepines or escalating doses are needed to alleviate delirium tremens
- Possess sedative and anticonvulsant properties
- Onset: 3–5 minutes, duration 15–45 minutes

Dosing and Administration

- Phenobarbital, 10 mg/kg IV loading dose
- Phenobarbital 60 mg q6h orally with taper to 30 mg twice daily in 5 days.
- Reduced dose recommended for patients with renal or hepatic dysfunction

Monitoring

- Respiratory depression if used with benzodiazepines
- Liver function tests
- Cardiac function tests
- Continuous infusion contains propylene glycol; monitor osmolar gap for toxicity

Side Effects

- Oversedation
- Respiratory compromise

Ketamine IV

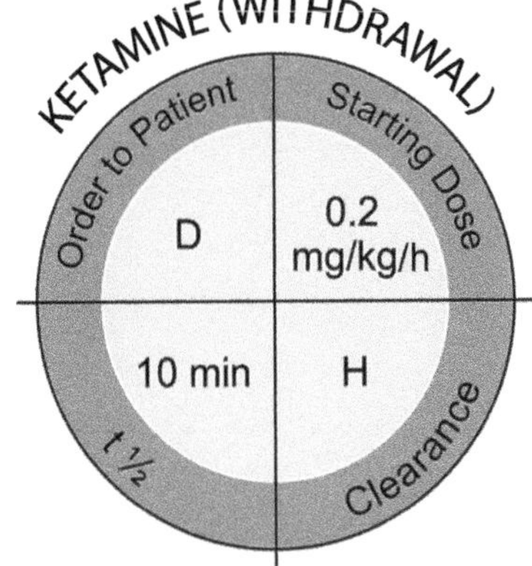

Pharmacologic Characteristics

- Beneficial in AWS because of NMDA receptor antagonism (20)
- Alcohol upregulates NMDA and downregulates GABA receptors
- Non-competitive NMDA receptor antagonist
- Produces analgesia at low doses
- Onset: <1 minute, duration: 5–10 minutes after bolus
- Hepatically metabolized to active metabolites
- Does not necessarily reduce benzodiazepine dosing

Dosing and Administration

- Mostly in intubated patients
- Bolus: 0.3 mg/kg IV
- Infusion: 0.2 mg/kg per hour

Monitoring

- Oversedation
- Blood pressure and heart rate

Side Effects

- Hallucinations and delirium reported in ~10% of patients
- Emergence reactions
- Hypertension
- Tachycardia
- Potential for increased intracranial pressure

Opioid Withdrawal

The current "fentanyl epidemic" on the Eastern Seaboard and in Canada will increase the likelihood that serious opioid withdrawal will occur in the ICU. The clinical features are nonspecific and can mimic those of an acute brain injury. The Clinical Opiate Withdrawal Scale (COWS) can be

Box 18.3 Clinical Opioid Withdrawal Scale (COWS)—Major Categories

- Pulse rate
- Sweating
- Restlessness
- Pupil size
- Bone or joint aches
- Runny nose or tearing
- Gastric upset
- Tremor
- Yawning
- Irritability
- Gooseflesh skin

used to help manage withdrawal symptoms (Box 18.3) (21). Opioid withdrawal starts with restlessness, myalgias, diarrhea, mydriasis, piloerection, and tachycardia ("cold turkey"). The severity of symptoms depends on the rapidity of withdrawal and the amount previously taken (causing tolerance).

Several drugs can be used to treat opioid withdrawal (23). In most cases, methadone 10 mg IM or 20 mg orally will provide rapid improvement of subjective and objective symptoms. Patients with more serious manifestations would need fluid resuscitation and treatment of nausea and vomiting.

Drug options for treating opioid withdrawal are as follows:

- Buprenorphine 0.3–0.9 mg IV/IM (for those patients who missed a dose of buprenorphine; not recommended for acute opioid withdrawal) (22–24)

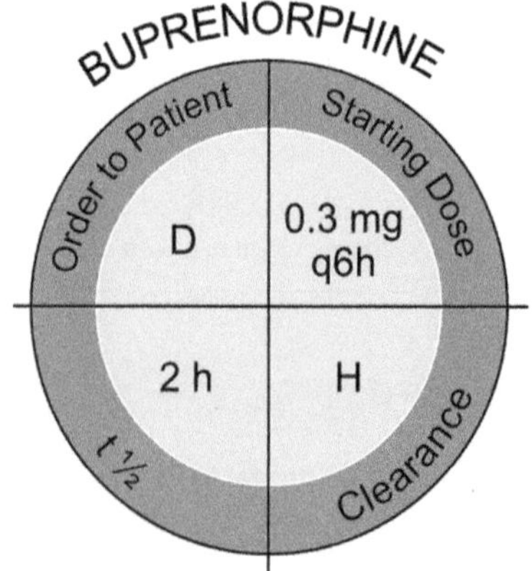

- Clonidine 0.1–0.3 mg orally hourly

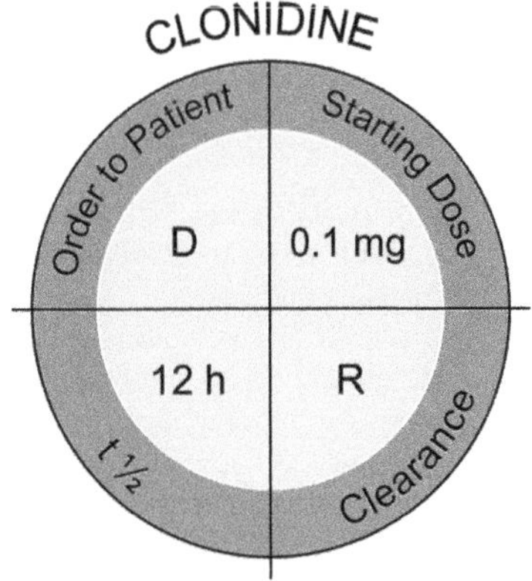

- Methadone 10 mg IV or IM.

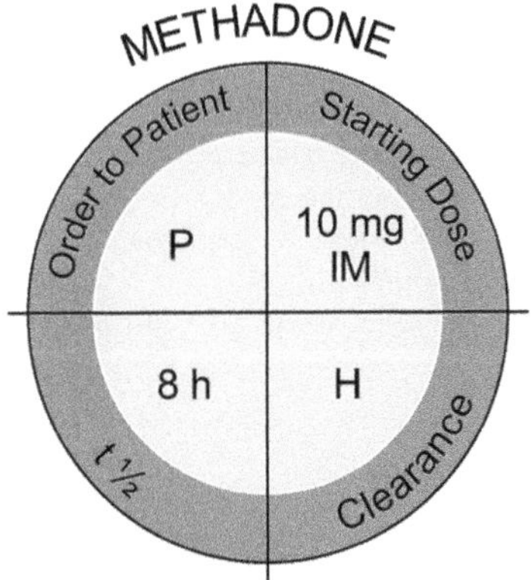

- Ondansetron 4 mg orally or IV (for nausea)
- Hydroxyzine 50–100 mg orally or IV (for nausea or anxiety)
- Diazepam 10–20 mg orally or IV (for anxiety)
- Promethazine 25 mg IV or IM (for nausea)
- Loperamide 4 mg orally (for diarrhea)
- Acetaminophen 650 mg (for pain)

Stimulant Withdrawal

Patients withdrawing from cocaine or amphetamines may experience restlessness, depression, and trouble sleeping. Most of the treatment involves symptomatic management. If delusions and hallucinations occur, brief treatment with chlordiazepoxide or haloperidol may be considered. There is little role for dopamine agonists (e.g., bromocriptine, pergolide) (25).

Baclofen Withdrawal

Acute baclofen withdrawal is usually seen with pump malfunction and rapidly can become an emergency. Patients demonstrate increased heart rate, labile blood pressures, variable temperatures or fever, hallucinations, agitation, and, eventually, a decline in the level of consciousness (26–32). A significant increase in muscle rigidity causing rhabdomyolysis, eventual multisystem failure, and possible seizures can be seen. Symptoms of withdrawal can become apparent as soon as 12 to 24 hours after baclofen pump failure.

The goal of treatment is to minimize muscle spasms, treat blood pressure variability, and prevent central nervous system complications. The alternative explanations to consider are autonomic dysreflexia, sepsis, serotonin syndrome, illicit drug abuse, neuroleptic malignant syndrome, and malignant hyperthermia.

Drugs for treatment of baclofen withdrawal are as follows:

- Oral replacement of baclofen with large doses (>120 mg/day), divided over six to eight doses; however, this may not be effective in the early management of withdrawal due to its slow onset (days)
- Benzodiazepines as adjuvant therapy (e.g., lorazepam, diazepam, midazolam)
  - Useful for muscle relaxation, normothermia, blood pressure stabilization, and no seizures
  - Other temporizing measures are cyproheptadine,dantrolene and tizanidine

Cyproheptadine PO

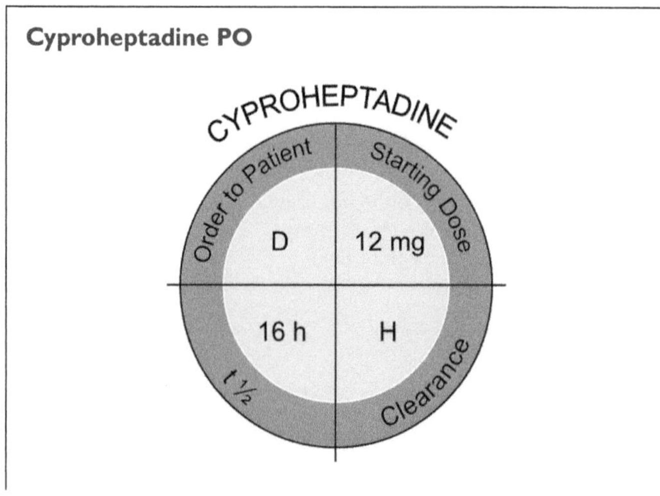

- Histamine-1 antagonist
- Treatment of spasticity
- 12-mg orally starting dose followed by 4–8 mg three or four times per day until improvement

Dantrolene PO

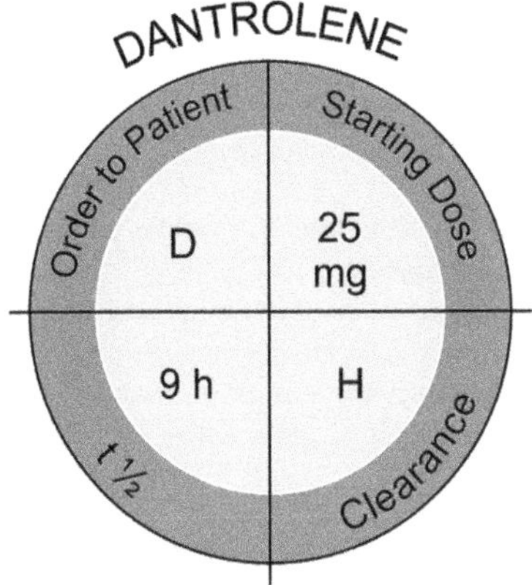

- Dantrolene blocks excitatory calcium-channel activity and prevents calcium release from endoplasmic reticulum, leading to a decrease in calcium-induced muscle contraction
- 10 mg/kg orally per day in three divided doses

Tizanidine PO

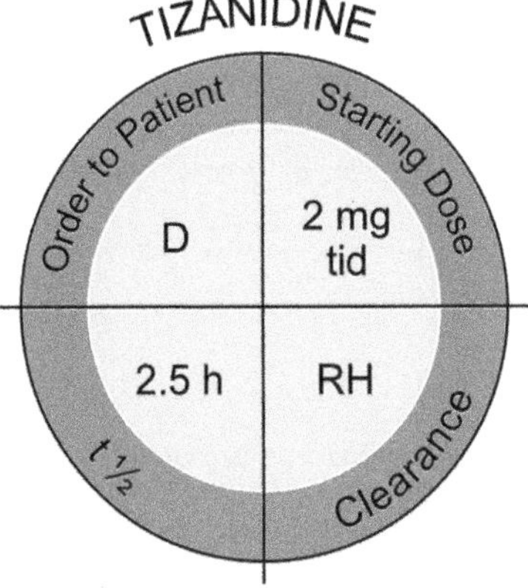

- Alpha-2 agonist, centrally active muscle relaxant that works by inhibiting presynaptic spinal neurons
- 8–12 mg/day in three or four divided doses
- Less effect on heart rate and blood pressure than clonidine (also an alpha-2 agonist)

Nicotine Withdrawal

- Estimated 25% to 50% of ICU patients are active smokers
- Symptoms begins 1–2 days after withdrawal and peak within 1 week
- Risk factor for increased frequency of agitation and incidental adverse events
- Signs include anger, irritability, frustration, anxiety, difficulty concentrating, and trouble sleeping
- Nicotine withdrawal has not been known to increase hospital mortality in ICU patients
- Few studies evaluating the effects of nicotine replacement therapy in ICU patients include oral replacement agents (e.g., bupropion and varenicline)
- Nicotine patch may cause headache, insomnia, and tachycardia
- Routine use of nicotine patch is not advised and may be harmful. Use only in selected symptomatic patients (33,34)
- Patches often contain metal and thus have to be removed prior to magnetic resonance imaging

Key Pointers

1. In alcohol withdrawal, diazepam or lorazepam is usually the first agent given before escalating to dexmedetomidine or propofol.
2. In opioid withdrawal, methadone, 10 mg IV will provide rapid improvement of subjective and objective symptoms.
3. Baclofen withdrawal is a life-threatening withdrawal syndrome requiring urgent treatment with oral replacement of baclofen in large doses (>120 mg/day).
4. Stimulant withdrawal involves symptomatic management, and many drugs are ineffective.
5. Nicotine and stimulant withdrawal are self-correcting and require little symptomatic intervention.

References

1. Adams, B. and K. Ferguson. *Pharmacologic Management of Alcohol Withdrawal Syndrome in Intensive Care Units*. AACN Adv Crit Care, 2017. **28**: 233–238.
2. Schmidt, K.J., et al., *Treatment of severe alcohol withdrawal*. Ann Pharmacother, 2016. **50**: 389–401.

3. Schuckit, M.A., *Recognition and management of withdrawal delirium (delirium tremens).* N Engl J Med, 2014. **371**: 2109–2113.
4. Jesse, S., et al., *Alcohol withdrawal syndrome: mechanisms, manifestations, and management.* Acta Neurol Scand, 2016. **135**: 4–16.
5. Perry, E.C., *Inpatient management of acute alcohol withdrawal syndrome.* CNS Drugs, 2014. **28**: 401–410.
6. Awissi, D.K., et al., *Alcohol, nicotine, and iatrogenic withdrawals in the ICU.* Crit Care Med, 2013. **41**: S57–68.
7. Sutton, L.J. and Jutel, A. *Alcohol withdrawal syndrome in critically ill patients: identification, assessment, and management.* Crit Care Nurse, 2016. **36**: 28–38.
8. Kosten, T.R. and P.G. O'Connor, *Management of drug and alcohol withdrawal.* N Engl J Med, 2003. **348**: 1786–1795.
9. Mayo-Smith, M.F., *Pharmacological management of alcohol withdrawal. A meta-analysis and evidence-based practice guideline. American Society of Addiction Medicine Working Group on Pharmacological Management of Alcohol Withdrawal.* JAMA, 1997. **278**: 144–151.
10. Bjorkqvist, S.E., et al., *Ambulant treatment of alcohol withdrawal symptoms with carbamazepine: a formal multicentre double-blind comparison with placebo.* Acta Psychiatr Scand, 1976. **53**: 333–342.
11. Malcolm, R., et al., *Double-blind controlled trial comparing carbamazepine to oxazepam treatment of alcohol withdrawal.* Am J Psychiatry, 1989. **146**: 617–621.
12. Turunen, H., et al., *Dexmedetomidine versus standard care sedation with propofol or midazolam in intensive care: an economic evaluation.* Crit Care, 2015. **19**: 67.
13. Wong, A., Smithburger, P.L. and Kane-Gill, S.L. *Review of adjunctive dexmedetomidine in the management of severe acute alcohol withdrawal syndrome.* Am J Drug Alcohol Abuse, 2015. **41**: 382–391.
14. Linn, D.D. and Loeser, K.C. *Dexmedetomidine for alcohol withdrawal syndrome.* Ann Pharmacother, 2015. **49**: 1336–1342.
15. Brotherton, A.L., et al., *Propofol for treatment of refractory alcohol withdrawal syndrome: a review of the literature.* Pharmacotherapy, 2016. **36**: 433–442.
16. Hammond, C.J., et al., *Anticonvulsants for the treatment of alcohol withdrawal syndrome and alcohol use disorders.* CNS Drugs, 2015. **29**: 293–311.
17. Martin, K. and Katz, A. *The role of barbiturates for alcohol withdrawal syndrome.* Psychosomatics, 2016. **57**: 341–347.
18. Mo, Y., Thomas, M.C. and Karras, Jr., G.E. *Barbiturates for the treatment of alcohol withdrawal syndrome: a systematic review of clinical trials.* J Crit Care, 2016. **32**: 101–107.
19. Rosenson, J., et al., *Phenobarbital for acute alcohol withdrawal: a prospective randomized double-blind placebo-controlled study.* J Emerg Med, 2013. **44**: 592–598 e592.
20. Wong, A., et al., *Evaluation of adjunctive ketamine to benzodiazepines for management of alcohol withdrawal syndrome.* Ann Pharmacother, 2015. **49**: 14–19.
21. Wesson, D.R. and Ling, W. *The Clinical Opiate Withdrawal Scale (COWS).* J Psychoactive Drugs, 2003. **35**: 253–259.
22. Gowing, L., et al., *Buprenorphine for managing opioid withdrawal.* Cochrane Database Syst Rev, 2017. **2**: CD002025.
23. Gowing, L., et al., *Alpha(2)-adrenergic agonists for the management of opioid withdrawal.* Cochrane Database Syst Rev, 2016: CD002024.

24. Royall, M., Garner, K.K., Hill, S.R. et al., *Alpha-adrenergic agonists for the management of opioid withdrawal.* Am Fam Physician, 2017. **95**: Epub ahead of print.

25. Moscovitz, H., Brookoff, D. and Nelson, L. *A randomized trial of bromocriptine for cocaine users presenting to the emergency department.* J Gen Intern Med, 1993. **8**: 1–4.

26. Coffey, R.J. and Ridgely, P.M. *Abrupt intrathecal baclofen withdrawal: management of potentially life-threatening sequelae.* Neuromodulation, 2001. **4**: 142–146.

27. Ross, J.C., et al., *Acute intrathecal baclofen withdrawal: a brief review of treatment options.* Neurocrit Care, 2011. **14**: 103–108.

28. Alden, T.D., et al., *Intrathecal baclofen withdrawal: a case report and review of the literature.* Childs Nerv Syst, 2002. **18**: 522–525.

29. Alvis, B.D. and Sobey, C.M. *Oral baclofen withdrawal resulting in progressive weakness and sedation requiring intensive care admission.* Neurohospitalist, 2017. **7**: 39–40.

30. Green, L.B. and Nelson, V.S. *Death after acute withdrawal of intrathecal baclofen: case report and literature review.* Arch Phys Med Rehabil, 1999. **80**: 1600–1604.

31. Greenberg, M.I. and Hendrickson, R.G. *Baclofen withdrawal following removal of an intrathecal baclofen pump despite oral baclofen replacement.* J Toxicol Clin Toxicol, 2003. **41**: 83–85.

32. Leo, R.J. and Baer, D. *Delirium associated with baclofen withdrawal: a review of common presentations and management strategies.* Psychosomatics, 2005. **46**: 503–507.

33. Pathak, V., et al., *Outcome of nicotine replacement therapy in patients admitted to ICU: a randomized controlled double-blind prospective pilot study.* Respir Care, 2013. **58**: 1625–1629.

34. Wilby, K.J. and Harder, C.K. *Nicotine replacement therapy in the intensive care unit: a systematic review.* J Intensive Care Med, 2014. **29**: 22–30.

Chapter 19

Treatment of Brain Injury-Associated Symptoms and Signs

Acute neurologic disease results in a myriad of minor and major symptoms, some of which are partly specific to the nature of the illness. In non-comatose patients, we can anticipate that acute brain injury may cause headache, nausea, vomiting, and difficulty with swallowing and managing secretions. (Drugs for headaches are discussed in Chapter 4.) Fever is common, and this vital sign not only requires immediate attention but also close control in acute brain injury. Fever management has become more defined and more complex and therefore is discussed in this chapter.

There are other symptoms that requires attention. Nausea is not often signaled by the patient, and management may suddenly become urgent with vomiting. Explosively large volumes of emesis can easily cause aspiration, mucus plugging of large bronchial branches, tachypnea, and acute hypoxemia.

Handling secretions is another major clinical problem. Typical examples are patients with a new brainstem ischemic or hemorrhagic stroke, and after posterior fossa craniotomy. Secretions are also commonly seen in patients with advanced Guillain-Barré syndrome, myasthenia gravis exacerbation, or advanced amyotrophic lateral sclerosis (ALS).

We can anticipate that hiccups are prominent in patients with a compressive mass or acute stroke in structures in the posterior fossa. Persistent hiccups are exhausting to the patient and often undertreated.

A cornucopia of drugs is available to manage these common, not trivial symptoms, however it should pointed out that many of them cause sedation and therefore common sense is advised.

Control of Nausea and Vomiting

It is an effect of vagal nerve activity. Any patient with an acute brain injury may start vomiting as a result of increased intracranial pressure (ICP) (1). Commonly seen in patients with aneurysmal subarachnoid hemorrhage during rupture or with the development of acute hydrocephalus, increased ICP may lead to vomiting and worsening headache. However, in the neurosciences ICU, the use of opioids for pain management is also a common cause of vomiting in patients susceptible to these drugs. Postoperative nausea and vomiting are common in patients who have had a neurosurgical procedure,

Box 19.1 Causes of Vomiting

- Acutely increased intracranial pressure
- Untreated pain
- Paralytic ileus
- Vertigo and early mobilization (posterior fossa surgery)

and it is most prevalent in patients with posterior fossa surgery. Even early mobilization will cause vertigo associated with vomiting. Frequent causes of vomiting are shown in Box 19.1 (2–7). Several drugs are available to control vomiting and are discussed here.

Ondansetron IV

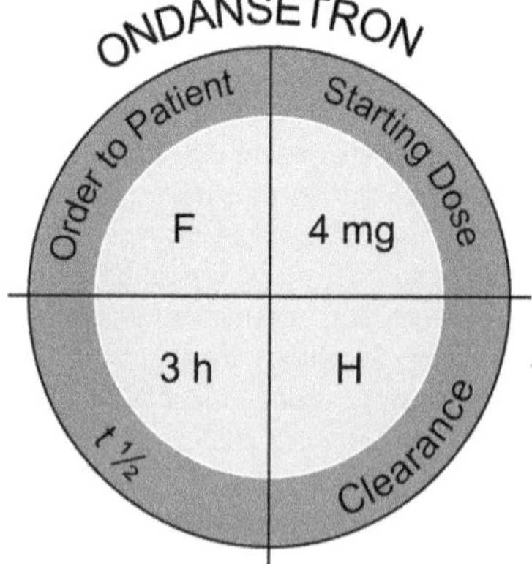

Pharmacologic Characteristics

- Selective 5-HT3 receptor antagonist
- Blocks serotonin (5-HT3) peripherally on vagal nerve terminus and centrally in the chemoreceptor trigger zone
- Peak effect: 10 minutes (IV)

Dosing and Administration

- 4 mg intravenously (IV) as a single dose
- Extensive hepatic metabolism; half-life is prolonged in patients with hepatic dysfunction

Monitoring

- Review other serotonergic and QT-prolonging agents
- Frequency of vomiting

- liver function tests
- Electrolytes

Side Effects

- QT-interval prolongation
- Drowsiness, sedation
- Acute, reversible dyskinesias and encephalopathy in high doses (8)
- Rare increase in liver function test results

Metoclopramide IV

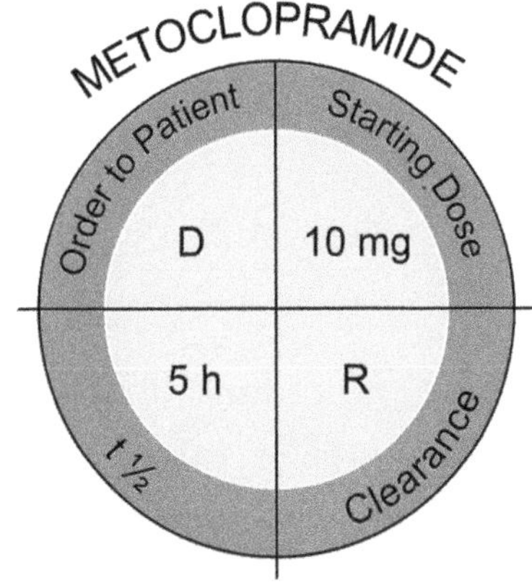

Pharmacologic Characteristics

- Prokinetic agent
- Dopamine antagonist (higher doses)
- Increases lower esophageal sphincter tone
- Promotes motility by sensitizing the gastrointestinal tract to acetylcholine
- Blocks serotonin receptors in the central nervous system chemoreceptor trigger zone
- Onset: 30 minutes orally, 1–2 minutes IV
- Duration: 1–2 hours (both oral and IV)

Dosing and Administration

- 10 mg IV (repeated four times daily)
- No dose adjustments are needed in patients with liver disease
- Give half the normal dose in patients with renal impairment
- Not dialyzable

Monitoring

- Extrapyramidal signs
- EKG

Side Effects

- Oculogyric crisis, dyskinesias, akathisia
- Mood disturbance
- Tachycardia and hypertension
- Drowsiness
- Arrhythmias (associated with rapid IV administration)
- Neuroleptic malignant syndrome
- Tardive dyskinesia

Droperidol IV

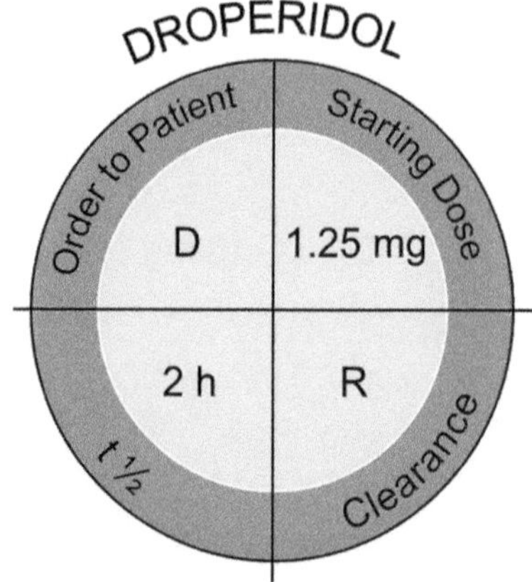

Pharmacologic Characteristics

- Butyrophenone dopamine antagonist
- Blockage of dopamine receptors in the chemoreceptor-trigger zone
- Usually given for postoperative vomiting
- Avoid use in Parkinson's disease
- Onset: 3–10 minutes
- Peak: 30 minutes
- Duration: 2–4 hours

Dosing and Administration

- Dose: 0.625–1.25 mg IV (maximum dose 2.5 mg)

Monitoring

- Considerable sedation
- EKG
- Extrapyramidal disturbances

Side Effects

- Hypotension at higher doses
- Cardiac arrhythmias and prolonged QT interval (at higher doses, more than 2.5mg/day)
- Neuroleptic malignant syndrome (rare)

Scopolamine Patch

Pharmacologic Characteristics

- Anticholinergic agent: blocks acetylcholine at parasympathetic smooth muscle
- Antagonizes histamine and serotonin
- Blocks muscarinic receptors on the sinoatrial node (resulting in decreased heart rate)
- Onset: 6 hours
- Peak: 24 hours
- Contraindicated in glaucoma

Dosing and Administration

- Dose: 1.5 mg transdermal patch placement every 3 days

Monitoring

- Touching the patch and eye-rubbing by patient causes mydriasis
- Patch may contain metal; may need to remove before magnetic resonance imaging (MRI)
- Signs of excessive anticholinergic effects
- Signs of ongoing vomiting

Side Effects

- Dizziness
- Dry mouth
- Bradycardia
- Hypotension
- Visual disturbance due to anticholinergic effect (common in elderly)
- Confusion (common in the elderly)

Dexamethasone IV

Pharmacologic Characteristics

- Mechanism of action is unclear for antiemetic effect
- Long-acting glucocorticoid with minimal mineralocorticoid properties
- Onset is rapid and duration is short

Dosing and Administration

- 4–8 mg IV

Monitoring

- Monitor closely for hyperglycemia
- Exacerbated hypertension
- Electrolytes
- May worsen cardiac failure
- Ongoing nausea

Side Effects

- Hyperglycemia
- Fluid retention
- Gastrointestinal symptoms
- Insomnia

Control of Hiccups

In the neurosciences ICU, lesions in the posterior fossa often cause persistent hiccups. Intractable hiccups are defined as nearly constant or prolonged periods of hiccups lasting more than 2 days. The causes of hiccups are shown in Box 19.2 (9).

Several drugs have been tested in clinical trials with mixed results. The first line of treatment is oral baclofen. Gabapentin is also considered in patients with acute neurologic illness (10,11). In refractory (and exhausting) hiccups, nonpharmacologic options are potentially successful and could be tried (Box 19.3).

Box 19.2 Causes of Hiccups

- Brainstem injury
- Cerebellar stroke
- Stomach distention
- Bowel obstruction
- Hyponatremia
- Hypocalcemia
- Diabetes mellitus
- Renal failure
- Medications (e.g., anesthetic drugs, diazepam, barbiturates, dexamethasone, chemotherapy, methyldopa)

Box 19.3 Nonpharmacologic Options to Treat Hiccups

- Inhalation of smelling salts
- Oropharyngeal stimulation with ice water
- Cold compress to face
- Breath holding
- Rebreathing hypercapnia
- Valsalva maneuver
- Trial of continuous positive airway pressure (CPAP)

Drugs Used for Hiccups

- Baclofen, 5–10 mg orally three times a day (maximum 75 mg/day in divided doses)

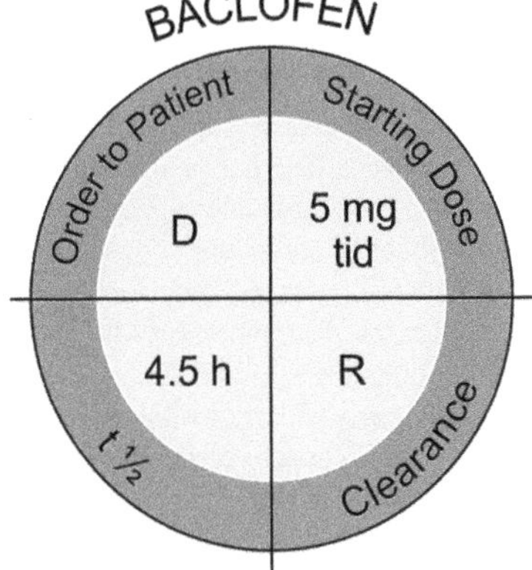

- Gabapentin, orally 300–600 mg/day (maximum 1,200 mg/day in divided doses)

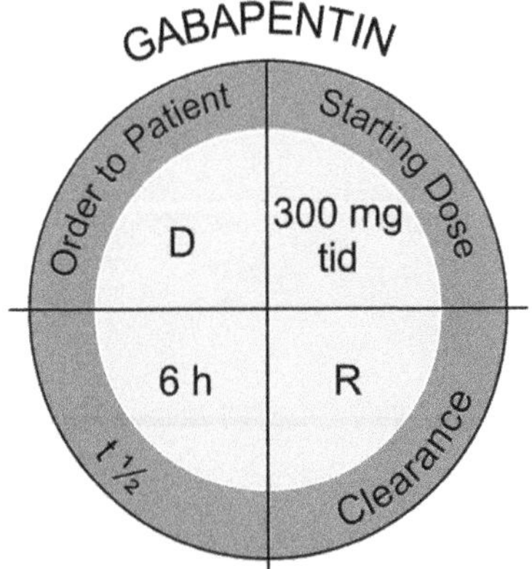

- Pregabalin orally 75–150 mg twice daily
- Metoclopramide orally 10 mg three times daily
- Chlorpromazine orally 25–50 mg three times daily
- Haloperidol orally 5–10 mg once daily at bedtime
- Carbamazepine orally 100–300 mg four times daily
- Valproate orally 15 mg/kg per day, divided three or four times per day
- Phenytoin orally 100 mg three times per day
- Nifedipine orally 60–180 mg daily, in divided doses

- Methylphenidate orally 10 mg once daily
- Amitriptyline orally 10–25 mg daily at bedtime

Control of Secretions

Secretion management is often necessary, and failure to do so causes mucous plugging and episodic hypoxemia. Secretions are particularly more common in patients with an endotracheal tube, and repeated episodes of suctioning are needed when the amount of secretions is significant. Suboptimal secretion management may lead to atelectasis, and bronchoscopy may be needed in the most recalcitrant cases. Secretions may be a result of a bacterial tracheobronchitis, and antibiotic treatment after positive culture is needed. Excessive secretions may occur with myasthenia gravis, usually as a result of high doses of pyridostigmine. Excessive secretions management occurs often in patients who require palliative care (12,13).

Secretions are best handled with a Yankauer suction catheter, which can be used by patients who have sufficient reach with their arms. If patients cannot handle their own secretions and are mechanically ventilated, presuctioning lavage with a saline solution ("saline bomb") while providing 100% oxygen through a manual bag is the best technique.

Drugs that can be used to reduce secretions are as follows:

- Amitriptyline, 100 mg at night (effect seen 4 hours after administration)

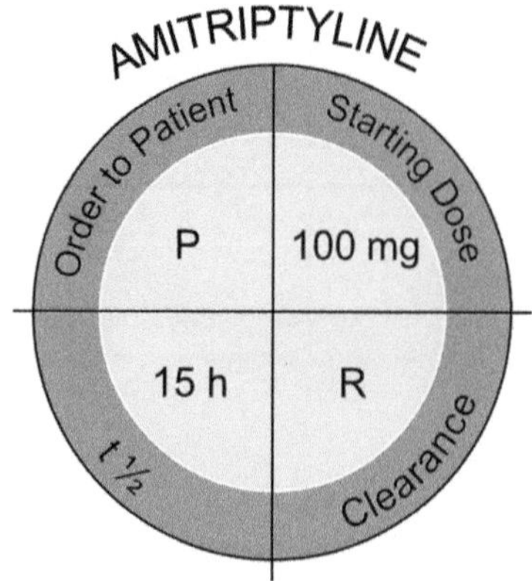

- Glycopyrrolate, 0.1 mg IV every 6 hours; 1 mg orally three times daily

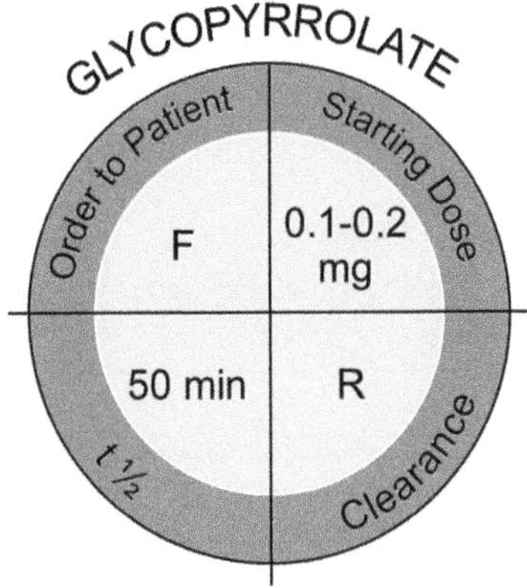

- Atropine, 0.5 mg subcutaneously every 4 hours as needed or 1 or 2 drops sublingually of 1% ophthalmic solution every 2–4 hours as needed
- Hyoscine hydrobromide, 0.25–0.5 mg IV every 4 hours, up to four times a day
- Scopolamine patch, 1.5 mg transdermal every 3 days
- Botulinum toxin type A, 100 MU (mostly in patients with ALS or Parkinson's disease) (14)
- External radiation of parotid glands (in ALS)

Control of Constipation and Dysmotility

Gastrointestinal dysmotility and constipation are common in the neurosciences ICU, and before treatment, a proximate cause must be established (Box 19.4).

Box 19.4 Causes of Intestinal Pseudo-obstruction

- Medication
  - Tricyclic antidepressants
  - Anticholinergic drugs
  - Anti-Parkinson drugs
  - Phenothiazine
  - Barbiturates
- Bed rest
- Hypothyroidism
- Dysautonomia (Guillain-Barré syndrome)
- Diabetes mellitus
- Spinal cord injury

Box 19.5 General Measures for Paralytic Ileus

- Nasogastric tube connected to intermittent suction
- Fluids for hydration
- Correction of metabolic alkalosis
- Pain management
- Rectal tube
- No oral intake for 24–48 hours
- Gastroenterology consultation for decompressive colonoscopy
- Surgery consultation to exclude obstruction

Complete absence of interstitial peristalsis is uncommon. Abdominal tenderness and distention are key physical findings, and widened loops showing involvement of the cecum and ascending or transverse colon. Diagnosis is confirmed by a plain radiograph of the abdomen showing significantly increased intestinal diameters. Air–fluid levels are present and can be demonstrated on an abdominal radiograph. Perforation is imminent when cecal dilatation reaches 10 cm on plain abdominal radiographs. Several measures (Box 19.5) and pharmacologic treatments should be considered for paralytic ileus (15,16), but not if there is a suspected acute surgical abdomen or gastrointestinal obstruction.

Drug that can be used for paralytic ileus are as follows:

- Methylnaltrexone for opioid-related ileus
  - 0.15 mg/kg subcutaneously once daily, usually 12 mg
  - Restoration of bowel function within 15 minutes of injection
  - With renal impairment (creatinine clearance [CrCl] <60 ml/min), reduce the dose to 6 mg
  - Half-life is 15 hours; time to peak is 30 minutes
  - Discontinue all laxatives prior to use; restart after 3 days if methylnaltrexone proves ineffective
- Senna, 10 ml once daily (contains 17.6 mg sennosides)
- Lactulose, 10–20 g (15–30 ml) once daily; 40 g daily as needed
- Erythromycin, 3 mg/kg (or 200 mg) IV every 8 hours
- Metoclopramide, 10 mg IV four times daily
- Neostigmine, 0.5 mg IV (contraindicated in patients with bradycardia, hypotension, recent myocardial infarction, previous beta-blocker therapy, bronchospasm, or renal failure)
- Octreotide, 50–100 mcg subcutaneously initially (range 200–900 mcg/day, in two or three divided doses)

Control of Fever and Shivering

Fever after acute brain injury is expected in many patients and often has noninfectious causes. Fever is a prognostic sign in patients with acute brain injury and increased ICP, and seizures may worsen with fever (17–20). Fever causes increased cardiac output that is therefore associated with increased oxygen consumption, increased carbon dioxide production, and generally increased energy expenditure. Oxygen consumption can increase by ~10% per degree Celsius. There is also a small increase brain oxygen consumption per degree of Celsius.

Fever is best controlled with mechanical devices and rarely is effectively and safely controlled with drugs. The severity of fever can be expressed by calculating fever burden, which is defined as a maximal temperature of 38°C summed from several days. Fever cannot and should not be attributed to a "central cause," and an aggressive search for an infectious or noninfectious source is mandatory. For example, if fever persists, all central access catheters should be removed and cultured. In a patient with diarrhea, stool culture and empiric antibiotics can be considered. Polymerase chain reaction (PCR) studies against *Clostridium difficile* and vancomycin-resistant *Enterococcus* toxins are warranted. An abdominal ultrasound for potential infectious sources should be considered as well as ultrasound scans for deep venous thrombosis.

Fever Management

Pharmacologic control of fever is notoriously difficult and seldom sustained. Temperature control with cooling devices has markedly improved practice. Acetaminophen is often used and is given orally (1,000 mg every

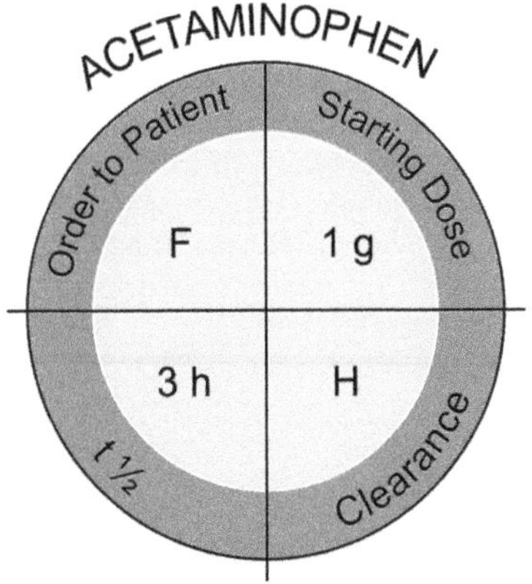

6 hours as needed; maximal dose of 4,000 mg per 24 hours). An infusion of acetaminophen 1 g IV through an infusion pump over 15 minutes reduces fever better than any oral dose but is associated with clinically significant blood pressure decreases (21). Its fever reducing effect is not sustained and rarely lasts beyond several hours. In a critical care population (the HEAT trial, which enrolled very small numbers of neurologic patients [22]), outcome or ICU stay was not improved with IV acetaminophen.

Another concern about using the IV route is the substantial price difference (factor of 50) between the IV and oral routes, although the cost has come down.

Shivering Management

- Mild shivering is best managed with IV dexmedetomidine, starting at a dose of 0.2 mcg/kg per hour titrated up to 1.5 mcg/kg per hour.
- Propofol (50–80 mcg/kg per minute) and fentanyl (25 mcg/hr) or meperidine (100 mg IM or IV) is equally helpful.
- Buspirone or magnesium infusion is rarely useful and only in mild presentations. Buspirone is 30 mg every 8 hours and magnesium sulfate is 1 g/hr IV infusion, aiming at serum magnesium levels of 4 mg/dl.
- If nothing else is successful, a neuromuscular blocker can be tried. The disadvantage of neuromuscular blockers is that there is a substantial risk of critical illness neuromyopathy after several days of use. Moreover, use of neuromuscular blockers requires continuous electroencephalographic monitoring in patients with prior seizures or those at risk of seizures.

Control of Rhabdomyolysis

Seizures may be associated with acutely severe rhabdomyolysis. Early clues are red (Coca-Cola)-tinted urine and an unexpected rise in the creatinine level (often >2 mg/dl). The creatinine phosphokinase level can rise dramatically and may exceed 100,000 units/L. Acute renal failure produces a non-anion gap metabolic acidosis and rising potassium values. The treatment is aggressive fluid resuscitation with 1,000 ml/hr for at least 2 hours and then slowing to 200 to 250 ml/hr. The infusate of choice is 0.45% NaCl + 75 mEq/L bicarbonate. Electrolytes, including calcium, potassium, and phosphate, need to be checked every 6 hours. Dialysis may be needed if the patient's creatinine and potassium levels are rising and urine output is less than 75 ml/hr. (Electrolyte correction is discussed in Chapter 15.) Most patients with rhabdomyolysis need extra fluids and nothing more.

Key Pointers

1. For nausea, ondansetron is preferred over metoclopramide due to its better safety profile.
2. Baclofen and gabapentin are first-line treatments for hiccups.
3. Amitriptyline may reduce secretions quickly.
4. Methylnaltrexone for opioid-related ileus may be rapidly effective.
5. Fever management is best achieved with cooling devices.

References

1. Hasler, W.L., *Pathology of emesis: its autonomic basis.* Handb Clin Neurol, 2013. **117**: 337–352.
2. Becker, D.E., *Nausea, vomiting, and hiccups: a review of mechanisms and treatment.* Anesth Prog, 2010. **57**: 150–157.
3. Lee, Y., et al., *Midazolam vs ondansetron for preventing postoperative nausea and vomiting: a randomised controlled trial.* Anaesthesia, 2007. **62**: 18–22.
4. Paech, M.J., et al., *A randomized, placebo-controlled trial of preoperative oral pregabalin for postoperative pain relief after minor gynecological surgery.* Anesth Analg, 2007. **105**: 1449–1453.
5. Shaikh, S.I., et al., *Postoperative nausea and vomiting: a simple yet complex problem.* Anesth Essays Res, 2016. **10**: 388–396.
6. Singh, P., Yoon, S.S. and Kuo, B. *Nausea: a review of pathophysiology and therapeutics.* Therap Adv Gastroenterol, 2016. **9**: 98–112.
7. Tramer, M.R., *Strategies for postoperative nausea and vomiting.* Best Pract Res Clin Anaesthesiol, 2004. **18**: 693–701.
8. Ritter, M.J., et al., *Ondansetron-induced multifocal encephalopathy.* Mayo Clin Proc, 2003. **78**: 1150–1152.
9. Steger, M., Schneemann, M. and Fox, M. *Systemic review: the pathogenesis and pharmacological treatment of hiccups.* Aliment Pharmacol Ther, 2015. **42**: 1037–1050.
10. Friedman, N.L. *Hiccups: a treatment review.* Pharmacotherapy, 1996. **16**: 986–995.
11. Thompson, D.F. and Brooks, K.G. *Gabapentin therapy of hiccups.* Ann Pharmacother, 2013. **47**: 897–903.
12. Newall, A.R., Orser, R. and Hunt, M. *The control of oral secretions in bulbar ALS/MND.* J Neurol Sci, 1996. **139**(Suppl): 43–44.
13. McGeachan, A.J. and McDermott, C.J. *Management of oral secretions in neurological disease.* Pract Neurol, 2017. **17**: 96–103.
14. Bhatia, K.P., Munchau, A. and Brown, *Botulinum toxin is a useful treatment in excessive drooling in saliva.* J Neurol Neurosurg Psychiatry, 1999. **67**: 697.
15. Elsner, J.L., Smith, J.M. and Ensor, C.R. *Intravenous neostigmine for postoperative acute colonic pseudo-obstruction.* Ann Pharmacother, 2012. **46**: 430–435.
16. Lauro, A., R. De Giorgio, and Pinna, A.D. *Advancement in the clinical management of intestinal pseudo-obstruction.* Expert Rev Gastroenterol Hepatol, 2015. **9**: 197–208.
17. Badjatia, N., *Hyperthermia and fever control in brain injury.* Crit Care Med, 2009. **37**(7 Suppl): S250–257.
18. Diringer, M.N., et al., *Elevated body temperature independently contributes to increased length of stay in neurologic intensive care unit patients.* Crit Care Med, 2004. **32**: 1489–1495.
19. Marik,E., *Fever in the ICU.* Chest, 2000. **117**: 855–869.
20. Naidech, A.M., et al., *Fever burden and functional recovery after subarachnoid hemorrhage.* Neurosurgery, 2008. **63**: 212–218.

21. Schell-Chaple, H.M., et al., *Effects of IV acetaminophen on core body temperature and hemodynamic responses in febrile critically ill adults: a randomized controlled trial.* Crit Care Med, 2017. **45**: 1199–1207.

22. Young, P., et al., *Acetaminophen for fever in critically ill patients with suspected infection.* N Engl J Med, 2015. **373**: 2215–2224.

Chapter 20

Drugs Used in Neurorehabilitation

Much neurorehabilitation is done without pharmaceuticals, but good drug options are available in patients with persistent disorders of consciousness, spasticity, and early depression after stroke. But, physicians should try to avoid drugs that have a depressant effect on the central nervous system, and there are many routinely used as a part of a patient's neurologic treatment (e.g., several antiepileptic agents, antispasmodics, antidepressants, and opioid analgesics).

Disorders of consciousness are major challenges in neurorehabilitation centers because they preclude entering in traditional rehabilitation programs. Improvement can be achieved with a neurostimulant, which potentially improves the patient's attention span and allows him or her to participate in therapy (1–3). This requires distinguishing a minimally conscious state (MCS) from a persistent vegetative state; in the latter, drug therapy likely is ineffective. In an MCS, verbal and motor responses to repeated commands are preserved. MCS with preserved language comprehension—albeit markedly abnormal—is best amenable to a trial of neurostimulants, although there may not be a long-lasting effect. No study has been able to resolve the major clinical dilemma—whether neurostimulants allow patients to gain effective and engaging communication and to make logical decisions rather than to lift them up to a situation where they become very much more aware of their incapability and become troubled by their extreme newly acquired disability (4).

Neurostimulants

Dopaminergic neurons may have a role in maintaining wakefulness, and this has been made more apparent after amphetamine studies showed more alertness. (Amphetamines enhance the release of dopamine and simultaneously inhibit the reuptake of dopamine.) Traumatic brain injury may damage but leave still functional dopaminergic tracts, so patients could respond to amantadine or other drugs. Enhancing wakefulness is not useful, however, if there is no enhanced awareness. Considerable remaining neuronal functional connectivity is needed, and a patient in a truly persistent vegetative state cannot be awakened. These drugs therefore have an effect only on patients in MCS. A major international randomized trial in patients with posttraumatic disorder of consciousness found that 4 weeks of treatment with amantadine (5–7) significantly improved functional outcomes as noted by improved communication and responses to commands; the patients' conditions worsened after drug discontinuation. There are no convincing data regarding the use of neurostimulants in patients with anoxic-ischemic encephalopathy; most recommendations apply only to those with traumatic brain injury (TBI). In most other reported studies, is it not possible to distinguish drug-associated improvement (e.g., increased verbalizations, pointing to objects, more consistency in following commands) from spontaneous improvement. Several dopaminergic drugs have been used in rehabilitation practices. Rehabilitation physicians may consider using dopaminergic or antidepressant drugs alone or in combination and amantadine in TBI for a 4-week trial. Zolpidem and lamotrigine have been used on a trial-by-trial basis. Dopaminergic drugs for disorders of consciousness are shown in table 20.1.

Table 20.1 Dopaminergic Agents for Disorders of Consciousness

Drugs	Mechanism	Dose Range (mg/day)	Comments
Levodopa/ carbidopa	Directly converted to dopamine (via dopa decarboxylase)	250–2000	Start at 25/100 mg three times a day; increase gradually to 25/250mg tablets.
Amantadine	Stimulates presynaptic release of dopamine; possible direct agonist effect	100–400	Start at 50 mg twice daily; increase by 100 mg weekly to 200 mg twice daily.
Bromocriptine	Direct agonist at receptor site	7.5–100	Start at 2.5 mg three times a day; increase weekly to 5 mg three times a day; then 10 mg three times a day; then by 15 mg per week.
Selegiline	Monoamine oxidase type B inhibitor	5–10	Initiate at 5 mg in the morning; can increase to 5 mg twice daily.

Zolpidem PO

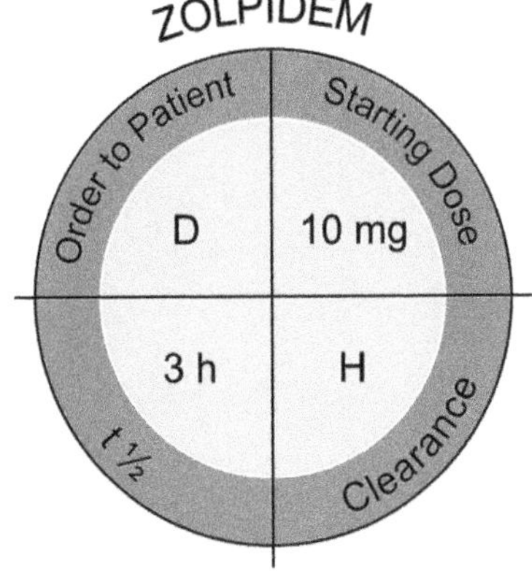

Pharmacologic Characteristics

- Sedative, hypnotic
- Action at GABA-A receptors via type I benzodiazepine receptor but with arousal, probable glutamine enhancement
- Insufficient evidence from published studies (8)
- Improvement in arousal and functional improvement in MCS within 1 hour of administration; effect lasts for ~4 hours, after which the peak level decreases (9,10)
- Incidental success in patients with TBI
- Lack of consistent improvement in anoxic-ischemic injury
- Rapid onset, short duration of action

Dosing and Administration

- 5–10 mg daily orally, up to 20 mg per dose

Monitoring

- Daytime alertness
- Improved cognition

Side Effects

- Major somnolence (most patients fall asleep)
- Abnormal thinking
- Suicidal behavior
- Behavioral changes
- Anaphylaxis

Methylphenidate PO

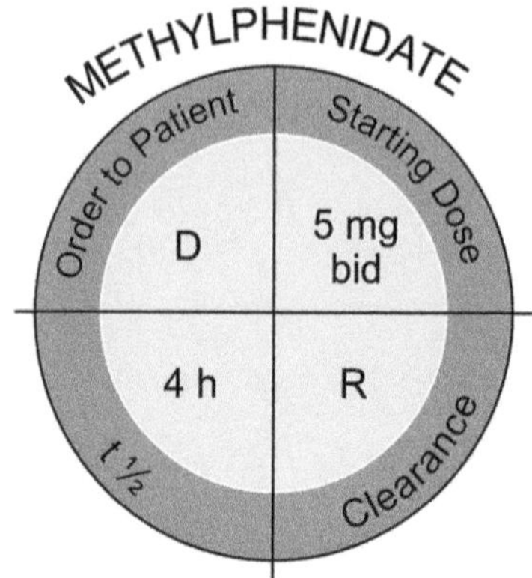

Pharmacologic Characteristics

- Increases dopamine and norepinephrine levels at synapses; blocks reuptake
- Facilitates arousal and improves attention span
- Little effect on motor recovery
- Only tested prospectively in TBI (11–13)

Dosing and Administration

- 0.3 mg/kg orally twice daily
- 5–30 mg/day (divided in one to three doses per day) for 4 weeks after stroke
- Administer last dose before/with evening meal to minimize risk of insomnia

Monitoring

- Blood pressure
- Signs and symptoms of depression

Side Effects

- At higher doses, headaches, anorexia, weight loss, insomnia
- May cause significant hypertension
- No evidence of recurrent brain hemorrhage

Amantadine PO

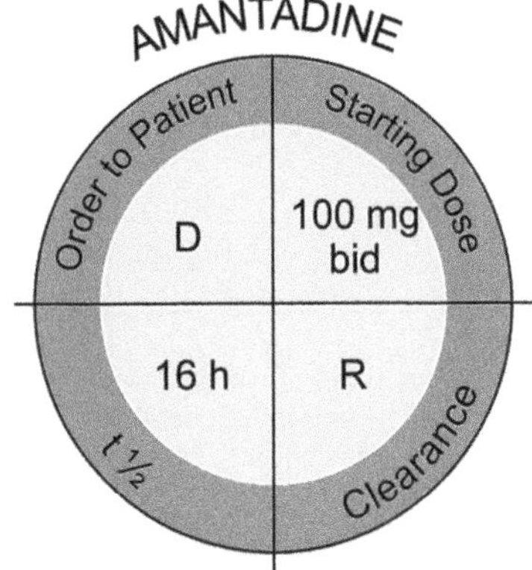

Pharmacologic Characteristics

- Enhances presynaptic dopamine release (5,6,14)
- Inhibits dopamine reuptake
- NMDA receptor antagonist
- Improves arousal and cognition
- May be combined with methylphenidate and sertraline (12)

Dosing and Administration

- 100 mg orally twice daily for 2 weeks
- 150 mg orally twice daily in week 3
- 200 mg orally twice daily in week 4
- Avoid abrupt withdrawal
- May need renal dose adjustment

Monitoring

- Daytime alertness
- Electroencephalogram for seizures
- Electrocardiogram (EKG)
- Blood pressure

Side Effects

- Anticholinergic effects
- Increased seizures (when evidence of prior seizures)
- May increase QT interval
- Hypotension (rare)

Bromocriptine PO

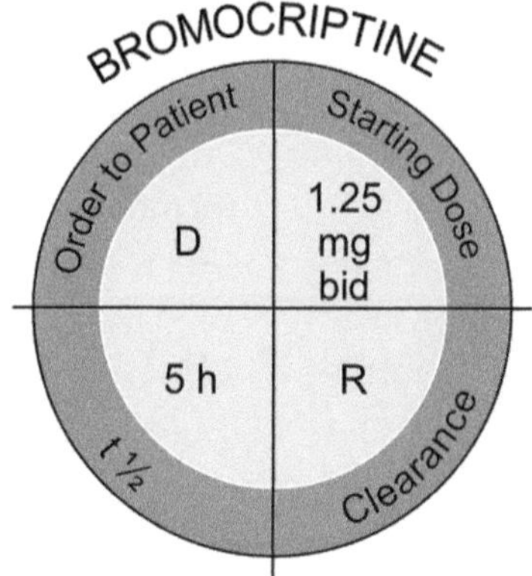

Pharmacologic Characteristics

- Dopamine agonist and semisynthetic ergot alkaloid (15–17)
- Improves motor function
- Improvement not sustained (15,16)

Dosing and Administration

- 1.25 mg twice daily orally increasing to 2.5–5 mg twice daily for 4 weeks, maximum dose 100 mg/day (in divided doses)
- Administer with food

Monitoring

- Response to therapy
- Blood glucose levels in diabetics
- Blood pressure

Side Effects

- Orthostatic hypotension
- Gastrointestinal (constipation, diarrhea, indigestion)
- Hypoglycemia

Modafinil PO

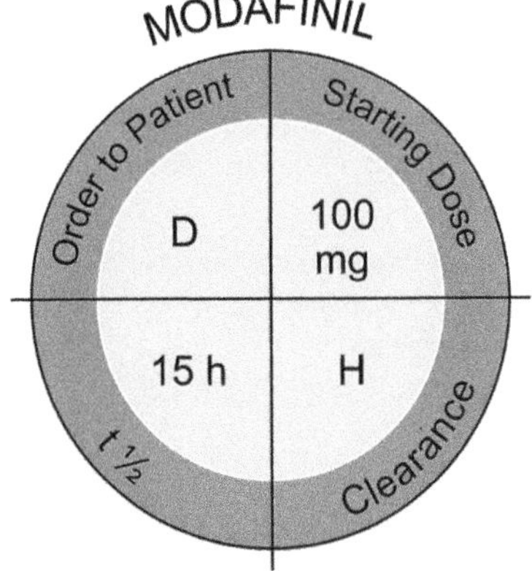

Pharmacologic Characteristics

- Central nervous system stimulant but does not alter norepinephrine or dopamine concentrations; possible GABA-mediated transmission
- Useful for excessive daytime sleepiness

Dosing and Administration

- 100–200 mg/day orally (once- or twice-daily dosing)
- Administer second dose of the day with noon meal (to avoid insomnia with late-day administration)

Monitoring

- Wakefulness
- Blood pressure, heart rate
- Dermatologic reactions
- Development of psychiatric symptoms

Side Effects

- Hypertension, tachycardia
- Headache
- Decreased appetite
- Anaphylactic reactions (some severe; e.g., Stevens-Johnson syndrome, drug rash with eosinophilia and systemic symptoms [DRESS])

Other Neurostimulants

Lamotrigine

- Sodium-channel blocker and antiepileptic
- Anti-glutamatergic effects may contribute to its psychotropic and neuroprotective effects
- Improved functional status in patients with severe TBI when started immediately after insult (18), but generally little improvement in disability

Tricyclic Antidepressants or Selective Serotonin Reuptake Inhibitors

- Improved arousal or initiation in MCS
- Stabilizes circadian rhythm
- Sertraline has no effect in patients with TBI (19,20)

Levodopa

- Precursor for dopamine
- Low levels of dopamine in cerebrospinal fluid after sustaining TBI
- More useful in patients with abulia, reduced speed, and extrapyramidal symptoms
- Promotes transition to improved level of consciousness
- Improves motor functioning in disorders of consciousness
- Maintains improvement 3 weeks after starting therapy for stroke

Drugs for Post-Stroke Depression

Annually in the United States, nearly 800,000 people experience a stroke. The vast majority of stroke patients have some rehabilitation needs, and those with major strokes require a comprehensive program. Rehabilitation includes both motor and cognitive recovery. Many rehabilitation physicians consider medication to be useful in post-stroke recovery.

Post-stroke depression but perhaps even more important boredom may start early and is common (estimated as 1 in 3 patients) (21–23). Predictive factors, in addition to a prior history of depression or an established psychiatric disorder, are prior angina pectoris and dependence in dressing. Depression after intracranial hemorrhage is strongly correlated with a worse 1-year outcome, but the relationship is not fully understood (24). Major studies have found that antidepressants are associated with significant improvement in terms of scores on functional scales (25,26), and most recent trials have included selective serotonin reuptake inhibitors (SSRIs). Several studies have found that dexamphetamine, but not methylphenidate, improved language comprehension and naming (27). Cholinergic drugs such as donepezil improve both aphasia and dysarthria (28,29). Use of these drugs is variable in practice but should be strongly considered in patients with clinical signs of depression or stalled improvement.

Donepezil PO

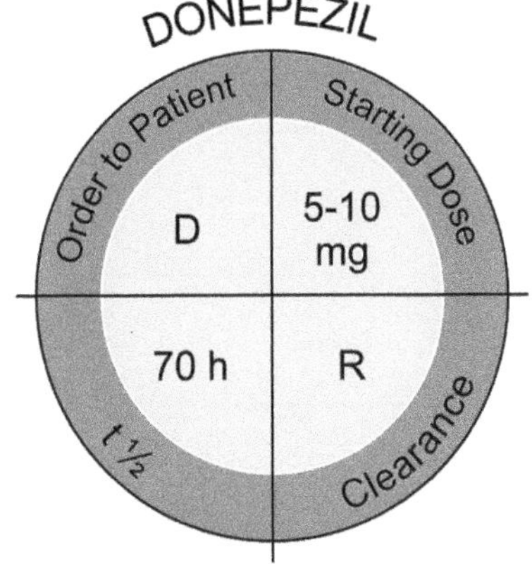

Pharmacologic Characteristics

- Reversible acetylcholinesterase inhibitor
- May lead to speech and language improvement

Dosing and Administration

- 5 mg daily for 30 days followed by 10 mg daily
- Usually prescribed for 3 months

Monitoring

- Increased risk of gastrointestinal bleeding if used concurrently with nonsteroidal anti-inflammatory drugs (NSAIDs)
- Clinical improvement
- Excessive cholinergic effects

Side Effects

- Diarrhea
- Loss of appetite
- Bradycardia (with high doses)
- Extrapyramidal signs (high doses, toxicity)
- Abnormal dreams, insomnia (less with morning dosing)

Fluoxetine PO

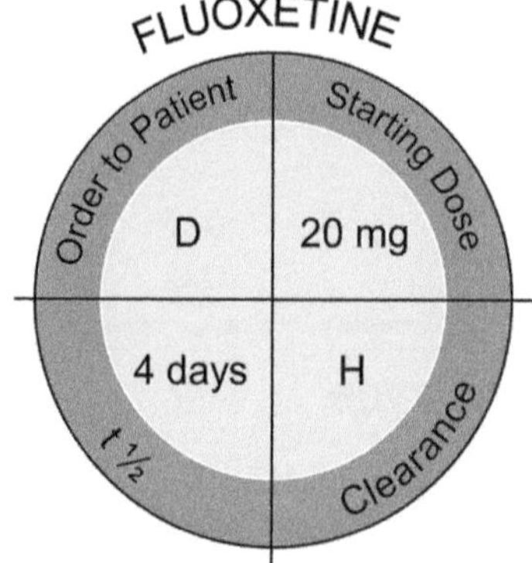

Pharmacologic Characteristics

- Selective serotonin reuptake inhibitor (SSRI)
- Onset: several weeks before clinical effect

Dosing and Administration

- 20 mg/day orally
- Treatment for at least 3 months
- Taper off to avoid withdrawal, though longer half-life decreases risk

Monitoring

- Weight gain
- Electrolytes
- Suicidal behavior
- EKG during first 48 hours
- Abnormal bruising or bleeding

Side Effects

- QT prolongation and torsades de pointes
- Risk of serotonin syndrome with other serotonergic drugs (Chapter 16)
- Erythema multiforme
- Hyponatremia
- Seizures (usually with overdose)
- Bleeding events

Citalopram PO

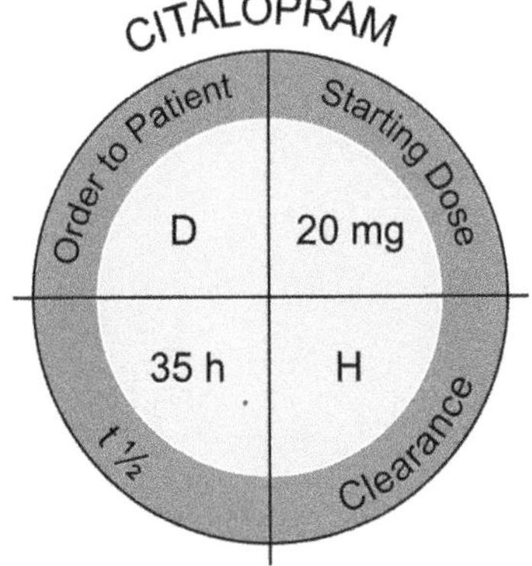

Pharmacologic Characteristics

- Selective serotonin reuptake inhibitor (SSRI)
- No effects on uptake of norepinephrine and dopamine

Dosing and Administration

- 20–40 mg orally (30)
- Maximum dose: 40 mg/day. Higher doses increase risk of prolonged QT interval and arrhythmias
- Taper off to avoid withdrawal symptoms (higher risk than with fluoxetine due to a shorter half-life)

Monitoring

- EKG
- Renal function
- Suicidal behavior
- Clinical response
- Electrolytes (potassium, magnesium, and sodium)

Side Effects

- Serotonin syndrome (Chapter 16)
- Seizures (increased risk in patients with epilepsy)
- QT prolongation, torsades de pointes
- Hyponatremia

Treatment of Spasticity

Spasticity decreases mobility, causing abnormal gait and painful spasms (often dystonias) and, equally important, bladder and sexual dysfunction. Treatment is targeted to GABA-ergic or adrenergic receptors (Fig. 20.1) (31).

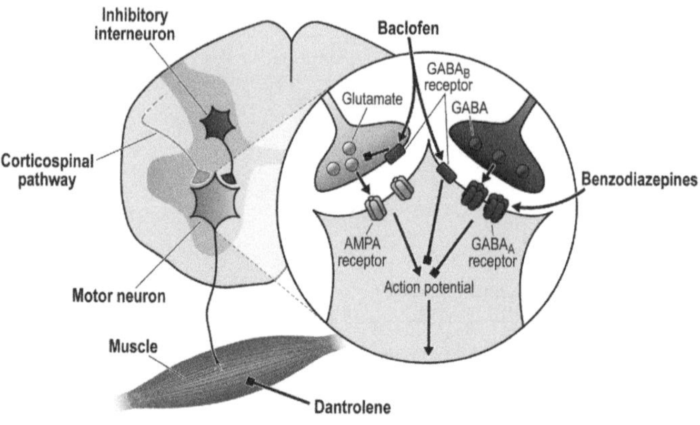

Figure 20.1 Mode of action for drugs to treat spasticity

Baclofen PO

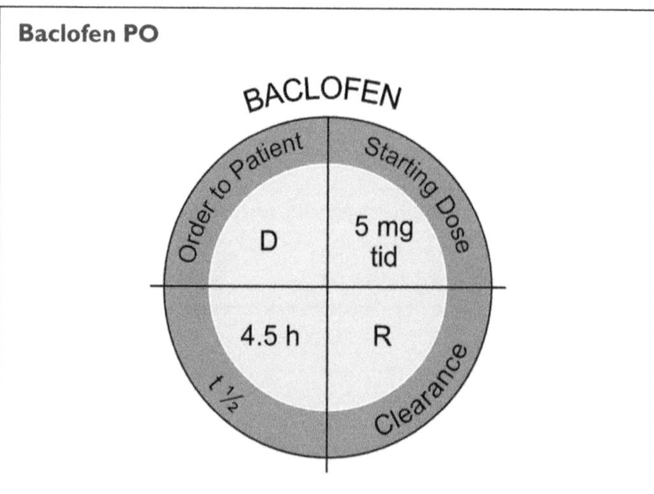

Pharmacologic Characteristics

- GABA-B receptor agonist, skeletal muscle relaxant; decreases calcium influx into cells, thus reducing excitatory neurotransmitter levels

- Modulation of impulse transmission from spine to cortex
- Inhibits monosynaptic and polysynaptic reflexes
- Mostly used in patients with muscle hypertonia of spinal origin
- Time to peak: 1 hour

Dosing and Administration

- Oral dosing: 5 mg orally three times a day, maximum dose 80 mg/day
- Decrease initial oral dosing regimen based on renal impairment; avoid use in patients on dialysis
- Intrathecal pump: 50–100 mcg screening dose; double screening dose for maintenance dose over 24 hours, then increase or decrease 5–10% of daily dose

Monitoring

- Muscle tone
- Painful cramps

Side Effects

- Sedation
- Hypotonia
- Headache
- Confusion
- Hypotension
- Vomiting

Tizanidine PO

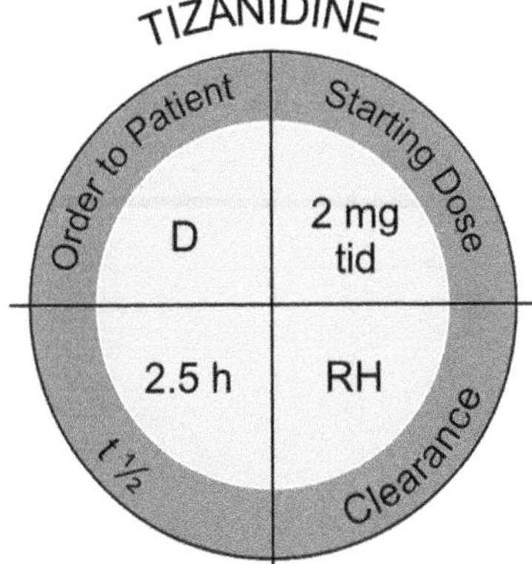

Pharmacologic Characteristics

- Central-acting alpha-2 adrenergic agonist
- Effects on polysynaptic and monosynaptic reflexes

- Anti-nociceptive effects
- Mostly for stroke-associated spasticity

Dosing and Administration

- Starting dose: 2 mg orally three times daily
- Titrate to optimal effect. Maximum dose is 36 mg/day in divided doses
- Gradually taper off when discontinuing therapy (decrease by 2–4 mg/day)
- Sudden discontinuation may lead to a hyperadrenergic symptom complex with anxiety, tremor, and tachycardia
- Avoid in patients with hepatic dysfunction; reduce dose if required

Monitoring

- Muscle tone
- Painful cramps
- Renal function
- Liver function tests

Side Effects

- May cause hypotension with rapid escalation
- Xerostomia (common)
- Potential drowsiness with high doses
- Hepatotoxicity

Dantrolene PO

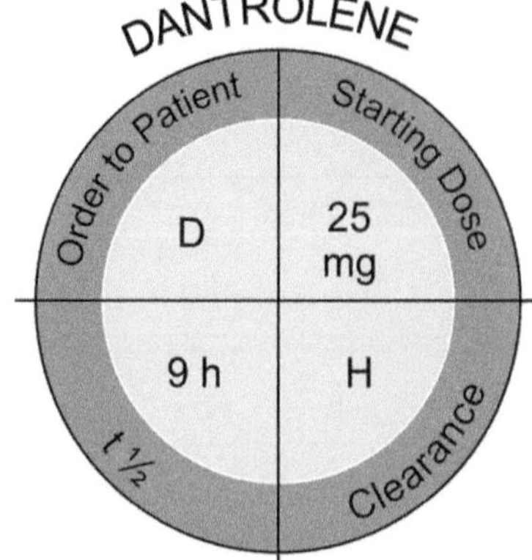

Pharmacologic Characteristics

- Skeletal muscle relaxant, less interaction with the spinal cord (compared to baclofen)
- Ceases excitatory-contraction coupling in cells; inhibits Ca^{2+} channels to block calcium release

- Used for spasticity associated with upper motor neuron disorders, but not if spasticity is needed to maintain upright posture when moving

Dosing and Administration

- Start with 25 mg once daily for 7 days; increase to 25 mg three times daily for 7 days, increase to 50 mg three times daily for 7 days, and then increase to 100 mg four times daily.

Monitoring

- Muscle tone
- Painful cramps
- Liver function tests (potential irreversible liver damage; incidence higher when taking doses >800 mg/day)

Side Effects

- Drowsiness
- Dizziness
- Dysphagia
- Nausea

Diazepam PO

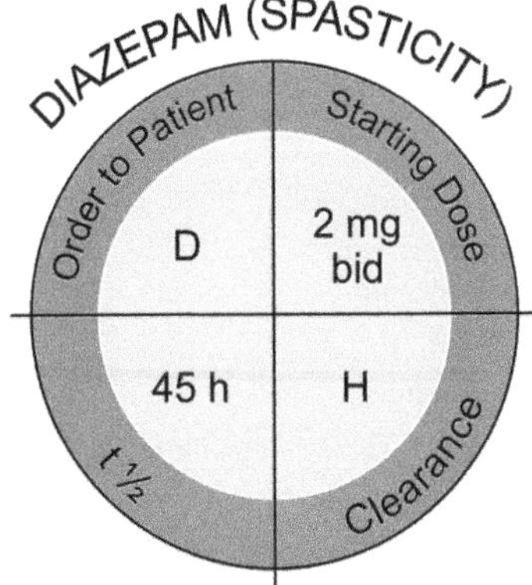

Pharmacologic Characteristics

- Central nervous system central-acting GABA-A agonist
- Used in conjunction with baclofen or tizanidine (as an adjunctive therapy)
- For spasticity associated with upper motor neuron dysfunction
- Useful in controlling nighttime spasms

Dosing and Administration

- 2 mg twice a day and 5 mg at night
- May increase to 40–60 mg/day in divided doses

Monitoring

- Heart rate and blood pressure
- Muscle tone
- Painful cramps

Side Effects

- Confusion, sedation
- Hypotension
- Potential for dependence and withdrawal

Clonidine PO

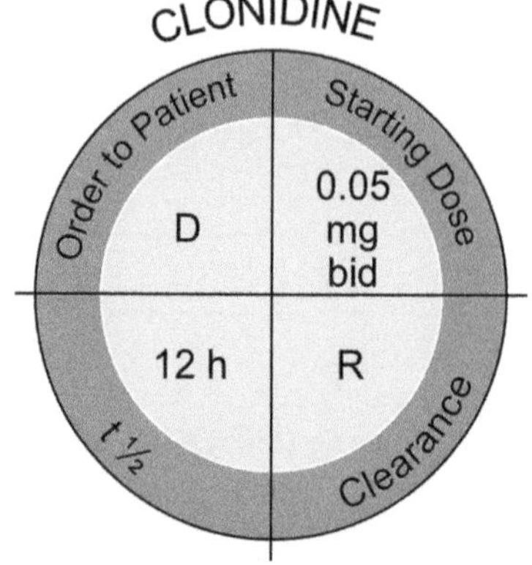

Pharmacologic Characteristics

- Central-acting alpha-2 agonist
- Analgesia at adrenoceptors in the spinal cord; prevents pain transmission to the brain

Dosing and Administration

- 0.05 mg orally twice daily, up to 0.1 mg four times daily

Monitoring

- Blood pressure, heart rate
- Renal function (increased hemodynamic adverse effects in patients with renal impairment)

Side Effects

- Hypotension, bradycardia
- Constipation
- Drowsiness
- Xerostomia
- Abdominal pain

Botulinum Toxin

Pharmacologic Characteristics

- Produces reversible paresis by blocking acetylcholine at neuromuscular junction
- Option for patients with disabling upper limb spasticity, bruxism with TBI, oropharyngeal dysphagia (e.g., focal spasticity)
- Recommended as first-line treatment for focal spasticity
- More effective than tizanidine at reducing tone, with fewer side effects

Dosing and Administration

- Start at 50 units/site for lower limb spasticity.
- The safety of doses >500 units has not routinely been studied.

Monitoring

- Treatment effect lasts for a few months; requires repeat injections.

Side Effects

- Anaphylaxis
- Severe respiratory failure (very rare)

Key Pointers

1. Neurostimulants may improve responsiveness in patients in MCS but likely only those on the higher end of the spectrum.
2. Amantadine has some effect on responsiveness in TBI.
3. Zolpidem is of questionable use in MCS.
4. Fluoxetine is indicated in post-stroke with clinical signs of depression.
5. Baclofen improves cramps with spasticity, not gait.

References

1. Ciurleo, R., Bramanti, P. and Calabro, R.S. *Pharmacotherapy for disorders of consciousness: are "awakening" drugs really a possibility?* Drugs, 2013. **73**: 1849–1862.
2. Clauss, R.P., *Neurotransmitters in coma, vegetative and minimally conscious states, pharmacological interventions.* Med Hypotheses, 2010. **75**: 287–290.
3. Pistoia, F., et al., *Awakenings and awareness recovery in disorders of consciousness: is there a role for drugs?* CNS Drugs, 2010. **24**: 625–638.
4. Cabrera, L.Y. and J. Illes. *Balancing ethics and care in disorders of consciousness.* Lancet Neurol, 2017. **pii**: S1474–4422.
5. Giacino, J.T., Katz, D.I. and Whyte, J. *Neurorehabilitation in disorders of consciousness.* Semin Neurol, 2013. **33**: 142–156.
6. Giacino, J.T., et al., *Placebo-controlled trial of amantadine for severe traumatic brain injury.* N Engl J Med, 2012. **366**: 819–826.

7. Meythaler, J.M., et al., *Amantadine to improve neurorecovery in traumatic brain injury-associated diffuse axonal injury: a pilot double-blind randomized trial.* J Head Trauma Rehabil, 2002. **17**: 300–313.
8. Bomalaski, M.N., et al., *Zolpidem for the treatment of neurologic disorders: a systematic review.* JAMA Neurol, 2017. **74**: 1130–1139.
9. Brefel-Courbon, C., et al., *Clinical and imaging evidence of zolpidem effect in hypoxic encephalopathy.* Ann Neurol, 2007. **62**: 102–105.
10. Cohen, L., Chaaban, B. and Habert, M.O. *Transient improvement of aphasia with zolpidem.* N Engl J Med, 2004. **350**: 949–950.
11. Moein, H., Khalili, H.A. and Keramatian, K. *Effect of methylphenidate on ICU and hospital length of stay in patients with severe and moderate traumatic brain injury.* Clin Neurol Neurosurg, 2006. **108**: 539–542.
12. Reynolds, J.C., Rittenberger, J.C. and Callaway, C.W. *Methylphenidate and amantadine to stimulate reawakening in comatose patients resuscitated from cardiac arrest.* Resuscitation, 2013. **84**: 818–824.
13. Whyte, J., et al., *Effects of methylphenidate on attention deficits after traumatic brain injury: a multidimensional, randomized, controlled trial.* Am J Phys Med Rehabil, 2004. **83**: 401–420.
14. Sawyer, E., Mauro, L.S. and Ohlinger, M.J. *Amantadine enhancement of arousal and cognition after traumatic brain injury.* Ann Pharmacother, 2008. **42**: 247–252.
15. Passler, M.A. and Riggs, R.V. *Positive outcomes in traumatic brain injury-vegetative state: patients treated with bromocriptine.* Arch Phys Med Rehabil, 2001. **82**: 311–315.
16. Patrick, P.D., et al., *Dopamine agonist therapy in low-response children following traumatic brain injury.* J Child Neurol, 2006. **21**: 879–885.
17. Whyte, J., et al., *The effects of bromocriptine on attention deficits after traumatic brain injury: a placebo-controlled pilot study.* Am J Phys Med Rehabil, 2008. **87**: 85–99.
18. Showalter, P.E. and Kimmel, D.N. *Stimulating consciousness and cognition following severe brain injury: a new potential clinical use for lamotrigine.* Brain Inj, 2000. **14**: 997–1001.
19. Meythaler, J.M., et al., *Sertraline to improve arousal and alertness in severe traumatic brain injury secondary to motor vehicle crashes.* Brain Inj, 2001. **15**: 321–331.
20. Reinhard, D.L., Whyte, J. and Sandel, M.E. *Improved arousal and initiation following tricyclic antidepressant use in severe brain injury.* Arch Phys Med Rehabil, 1996. **77**: 80–83.
21. de Man-van Ginkel, J.M., et al., *In-hospital risk prediction for post-stroke depression: development and validation of the Post-stroke Depression Prediction Scale.* Stroke, 2013. **44**: 2441–2445.
22. Hackett, M.L., et al., *Frequency of depression after stroke: a systematic review of observational studies.* Stroke, 2005. **36**: 1330–1340.
23. Robinson, R.G. and Spalletta, G. *Poststroke depression: a review.* Can J Psychiatry, 2010. **55**: 341–349.
24. Stern-Nezer, S., et al., *Depression one year after hemorrhagic stroke is associated with late worsening of outcomes.* NeuroRehabilitation, 2017. **41**: 179–187.
25. Chollet, F., et al., *Pharmacological therapies in post-stroke recovery: recommendations for future clinical trials.* J Neurol, 2014. **261**: 1461–1468.

26. Chollet, F., et al., *Fluoxetine for motor recovery after acute ischemic stroke (FLAME): a randomized placebo-controlled trial.* Lancet Neurol, 2011. **10**: 123–130.

27. Walker-Batson, D., et al., *Amphetamine and other pharmacological agents in human and animal studies of recovery from stroke.* Prog Neuropsychopharmacol Biol Psychiatry, 2016. **64**: 225–230.

28. Barrett, K.M., et al., *Enhancing recovery after acute ischemic stroke with donepezil as an adjuvant therapy to standard medical care: results of a phase IIA clinical trial.* J Stroke Cerebrovasc Dis, 2011. **20**: 177–182.

29. Berthier, M.L., et al., *A randomized, placebo-controlled study of donepezil in poststroke aphasia.* Neurology, 2006. **67**: 1687–1689.

30. Zittel, S., Weiller, C. and Liepert, J. *Citalopram improves dexterity in chronic stroke patients.* Neurorehabil Neural Repair, 2008. **22**: 311–314.

31. Hesse, S. and Werner, C. *Poststroke motor dysfunction and spasticity: novel pharmacological and physical treatment strategies.* CNS Drugs, 2003. **17**: 1093–1107.

List of Graphs

The following abbreviations are used in the graphs:

Order to the Patient:
The estimated time from when the physician orders a medication to the time it is available to be administered

F: Fast and readily available in the intensive care unit. These drugs either do not require a pharmacist review because delay of review could be detrimental to the patient or are universal ("standard stock") to all care floors after pharmacist order review.

D: Delayed (<15 minute). These drugs need a pharmacist review and could be urgent. Minimal or no drug preparation is required, and these medications may not be available in a drug storage device.

P: Protracted (>30 minutes for dosing). These are largely drugs that have individualized doses for them, requiring preparation, and could include potentially controlled substances that require hand delivery and a paper trail to dispense to the floor.

Starting Dose:
Single starting dose—oral, IV, or infusion

Half-life:
Time in hours and minutes (and weeks in some)

Clearance:
R is renal, H is hepatic, and RH both renal and hepatic

Abciximab 135
Acetaminophen 52
Acyclovir 178
Alteplase 122
Amantadine 313
Amiodarone 218
Amitriptyline 302
Amlodipine 209
Ampicillin 167
Apixaban 102
Argatroban 107
Aspirin 129
Atracurium 27
Atropine 220
Azathioprine 158
Baclofen 320
Bilvalirudin 106
Bisacodyl 276
Bromocriptine 314
Buprenorphine 288
Carbamazepine 58, 283
Cefepime 168
Cefotaxime 169
Ceftriaxone 170
Celecoxib 57
Cilostazol 134
Cimetidine 268
Cisatracurium 26
Citalopram 319
Clevidipine 208
Clonidine 215, 324
Clopidogrel 131

Codeine 53
Conivaptan 241
Cyclophosphamide 147
Cyproheptadine 290
Dabigatran 105
Dantrolene 322
Dantrolene NMS 258
Daptomycin 171
Desmopressin 244
Dexamethasone 150
Dexmedetomidine 13
Diazepam 283, 323
Diltiazem 217
Dipyridamole/Aspirin 133
Dobutamine 192
Donepezil 41, 317
Dopamine 191
Droperidol 298
Edoxaban 103
Enalaprilat 212
Enoxaparin (therapeutic) 98
Enoxaparin (prophylactic) 262
Epinephrine 189
Epsilon-Aminocaproic Acid 118
Eptifibatide 136
Esmolol 204
Etomidate 18
Famotidine 266
Fentanyl 20
Flucytosine 181
Fludrocortisone 243
Flumazenil 253
Fluoxetine 318
Fondaparinux 104, 263
Fosphenytoin 82
Fresh Frozen Plasma 109
Gabapentin 57
Ganciclovir 179
Gentamicin 172
Glycopyrrolate 303
Haloperidol 36
Heparin (prophylactic) 260
Heparin (therapeutic) 96
Hydralazine 205
Hydrochlorothiazide 214
Hypertonic saline 14.6% 71
Hypertonic saline 23.4% 72
Isoproterenol 194
IVIG 151
Ketamine 85, 287
Ketorolac 56
Labetalol 203
Lacosamide 88
Lansoprazole 271
Levetiracetam 83
Lisinopril 210
Lorazepam (infusion) 40
Lorazepam 17
Losartan 211
Mannitol 20% 69
Melatonin 41
Meropenem 173
Methadone 289
Methylphenidate 312
Methylprednisolone 146
Metoclopramide 297
Metoprolol 219
Midazolam (sedation) 41
Midazolam 81
Milrinone 193
Modafinil 315
Morphine 19
Mycophenolate Mofetil 159
Naloxone 252
Nicardipine 206
Nimodipine 277
Nitroprusside 207
Norepinephrine 187
Olanzapine 37
Omeprazole 270
Ondansetron 296
Oxycodone 55
Pancuronium 25
Pantoprazole 269
Pentobarbital 87
Phentolamine 254
Phenylephrine 188
Physostigmine 255
Pralidoxime 257
Prednisone 145
Propofol 14
PCC 110
Pyridostigmine 157
Quetiapine 37
Ranitidine 267
Recombinant Factor VIIa 112

Rituximab 149
Rivaroxaban 101
Rocuronium 26
Succinylcholine 24
Sucralfate 272
SMZ/TMP 175
Ticagrelor 132
Tirofiban 137
Tizanidine 321
Tolvaptan 242
Topiramate 89
Tramadol 58
Tranexamic Acid 117
Valproate 84
Vancomycin 176
Vasopressin 190
Vecuronium 25
Verapamil 213
Vitamin K 108
Warfarin 100
Zolpidem 311

Index

Page numbers followed by *b*, *f*, and *t* refer to boxes, figures, and tables, respectively.

A

Abciximab, 135–36
ACE (angiotensin-converting enzyme) inhibitors, 202*f*
Acetaminophen, 50, 53, 305–6
Acidosis
  metabolic, 248*t*
  neuromuscular blockers and, 27
Activated charcoal, for treatment of overdose, 250
Activated partial thromboplastin time (aPTT), 95
Acute brain injury
  analgosedation, 12
  blood pressure treatment, 199–200, 200*t*
  fluid therapy, 223
  See also Brain injury
Acyclovir, 178–79
ADH (antidiuretic hormone), 223
AEDs. *See* Antiepileptic drug(s)
Age, neuromuscular blockers and, 27
Agitation
  and delirium, 31, 35–36
  refractory, 32
Alcohol intoxication, 247
Alcoholism, 280
Alcohol withdrawal syndrome (AWS), 280–83, 281*b*
Allodynia, 50
Alpha$_1$ blockers, 202*f*
Alpha $_1$ receptors, 185–86
Alpha-agonists, 10*t*, 202*f*
Alteplase, 122–23
  contraindications, 121*b*
Amantadine, 313
Amiodarone, 218–19
Amitriptyline, 302
Amlodipine, 209–10
Amphetamines, 248*t*, 289–90
Amphotericin B, 180–81
Ampicillin, 167–68
Analgesic agents
  analgosedation with, 18–23
  drug interactions, 7*t*
Analgosedation, 12–29
  analgesic agents, 18–23
  deciding to use, 12–13
  and neuromuscular blockers, 23–28
  sedatives, 13–18
Aneurysm, ruptured, 49
Angioedema, tPA associated, 123*b*
Angiotensin-converting enzyme (ACE) inhibitors, 202*f*
Angiotensin receptor blockers, 202*f*
Antiarrhythmic drugs, 216–21, 217*t*
  amiodarone, 218–19
  atropine, 220–21
  diltiazem, 217–18
  metoprolol, 219–20
Antibiotic(s), 162–63
  ampicillin, 167–68
  antimicrobial therapy, 163*t*, 167–78
  cefepime, 168–69
  cefotaxime, 169–70
  ceftriaxone, 170–71
  daptomycin, 171–72
  gentamicin, 172–73
  meropenem, 173–74
  penicillin G, 174
  pneumonia treatment, 273*t*
  prophylactic use, 272
  rifampin, 174–75
  sulfamethoxazole/ trimethoprim, 175–76
  vancomycin, 176–78
Anticholinergic toxidrome, 255–56
Anticoagulation management, 93–113
  factor Xa inhibitors, 101–5
  hemorrhage from anticoagulants, 108
  heparin and warfarin, 94–101
  reversal of vitamin K antagonists, 108–13
  targets of anticoagulants, 94*f*
  thrombin inhibitors, 105–7
Antidepressants, tricyclic, 10*t*, 316
Antidiuretic hormone (ADH), 223
Antidotes
  atropine, 256–57
  cyproheptadine, 258*t*
  dantrolene, 258*t*
  flumazenil, 253
  naloxone, 252
  overdose detoxification, 247–59, 249*t*
  phentolamine, 254–55
  physostigmine, 255–56
  pralidoxime, 257
Antiepileptic drug(s) (AEDs), 77–91
  consequences of stopping, 10*t*
  dose adjustments with dialysis, 90, 91, 91*f*
  drug interactions, 7, 90, 90*t*
  fosphenytoin, 79*f*, 82–83
  ketamine, 79*b*, 85–86
  lacosamide, 79*b*, 88–89
  levetiracetam, 77–78, 79*f*, 83–84
  lorazepam, 79*f*, 80–81
  midazolam, 79, 79*b*, 81–82
  pentobarbital, 79*b*, 87–88
  propofol, 79, 79*b*, 86–87
  topiramate, 89–90
  treatment protocols, 77–80
  valproate, 84–85
Anti-factor Xa, 95
Antifibrinolytic(s), 115–19
  basic mechanisms and targets, 115–16
  characteristics, 116
  epsilon-aminocaproic acid, 118–19
  tranexamic acid, 115–18, 116*b*–117*b*

Antifungals, 180–84
amphotericin B, 180–81
fluconazole, 182–83
flucytosine, 181–82
voriconazole, 183–84
Antihypertensives, 201–16
amlodipine, 209–10
clevidipine, 208–9
clonidine, 215–16
enalaprilat, 212–13
esmolol, 204–5
hydralazine, 205–6
hydrochlorothiazide, 214–15
labetalol, 203–4
lisinopril, 210–11
losartan, 211–12
mechanisms, 202*f*
nicardipine, 206–7
nitroprusside, 207–8
verapamil, 213–14
Antimicrobial therapy, 162–84
antibiotics, 167–78
antifungals, 180–84
antivirals, 178–80
for bacterial meningitis, 162–65
for viral, fungal, and parasitic infections, 165–67
Antimuscarinics, 28
Antiplatelet agents, 127–40
abciximab, 135–36
after stroke, 127–28
aspirin, 129–30
characteristics, 129
cilostazol, 134–35
clopidogrel, 131
dipyridamole/aspirin, 133
discontinuing, 139
dosing recommendations, 128
eptifibatide, 136–37
glycoprotein IIb/IIIa inhibitors, 135–38
resistance to, 138–39, 138*b*
testing platelet function, 138
ticagrelor, 132
tirofiban, 137–38
Antipsychotic drugs, 36, 258
Antivirals, 178–80
for acute viral encephalitis, 166
acyclovir, 178–79
ganciclovir, 179–80
Apheresis, 150, 150*t*, 151
Apixaban, 102–3
aPTT (activated partial thromboplastin time), 95
Arboviruses, 165–66
Argatroban, 107–8
Arrhythmias, cardiac, 216*t*
Aspergillus, 166, 167*t*
Aspirin, 129–30, 138–39
Atracurium, 27
Atropine, 220–21, 256–57
Autoimmune encephalitis, 32
Azathioprine, 158–59

B

Baclofen, 10*t*, 301, 320–21
Baclofen withdrawal, 290–92
Bacterial meningitis, 162–65
Barbituates, 248*t*, 286
blood-brain barrier, 3
Behavioral Pain Scale (BPS), 48, 49*t*
Benzodiazepines
consequences of stopping, 10*t*
delirium treated with, 35–36, 40–42
drugs inhibiting metabolism of, 7
lorazepam, 42
midazolam, 41
withdrawal syndromes treated with, 282
Beta-adrenergic receptors, 185
Beta-blockers, 10*t*, 202*f*
Bioavailability, drug, 1–4
Bisacodyl, 276–77
Bivalirudin, 106–7
Bleeding
life-threatening (*see* Life-threatening bleeding, treatment of)
postoperative, 139
Blood–brain barrier , 3
Blood pressure treatments, 199–221
after urgent hypertension control, 216
antiarrhythmic drugs, 216–21
antihypertensives, 201–16
and hypertension, 199–201
monitoring tests after, 201*b*
Body movement, as pain indicator, 47*f*
"Body packers," 250
Body water, 223
Botulinum toxin, 325
Bowel irrigation, 250
Brain injury-associated symptoms/signs, 295–307
constipation and dysmotility, 303–4
fever and shivering, 304–6
hiccups, 300–302
nausea and vomiting, 295–300
rhabdomyolysis, 306
secretions, 302–3
Brain volume, and osmotic therapy, 66–67
Broad-spectrum antibiotics, 162
Bromocriptine, 314
"Bundle strategies," 49
Buprenorphine, 288

C

Caffeine, for pain management, 52
Calcium channel blockers, 202*f*
CAM-ICU (Confusion Assessment Method for the Intensive Care Unit), 33, 34*t*–35*t*
Carbamazepine, 62–63, 283
Cardiac arrhythmias, 216*t*
Cardiogenic shock, 195
Catheter-associated urinary tract infections (CAUTI), 273, 274*b*
Catheter-related bloodstream infections (CRBSI), 274
Catheters, 6, 186, 227, 273
Cefepime, 168–69
Cefotaxime, 169–70
Ceftriaxone, 170–71
Celecoxib, 60
Central intravenous catheter, 6, 186
Central line-associated blood stream infections (CLABSI), 274
Central nervous system infections
antimicrobial therapy for, 162–84
of transplant recipients, 167*t*
Cerebral hematoma, tPA-associated, 123*b*
Cerebral salt wasting, 234
Cerebral vasoconstriction syndrome, 52

Cerebral vasospasm, 277–78
Cerebrospinal fluid (CSF), bacterial meningitis diagnosis from, 163, 163*t*
Cerebrospinal fluid hypovolemia syndrome, 52
Charcoal, activated, 250
Checkpoint inhibitor immunotherapy, 156
Cholinergic drugs, 316–19
Cholinergic syndrome, 256–57
Cilostazol, 134–35
Cimetidine, 268
Cisatracurium, 26
Citalopram, 319
Clevidipine, 208–9
Clinical Institute Withdrawal Assessment (CIWA), 281, 281*b*, 282
Clinical Opiate Withdrawal Scale (COWS), 288, 288*b*
Clonidine, 215–16, 289, 324
Clopidogrel, 131, 138
Clostridium difficile, 305
Cocaine, 248*t*, 289–90
Coccidioides immitis, 166
Codeine, 54
Colloids, 225, 226*f*, 229–30
Complications, preventing, 260–78
  cerebral vasospasm, 277–78
  constipation, 275–77
  deep venous thrombosis, 260–64
  hyperglycemia, 264
  infections, 272–75
  stress ulcers, 264–72
Confusion Assessment Method for the Intensive Care Unit (CAM-ICU), 33, 34*t*–35*t*
Conivaptan, 241
Constipation, 275–77, 303–4
Corticosteroids
  for bacterial meningitis treatment, 163
  cyclophosphamide, 147–48
  dexamethasone, 142–45, 143*t*
  immune modulation with, 142, 143, 143*b*
  methylprednisolone, 146–47
  prednisone, 145–46
  rituximab, 149–50
Critical-Care Pain Observation Tool (CPOT), 48, 48*t*
Cryptococcal meningitis, 166*t*
Cryptococcus neoformans, 166, 167*t*
Crystalloids, 225, 226*f*, 228–29
CSF (cerebrospinal fluid), bacterial meningitis diagnosis from, 163, 163*t*
Cyclophosphamide, 147–48
Cyproheptadine, 258*t*, 290–91

D

Dabigatran, 105–6
Dantrolene, 258*t*, 291, 322–23
Daptomycin, 171–72
Decontamination
  gastric, 249*t*
  gastrointestinal, 249–51
Deep venous thrombosis prevention, 260–64
  enoxaparin, 262
  fondaparinux, 263
  heparin, 260–61
  low-molecular-weight heparin, 260–62
Delirium, 31–44
  benzodiazepines for treatment of, 35–36, 40–42
  causes of, 31–33
  clinical features of, 33–35
  hyperactive, 31
  hypoactive, 31
  neuroleptics for treatment of, 36–40
  prevention of, 43–44
  refractory withdrawal, 284–87
  and treatment of agitation, 35–36
Depolarizing neuromuscular blockers, 23, 23*f*
Depression, post-stroke. See Post-stroke depression treatments
Desmopressin, 244
Detoxification, 249–51, 249*t*
Dexamethasone
  in antimicrobial therapy, 165
  controlling vomiting with, 299–300
  for immunosuppression, 144–45
  for pain management, 52
  in patients with primary brain tumors, 142, 143*t*
Dexmedetomidine, 13–14, 39–40, 284–85
Dextrans, 230
Dextrose-based solutions, 230
Diabetes insipidus, 240*b*
Diagnostic and Statistical Manual of Mental Disorders (DSM- 5), 280, 281*b*
Diazepam
  interfering agent of, 7*t*
  as spasticity treatment, 323–24
  withdrawal syndromes treated with, 282, 283
Diltiazem, 217–18
Dipyridamole/aspirin, 133
Direct oral anticoagulants (DOACs), 93
Direct vasodilators, 202*f*
Diuresis, forced, 250
Diuretics, 10*t*, 202*f*
DOACs (direct oral anticoagulants), 93
Dobutamine, 192–93
Docusate sodium, 276
Donepezil, 43, 317
Dopamine, 191–92
Dopaminergic agents, 310*t*
Dopaminergic neurons, 309
Droperidol, 298–99
Drug delivery, 1–11
  absorption and distribution, 3–4
  administration routes, 4–6
  bioavailability, 1–4
  drug interactions, 7–8
  and medication errors, 8–9
  and pharmacogenomics, 9
  and pharmacology, 9, 10
Drug interactions, 7–8, 7*t*, 90, 90*t*
DSM-5 *(Diagnostic and Statistical Manual of Mental Disorders)*, 280, 281*b*
Dysautonomias, 257–58
Dysmotility, 303–4

E

Edoxaban, 103–4
Electrolyte disorders, 234–45
  of sodium, 240–45
  treatment of, 234–35
  and water homeostasis, 235–40

Electrolyte replacements, 234–35, 236*t*
Emulsions, detoxification, 249*t*, 251
Enalaprilat, 212–13
Encephalitis, 32, 162, 165–66, 166*t*
Enoxaparin, 98–99, 262
Enteral administration, 3
Enteral nutrition, 264
Enteric tube binding, 5
Enterobacteriaceae, 165
Enterococcus species, 305
Epinephrine, 189
Epsilon-aminocaproic acid, 118–19
Eptifibatide, 136–37
Escherichia coli, 165
Esmolol, 204–5
Etomidate, 18
Extended-release formulations, 5
Eye, indicators of intoxication, 249*t*

F

Facial expression, as pain indicator, 47*f*
Factor VIIa, 112–13
Factor X, 94
Factor Xa inhibitors, 101–5
  apixaban, 102–3
  edoxaban, 103–4
  fondaparinux, 104–5
  rivaroxaban, 101–2
Famotidine, 266
Fentanyl, 7*t*, 20–21, 56, 247
Fever, 295, 304–6
Fever burden, 305
Fibrinolytics, 115, 119–21
"Five rights," of medication administration, 8
Fluconazole, 182–83
Flucytosine, 181–82
Fludrocortisone, 243
Fluid intake, 224, 224*f*
Fluid loss, 224, 224*f*
Fluid overload, 232
Fluid resuscitation, 227
Fluids
  colloids, 225, 226*f*, 229–30
  crystalloids, 225, 226*f*, 228–29
  daily requirements, 226*f*
  dextrans, 230
  distribution, 4
  excessive loading, 231
  hyperosmolar, 67–73
  infusion rates, 227*b*
  IV catheter-administered, 227, 228*t*
  ringers lactate, 228
  solutions from, 227*t*
Fluid status, 223–24
Fluid therapy, 223–32
  and fluid overload prevention, 232
  principles, 224–25, 230–31
  regulation of fluid status, 223–24
  types of fluids and administration, 225–30
  volume depletion, 231–32
Flumazenil, 253
Fluoxetine, 318
Fondaparinux, 104–5, 263
Forced diuresis, 250
Fosphenytoin, 79*f*, 82–83
Free drugs, 4
Fresh-frozen plasma (FFP), 109–10
Fungal infections, 162, 165–67

G

Gabapentin, 61, 301
Ganciclovir, 179–80
Gastric decontamination, 249*t*
Gastric lavage, 250
Gastrointestinal decontamination, 249–51
Gastrointestinal dysmotility, 303
Gentamicin, 172–73
Glomerular filtration rate (GFR), 4
Glycoprotein IIb and IIIa inhibitors, 135–38
Glycopyrrolate, 303

H

H2RBs (histamine-2 receptor blockers), 265
Haemophilus influenzae, 144, 164
Hallucinogens, 248*t*
Haloperidol, 36–37
Headaches
  conditions associated with, 49–50
  pain management for, 51–63
Headache treatments, 50*b*
  acetaminophen, 53
  caffeine, 52
  carbamazepine, 62–63
  celecoxib, 60
  codeine, 54
  dexamethasone, 52
  fentanyl, 56
  gabapentin, 61
  ketamine, 63
  ketorolac, 59
  morphine, 55
  nimodipine, 52
  oxycodone, 57
  propranolol, 51
  tramadol, 58
  valproic acid, 51
  verapamil, 52
Hematoma
  subdural, 117, 117*b*
  tPA-associated, 123*b*
Hemodialysis, for overdose detoxification, 249*t*
Hemodynamic instability, hypotension with, 195
Hemorrhage
  from anticoagulants, 108
  antifibrinolytics for treatment of, 116
  and antiplatelet agents, 139
  See also Subarachnoid hemorrhage (SAH)
Heparin, 96–97, 260–61
  for anticoagulation management, 94–101
  dosage of, 95*b*–96*b*
  low-intensity, 96*b*
  subcutaneous, 260
  unfractionated, 93–95
  See also Low-molecular-weight heparin (LMWH)
Heparin-induced thrombocytopenia, 95, 97*t*
Hiccups, 300–302, 300*b*
Histamine-2 receptor blockers (H2RBs), 265
Histoplasma capsulatum, 166
HSV-1, 165
Hydralazine, 205–6
Hydrochlorothiazide, 214–15
Hydromorphone, 21–22
Hyperalgesia, 50
Hyperammonemia, 248*t*
Hypercalcemia, 27, 236*t*
Hyperglycemia, 248*t*, 264, 265*b*
Hyperhydration, 231
Hyperkalemia, 236*t*
Hypermagnesemia, 27, 236*t*
Hypernatremia, 235, 237, 239
  causes of, 238*t*
  in diabetes insipidus, 240
  treatment of, 239, 239*t*
Hyperosmolar fluids, 67–73

hypertonic saline, 68, 68*b*, 71–74
mannitol, 68–71, 68*b*, 73–74
Hyperosmotic solutions, 225
Hyperphosphatemia, 236*t*
Hypertension, 199–201
Hypertonic saline, 68, 68*b*, 71–74
Hypertonic solutions, 230
Hypervolemia, 237*t*
Hypocalcemia, 236*t*
Hypoglycemia, 248*t*
Hypokalemia, 27, 234, 236*t*
Hypomagnesemia, 235, 236*t*
Hyponatremia, 234–35, 237
causes of, 237*t*
laboratory abnormalities with, 248*t*
treatment of, 238*t*
Hypophosphatemia, 235, 236*t*
Hypotension, 185, 195
Hypothermia, 27
Hypovolemia, 223–24, 231, 238*t*
Hypovolemic hyponatremia, 234
Hypovolemic shock, 195

I

ICP. *See* Intracranial pressure
Illicit drugs, overdose of, 247–48
Immune modulation, 142–61
Immunoglobulin, 151–56, 151*b*–154*b*
Immunosuppression, 142–56
corticosteroids for, 142–50
intravenous immunoglobulin for, 151–56
plasma exchange in, 150–51
Immunotherapy, 156–60
autoimmune targets, 157–60
checkpoint inhibitor, 156
Infections
of bloodstream, 274
of central nervous system, 162–84, 167*t*
fungal, 162, 165–67
opportunistic, 166
parasitic, 166–67
prevention of, 272–75
of shunts, 275*t*
of urinary tract, 273, 274*b*
of vascular access locations, 274
viral, 165–66
Infusion rates, fluid, 227*b*
Infusions
hypertonic saline, 74
mannitol, 69
Inotrope(s), 185–86, 191–97
characteristics, 191
dobutamine, 192–93
dopamine, 191–92
effects, 194–97, 196*t*
isoproterenol, 194
mechanisms of action, 185–86, 186*t*
milrinone, 193
International Normalized Ratio (INR), 93, 95
Interosseous administration, 6
Interstitial peristalsis, 304
Intestinal pseudo-obstruction, 303*b*
Intoxication, alcohol, 247
Intra-arterial routes of administration, 6
Intracranial pressure (ICP)
brain injury-associated symptom/sign, 295
increased, 66, 67*b*
and osmotic therapy, 73–75
Intranasal route of administration, 6
Intravenous administration, 5, 228*t*
Intravenous (IV) catheters, 6, 186, 227
Intravenous immunoglobulin (IVIG), 151–56, 151*b*–154*b*
Intraventricular route of administration, 6
Ischemic stroke, 121*b*, 231
Isoproterenol, 194
IV (intravenous) administration, 5, 228*t*

K

Ketamine
analgosedation with, 22–23
as antiepileptic drug, 79*b*, 85–86
pain management with, 63
refractory withdrawal delirium treatment with, 287
Ketorolac, 59
Klebsiella pneumoniae, 165

L

Labetalol, 203–4
Lacosamide, 79*b*, 88–89
Lamotrigine, 316
Lansoprazole, 271
Levetiracetam, 77–78, 79*f*, 83–84
Levodopa, 316
Life-threatening bleeding, treatment of, 108–13
fresh-frozen plasma, 109–10
prothrombin complex concentrate, 110–11
recombinant factor VIIa, 112–13
vitamin K, 108–9
Liquid formulations, 5
Lisinopril, 210–11
Listeria monocytogenes, 164, 167*t*
LMWH. *See* Low-molecular-weight heparin
Lorazepam
analgosedation with, 17
as antiepileptic drug, 79*f*, 80–81
delirium treatment with, 42
interfering agent of, 7*t*
withdrawal syndromes treated with, 282
Losartan, 211–12
Low-intensity heparin, 96*b*
Low-molecular-weight heparin (LMWH)
as anticoagulant, 93–95, 98–99
for deep venous thrombosis prevention, 261–62
prophylactic use, 260

M

Magnesium, 235
Maintenance medications, 10*t*
Mannitol, 68–71, 68*b*, 73–74
MAP (mean arterial pressure), 185
Mean arterial pressure (MAP), 185
Medication errors, 8–9
Melatonin, 44
Meningitis
acute syphilitic, 166*t*
bacterial, 162–65
cryptococcal, 166*t*
nosocomial, 275*t*
pneumococcal, 162
tuberculous, 166*t*
Meropenem, 173–74

Metabolic acidosis, 248*t*
Methadone, 289
Methylphenidate, 312
Methylprednisolone, 146–47
Metoclopramide, 297–98
Metoprolol, 219–20
Midazolam
as antieplipetic drug, 79, 79*b*, 81–82
as delirium treatment, 41
interfering agent of, 7*t*
sedation with, 16
Milrinone, 193
Minimally conscious state (MCS), 309–10
Modafinil, 315
Morphine, 7*t*, 19–20, 55
Multi-drug–resistant organisms, 273
Muscle tension, as pain indicator, 47*f*
Myasthenia gravis treatments, 156–60
azathioprine, 158–59
mycophenolate, 159–60
pyridostigmine, 157–58
Mycophenolate mofetil, 159–60
Myocardial dysfunction, inotrope treatments for, 191

N

Naloxone, 252
Narcotic analgesics, 50
Nausea, 295–300
Neisseria meningitidis, 144, 164
Neostigmine, 28
Neuroleptic malignant syndrome (NMS), 257–58, 258*t*
Neuroleptics, 36–40
dexmedetomidine, 39–40
haloperidol, 36–37
olanzapine, 38–39
quetiapine, 37–38
Neurologic complications, with drugs, 248*t*
Neurologic disease, acute, 295
Neuromuscular blockers, 12, 23–29
atracurium, 27
characteristics, 24
cisatracurium, 26
classes, 23–24
pancuronium, 25
reversal of, 28
rocuronium, 26
side effects, 27–28
succinylcholine, 24–25
vecuronium, 25
Neurorehabilitation, 309–25
neurostimulants for, 309–16
and post-stroke depression, 316–19
spasticity treatments in, 320–25
Neurostimulants, 309–16
amantadine, 313
bromocriptine, 314
lamotrigine, 316
levodopa, 316
methylphenidate, 312
modafinil, 315
tricyclic antidepressants, 316
zolpidem, 311
Neurosurgery, pain management for patients after, 51*b*–52*b*
Nicardipine, 206–7
Nicotine withdrawal, 292
Nimodipine, 52, 277–78
Nitroprusside, 207–8
NMDA (*N*-methyl-D-aspartate) hypofunction model, 32
NMS (neuroleptic malignant syndrome), 257–58, 258*t*
Nocardia species, 166
Nocardia asteroïdes, 167*t*
Nondepolarizing neuromuscular blockers, 23, 23*f*
Norepinephrine, 187, 223
Normovolemia, 237*t*
Nosocomial meningitis, 275*t*
Numerical pain rating scale, 47*f*

O

Olanzapine, 38–39
Omeprazole, 270
Ondansetron, 296–97
Opioids
for analgosedation, 18–23
consequences of stopping, 10*t*
fentanyl, 20–21
hydromorphone, 21–22
ketamine, 22–23
morphine, 19–20
neurologic complications with, 248*t*
for pain management, 49
remifentanil, 21
toxidrome of, 251–52
Opioid withdrawal, 287–89
Opportunistic infections, 166
Oral administration, 5, 216
Oral disintegrating tablets, 5
Organ dysfunction, neuromuscular blockers causing, 27
Osmolar gap, 248*t*
Osmolarity, 68*b*, 235
Osmotic fluids, 67*b*. *See also* Hyperosmolar fluids
Osmotic pressure, 225
Osmotic therapy, 66–75
agents, 73–75
and brain volume, 66–67
hyperosmolar fluids, 67–73
Overdose, 247–59
agents for detoxification, 250–51
first treatment considerations, 249–50
major toxidromes, 251–57
neurology of, 248–49
toxic dysautonomias, 257–58
toxins and laboratory abnormalities, 247–48
Oxycodone, 57

P

Pain management, 47–64
drugs, 50–51
grading of pain, 47–49
for headaches, 51–63
patient-controlled, 64
and types of pain, 49–50
Pancuronium, 25
Pantoprazole, 269
Paralytic ileus, 304, 304*b*
Parasitic infections, 166–67
Parkinson's disease, 10*t*
Paroxysmal hyperactivity syndrome, 201
Patient-controlled analgesia, 64, 64*b*
PCR (polymerase chain reaction), bacterial meningitis diagnosis by, 164
Penicillin G, 174
Pentobarbital, 79*b*, 87–88
Peripheral intravenous catheters, 6
Permeability, drug, 3
Permissive hypotension, 232
pH, urinary, 250
Pharmacodynamics, 1
Pharmacogenomics, 9
Pharmacokinetics, 1, 2*b*
Phentolamine, 254–55
Phenylephrine, 188

Phosphate, as electrolyte disorder treatment, 235
Physostigmine, 255–56
Phytonandione (vitamin K), 108–9
Plasma exchange, 150–51
Platelet function testing, 138
Pneumococcal meningitis, 162
Pneumonia, ventilator-associated, 272
Polymerase chain reaction (PCR), bacterial meningitis diagnosis by, 164
Postoperative bleeding, 139
Post-stroke depression treatments, 316–19
  citalopram, 319
  donepezil, 317
  fluoxetine, 318
Posttraumatic headache, 51–52
Potassium, as electrolyte disorder treatment, 234
Pralidoxime, 257
Prednisone, 145–46
Preeclampsia, 202
Pregnancy, blood pressure and, 202
Privigen, 154*b*
Prophylactic. *See* Low-molecular-weight heparin (LMWH)
Propofol
  analgosedation with, 14–15
  as antiepileptic drug, 79, 79*b*, 86–87
  interfering agent of, 7*t*
  refractory withdrawal delirium treatment with, 285–86
Propranolol, 51
Propylene glycol, 5
Prothrombin complex concentrate (PCC), 110–11
Prothrombin time (PT) test, 95
Proton pump inhibitors, 265
Pseudo-hyponatremia, 235
Pseudomonas species, 273
Pseudomonas aeruginosa, 165
PT (prothrombin time) test, 95
Pyridostigmine, 157–58

Q

Quetiapine, 37–38

R

Ranitidine, 267
RASS (Richmond Agitation Sedation Scale), 13
Recombinant factor VIIa, 112–13
Rectal administration, 6
Refeeding syndrome, 235
Refractory agitation, 32
Refractory withdrawal delirium treatment, 284–87
  barbituates, 286
  dexmedetomidine, 284–85
  propofol, 285–86
  ketamine, 287
Remifentanil, 21
Replacement fluid volume, 240
Respiratory alkalosis, 248*t*
Restlessness, sedation used for, 12
Reversal drugs
  for anticoagulants, 93–95, 108
  for antiplatelet agents, 139
  for neuromuscular blockers, 28
  for vitamin K antagonists, 108–13
Reversible cerebral vasoconstriction syndrome, 52
Rhabdomyolysis, 234, 306
Richmond Agitation Sedation Scale (RASS), 13
Rifampin, 174–75
Ringers lactate, 228
Rituximab, 149–50
Rivaroxaban, 101–2
Rocuronium, 26, 28
Ruptured aneurysm, 49

S

SAH. *See* Subarachnoid hemorrhage
Saline, hypertonic, 68, 68*b*, 71–74
Salt tablets, 245
Sandoglobulin, 154*b*
Sandoz, 154*b*
Scopolamine, 299
Sedation, 12, 13*b*. *See also* Analgosedation
Sedative-hypnotic toxidrome, 252–53
Sedatives, 13–18
  analgosedation with, 13–18
  dexmedetomidine, 13–14
  in drug interactions, 7*t*
  etomidate, 18
  lorazepam, 17
  midazolam, 16
  propofol, 14–15
Seizures, 77, 78*t*, 282
Selective serotonin reuptake inhibitors (SSRIs), 10*t*, 316
Senna, 275
Serotonergic medications, 10*t*
Serotonin syndrome, 257–58, 258*t*
Shivering, as brain injury-associated symptom/sign, 304–6
Shock, 195
Shunt infection, 275*t*
SMZ/TMP (sulfamethoxazole/trimethoprim), 175–76
Sodium, in fluid therapy, 223–24
Sodium chloride tablets, 245
Sodium electrolyte disorders, 235–45
  about, 235–40
  conivaptan for treatment of, 241
  desmopressin for treatment of, 244
  fludrocortisone for treatment of, 243
  sodium chloride tablets for treatment of, 245
  tolvaptan for treatment of, 242–43
Spasticity treatments, 320–25, 320*f*
  baclofen as, 320–21
  botulinum toxin as, 325
  clonidine as, 324
  dantrolene as, 322–23
  diazepam as, 323–24
  tizanidine as, 321–22
Spinal cord compression, 144
SSRIs (selective serotonin reuptake inhibitors), 10*t*, 316
Staphylococcus aureus, 164, 273
Staphylococcus epidermis, 164
Status epilepticus, 78–80, 79*f*, 80*b*
Stimulant withdrawal, 289–90
Streptococcus pneumoniae, 143, 144, 164
Stress ulcer prevention, 264–72
  cimetidine, 268
  famotidine, 266
  lansoprazole, 271
  omeprazole, 270
  pantoprazole, 269
  ranitidine, 267
  sucralfate, 272

Stroke, 121*b*
antiplatelet agents in, 127–28
and blood pressure treatments, 200, 216
ischemic, 121*b*, 231
See also Post-stroke depression treatments
Subarachnoid hemorrhage (SAH), 295
antifibrinolytics for prevention of, 116, 117*b*
electrolyte disorders with, 237
and fluid therapy, 230
pain management for, 51*b*
vasopressors and inotropes for treatment of, 197
Subcutaneous (SQ) heparin, 260
Subdural hematoma, 117, 117*b*
Succinylcholine, 24–25
Sucralfate, 272
Sugammadex, 28
Sulfamethoxazole/trimethoprim (SMZ/TMP), 175–76
Super-refractory status epilepticus, 79
Sustained-release formulations, 5
Sympathetic storms, 201
Sympathomimetic toxidrome, 254–55
Syphilitic meningitis, acute, 166*t*

T

Taxoplasma gondii, 167*t*
Thiamine therapy, for alcohol withdrawal, 282
Thrombin, 94, 94*f*
Thrombin inhibitors, 105–7
argatroban, 107–8
bivalirudin, 106–7
dabigatran, 105–6
Thrombocytopenia, heparin-induced, 95, 97*t*
Thrombolytics, 115–16, 119–24
alteplase, 122–23
fibrinolytics as, 119–21
post-alteplase care, 123–24
risks vs. benefits, 121*b*
Thunderclap headache, 49, 50
Ticagrelor, 132
Tirofiban, 137–38
Tissue plasminogen activator (tPA), 115, 119, 123*b*. *See also* Alteplase
Tizanidine, 291–92, 321–22
Tolvaptan, 240, 242–43
Tonicity, 223
Topiramate, 89–90
Toxic dysautonomias, 257–58
Toxicity, 7, 77, 78*t*
Toxins
botulinum, 325
neurologic signs of exposure, 249*t*
and overdose, 247–48
Toxoplasma encephalitis, 166*t*
Toxoplasma gondii, 166
tPA (tissue plasminogen activator), 115, 119. *See also* Alteplase
TPA-associated angioedema, 123*b*
TPA-associated cerebral hematoma, 123*b*
Tramadol, 58
Tranexamic acid (TXA), 115–18, 116*b*–117*b*
Traumatic brain injury (TBI), 310. *See also* Brain injury
Tricyclic antidepressants, 10*t*, 316
Tuberculous meningitis, 166*t*

U

Unfractionated heparin (UFH), 93–95
Urinary pH, 250
Urinary tract infections, 273, 274*b*
Urine alkalization, 249*t*

V

Valproate, 84–85
Valproic acid, 51
Vancomycin, 176–78
Vaptans, 240
Varicella zoster virus (VZV), 165
Vascular access infections, 274
Vasodilators, direct, 202*f*
Vasodilatory shock, 195
Vasopressin, 190
Vasopressor(s), 185–90, 194–97
characteristics, 186
effects, 194–97, 196*t*
epinephrine, 189
mechanisms of action, 185–86, 186*t*
norepinephrine, 187
phenylephrine, 188
vasopressin, 190
Vasospasm, cerebral, 277–78
Vecuronium, 25
Ventilator-associated pneumonia, 272
Ventilator compliance, as pain indicator, 47*f*
Ventriculitis, 274
Verapamil, 52, 213–14
Viral encephalitis, 162
Viral infections, 165–66
Vitamin K (phytonandione), 108–9
Vitamin K antagonists, reversal of, 108–13
Volume depletion, in fluid therapy, 231–32
Vomiting
as brain injury-associated symptom/sign, 295–300
causes of, 296*b*
dexamethasone for control of, 299–300
droperidol for control of, 298–99
metoclopramide for control of, 297–98
ondansetron for control of, 296–97
scopalamine for control of, 299
Voriconazole, 183–84

W

Warfarin, 93–101, 94*f*
Water, body, 223
Water homeostasis, 235–40
Weight, drug dosing and, 3
West Nile virus, 165–66
Withdrawal syndrome(s), 280–92
alcohol, 280–83
baclofen, 290–92
nicotine, 292
opioid, 287–89
and refractory withdrawal delirium, 284–87
stimulant, 289–90

Z

Zolpidem, 311